Hand
Pearls

Hand Pearls

MATTHEW J. CONCANNON, MD, FACS
Director, Hand & Microsurgery
Division of Plastic and Reconstructive Surgery
University of Missouri Health Sciences Center
Columbia, Missouri

JACK HUROV, PHD, MSPT, CHT
Hand Therapist
Clifford V. Abbott Health and Rehabilitation Pavilion
Baptist Medical Center–Health MidWest
Kansas City, Missouri

HANLEY & BELFUS, INC. / Philadelphia

Publisher: HANLEY & BELFUS, INC.
                Medical Publishers
                210 S. 13th Street
                Philadelphia, PA 19107
                (215) 546-7293, 800-962-1892
                FAX (215) 790-9330
                Website: http://www.hanleyandbelfus.com

Library of Congress Cataloging-in-Publication Data

Hand pearls / edited by Matthew J. Concannon, Jack Hurov.
    p. ; cm.—(The Pearls series)
  Includes index.
  ISBN 1-56053-463-X
    1. Hand—Diseases—Case studies—Problems, exercises, etc. 2. Hand—Wounds and
injuries—Case studies—Problems, exercises, etc. I. Concannon, Matthew J., 1962–
II. Hurov, Jack, 1955– III. Series.
    [DNLM: 1. Hand—Case Report. 2. Hand—Problems and Exercises. 3. Hand
Deformities—Case Report. 4. Hand Deformities—Problems and Exercises. 5. Hand
Injuries—Case Report. 6. Hand Injuries—Problems and Exercises. WE 18.2 H2357
2001]
  RD559 .H35938 2002
  617.5′75′0076—dc21

                2001024183

Printed in Canada

HAND PEARLS   ISBN 1-56053-463-X

Last digit is the print number: 9 8 7 6 5 4 3 2 1

CONTENTS

Patient   **Page**

PREFACE

You have much to teach and learn from your peers.
Chinese proverb
May you live in interesting times.
Chinese curse

The organization of this book reflects the unique relationship between hand therapy and hand surgery. There is simply no substitute to having an integrated team examine and treat the patient with an injury, degenerative disease, or pediatric condition affecting the hand or arm.

Particularly in the treatment of hand problems, the collaboration of surgeon and therapist is critical to achieve the best possible result and obtain (or regain) the maximal amount of function. This working relationship is unique in the field of medicine, and failure to appreciate a cooperative endeavor can result in a significant disservice to the patient.

Multiple approaches to hand and upper extremity treatment have evolved since the mid-1970s, when hand therapists and hand surgeons first met, as a group, to discuss problems of mutual importance. While many of the therapy treatment guidelines described in this book will be well-known, some may be less familiar. Keep in mind that none of the therapeutic approaches described in this work should be regarded as restrictive; they are based on the authors' backgrounds and training. The occasional repetition of approaches and methods in the clinical and therapy sections of the same case serves to dramatize the parallel experiences shared by the hand surgeon and hand therapist.

There is ample published evidence on impairment and functional outcomes to support the basic principle of early referral of postoperative patients to hand therapy for supervised exercise. Exceptions do exist, however. For example, in replantation and skin grafting cases, the patient's vascular status may be tentative for several weeks and, where fracture reduction is tenuous, early mobilization would violate uneventful wound healing. The value of *Hand Pearls* resides in its explicit appreciation of the mutual concerns of hand therapist and hand surgeon regarding these issues. Each treatment plan therefore needs to be devised by surgeon, therapist, and patient as a triumvirate and tempered by the realities of the patient's physical, cognitive, and socioeconomic condition.

It is with pride that we have created this book. It is our hope that it will be of value in your practice as a clinical tool—"a curbside consultation on a shelf."

~MC/JH

Dedication

This book is dedicated to our first teachers and most demanding role models (our fathers):
Len Hurov and Jerry Concannon.

ACKNOWLEDGMENTS

I am lucky to have been able to collaborate on this project with my friend Jack Hurov, whose objective and intellectual approach to hand problems and their therapeutic solutions has more than once prompted me to re-evaluate my own approach and "dogma."

~MC

Matt Concannon provides an environment in the clinic that epitomizes the working relationship between the hand surgeon and the hand therapist. The opportunity to participate in this project is my way of acknowledging those hand surgeons and hand therapists who have trained me, and it is my way of providing a stepping stone for those clinicians who follow.

~JH

We gratefully acknowledge the volunteer hand models who graciously posed for various pictures at the drop of a hat: Kathy Concannon, Karla Damm-Hurov, Jeanette Brown, Carlos Farias, Karla Malaney, RN, MA, CNS, York Yates, and G. Jackie Yee.

Denise Boland and Karla Damm-Hurov deserve special thanks for their invaluable assistance with manuscript preparation. The references are correctly cited largely as a result of Ms. Boland's tireless efforts.

We are indebted to the staff of Hanley & Belfus, Inc., whose suggestions regarding the direction and focus of this book greatly improved the final outcome. We are particularly indebted to Jacqueline Mahon, who masterfully converted the original text into readable English.

Finally, as always, we would like to acknowledge the love and support of our families: Kathy, Meghan, Chaeleigh, Ryan, Bridget, and Erin Concannon (the mobile chaos unit) and Karla Damm-Hurov.

GLOSSARY

ADLs	activities of daily living
APB	abductor pollicis brevis
APL	abductor pollicis longus
CMC	carpometacarpal
DIP	distal interphalangeal
EDC	extensor digitorum communis
EIP	extensor indicis proprius
EPB	extensor pollicis brevis
EPL	extensor pollicis longus
FDP	flexor digitorum profundus
FDS	flexor digitorum superficialis
FPB	flexor pollicis brevis
FPL	flexor pollicis longus
MCP	metacarpophalangeal
ORIF	open reduction and internal fixation
ORL	oblique retinacular ligament
PIP	proximal interphalangeal
ROM	range of motion

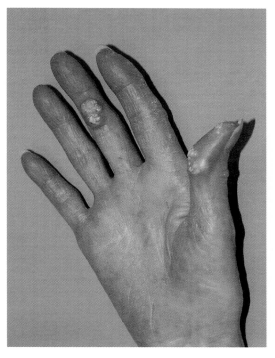

See Case 1.

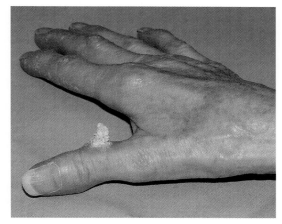

See Case 1.

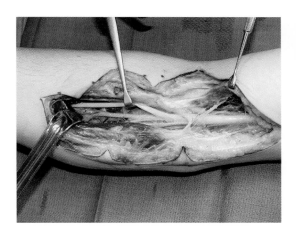

See Case 12.

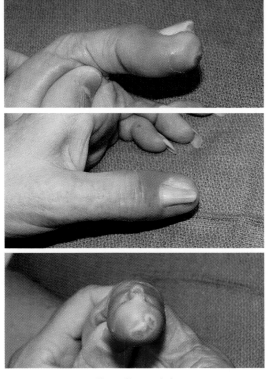

See Case 14.

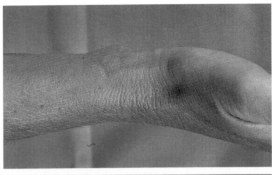

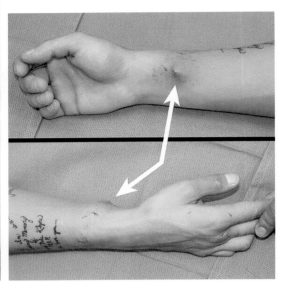

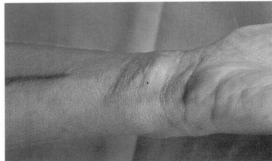

See Case 17.

See Case 42.

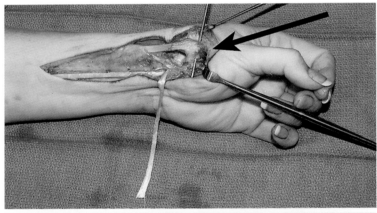

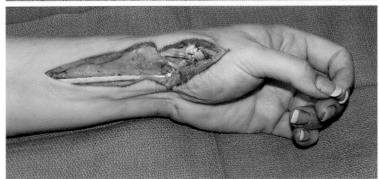

See Case 18.

PATIENT 1

An 83-year-old woman with scleroderma and longstanding lesions on her hands

An 83-year-old woman with scleroderma presents with a several-year history of gradually worsening lesions on both of her hands. The lesions are located on both the palmar and dorsal aspects. According to the patient they arose in the subcutaneous tissue, but as they increased in size they began to "pop through" the skin. The lesions are not tender, but they do cause discomfort when she hits or catches them on surfaces.

Physical Examination: Vital signs: normal. Skin: some telangiectasias over face and hands. Chest: fine crackles in all fields. Hands: neurovascular exam normal; numerous subcutaneous, multilobular, hard nodules on dorsal and volar aspects of hands and fingers (see figures); all lesions nontender; no surrounding erythema.

Laboratory Findings: ESR 35 mm/hr (0–30 normal). CBC and chemistry panels: normal. Parathyroid hormone, calcium, and phosphate levels: normal. Radiograph: see figure, *next page*.

Question: What is the diagnosis?

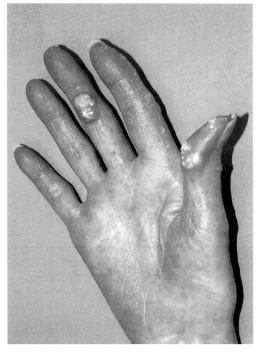
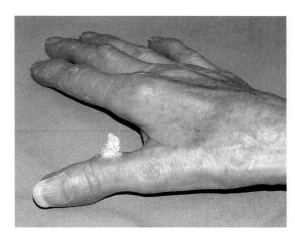

See color panels.

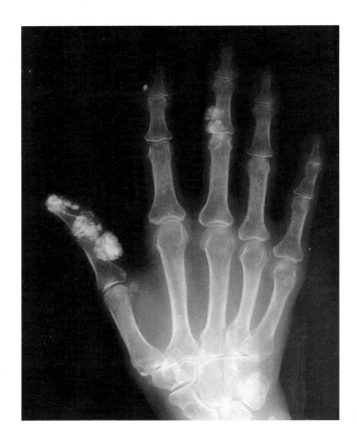

Diagnosis: Calcinosis of the hands (CREST variant of scleroderma)

Discussion: Scleroderma ("hard skin") is a rare, chronic autoimmune disease that affects primarily women (four times more frequently than men). It most commonly strikes between the ages of 30 and 60. The disease causes thickening and hardening of the skin, and also affects and damages arteries, joints, and internal organs, including the lungs and kidneys.

The hallmark of the vascular component of scleroderma is Raynaud's phenomenon. This is a blanching of the fingers when exposed to cold, followed by a skin-color change to purple-blue and/or red. It is generally the first manifestation of the disease.

This patient has the *limited* form of scleroderma, also called the CREST variant. The acronym "CREST" comes from its symptoms: **C**alcinosis, **R**aynaud's, **E**sophageal problems, **S**clerodactyly, and **T**elangiectasias. It takes only two of the five CREST symptoms for a diagnosis of CREST to be made.

Calcinosis appears as hard, whitish areas in the superficial skin, commonly overlying the elbows, knees, or fingers. Sometimes it is not visible, and is detected only by x-ray. The lumps may break through the skin and leak a chalky, white liquid. These firm deposits can be tender, become infected, or may require surgical removal. Calcinosis is *not* caused by too much calcium in the diet. Usually, no treatment is required, although surgical excision is sometimes done for extensive or very painful cases. A few conditions other than scleroderma may also cause calcinosis, such as dermatomyositis, hyperparathyroidism, tumors, or parasitic infections. Patients with severe sclerodactyly and vascular spasm may be at a higher risk for postoperative wound-healing problems than the general population. Although there are several case reports in the literature touting possible benefits of various medical regimens in the treatment of calcinosis in CREST syndrome (e.g., diltiazem, warfarin), controlled trials demonstrating real benefits to the patient have yet to be performed.

It is more common for these patients to come to the physician for treatment of Raynaud's phenomenon. Scleroderma and Raynaud's syndrome can cause painful ischemic ulcers on the fingers. The treatment for these ischemic changes includes sympathectomy of the common and proper digital arteries, and possible vascular bypass surgery if needed.

Sclerodactyly refers to localized thickening and tightness of the skin of the fingers or toes, which can give them a "shiny" appearance. The tightness can cause severe limitation of motion of the fingers and toes. These skin changes generally progress much more slowly in patients with CREST variant than in patients with the diffuse form of scleroderma.

Clinical Pearls

1. Colchicine can reduce the inflammation associated with calcinosis.
2. Other causes of calcinosis are: dermatomyositis, derangements in vitamin D metabolism, hyperparathyroidism, tumors, and parasitic infections.
3. Patients with this disease who are troubled by distal finger ischemia may experience great improvement with distal sympathectomy. Occasionally, vascular bypass surgery of the arm or palm may also improve the blood supply to the hand and fingers.

REFERENCES
1. Dolan AL, Kassimos D, Gibson T, Kingsley GH. Diltiazem induces remission of calcinosis in scleroderma. Br J Rheumatol 34:576–578, 1995.
2. Flatt AE. Digital artery sympathectomy. J Hand Surg 5:550–556, 1980.
3. Jones NF, Imbriglia JE, Steen VD, Medsger TA. Surgery for scleroderma of the hand. J Hand Surg 12:391–400, 1987.
4. McCall TE, Petersen DP, Wong LB. The use of digital artery sympathectomy as a salvage procedure for severe ischemia of Raynaud's disease and phenomenon. J Hand Surg 24:173–177, 1999.
5. Ward WA, Van Moore A. Management of finger ulcers in scleroderma. J Hand Surg 20:868–872, 1995.

Perspectives For Therapy

Fibrosis of the soft tissues of the hands, associated with scleroderma, can result in severely limited hand function. In pediatric patients, soft tissue fibrosis may result in altered bone growth.

When evaluating patients with scleroderma, the hand therapist should address **three basic components: (1)** thorough visual appraisal of the hands, coupled with palpation, **(2)** objective measurement of hand motion, and **(3)** practical assessment of hand function.

It is important to quantify and document the presence of edema. Frank joint swelling may be associated with rheumatoid arthritis and cause significant joint pain. Obliteration of dorsal skin creases, wrinkles, and folds is the hallmark of edema and is consistent with decreased skin mobility. Although it is difficult to quantify precisely, dorsal edema will limit hand motion and this provides an indirect measure of the topographic anatomy of the skin.

The presence of digital ischemic ulcers and calcium deposits that erupt through the skin should be documented. Digit ulceration may be caused by PIP joint flexion contractures in which prolonged positioning of the joints results in decreased nutritional flow and skin breakdown due to mechanical pressure.

The primary impairments associated with progressive fibrosis are loss of MCP joint flexion, decreased PIP joint extension, and diminished thumb opposition (combining CMC joint flexion, abduction, and axial rotation). The observed mechanical faults are therefore extension of the MCP joints, flexion of the PIP joints, and adduction of the thumb. These may be fixed contractures or passively correctable.

Practical assessment of hand function may be conducted through interview, questionnaire, or quantitative analysis and includes the patient's ability to write, dress, and groom, perform hygiene tasks, and use utensils for eating. These are essential components of self-care and permit the assessment of object manipulation, prehension patterns, and dexterity.

The specific impairment and functional problems to be addressed by the hand therapist and patient are premised on the results of these three basic components of the hand evaluation. Foremost among the goals for hand therapy is **patient education,** emphasizing behavioral methods to enhance peripheral circulation and tissue temperature. Meticulous skin and wound care is indicated and includes protection of healing digital ulcers, pressure reduction, and skin moisturization. Exercise, joint and soft tissue mobilization, and splinting are appropriate modalities used to improve MCP joint flexion, PIP joint extension, and thumb abduction. Assistive devices and adapted equipment may also be offered to the patient with scleroderma. Splints that protect healing digital ulcers will promote pain-free hand function, while adapted equipment compensates for limitations in motion, strength, and coordination.

Hand Therapy Pearls

1. Patient education plays a central role in the hand therapist's treatment of scleroderma. Patients should be instructed in methods that promote optimal wound healing, increase tissue temperature, and enhance skin mobility.

2. Exercise, joint and soft tissue mobilization, and splinting are appropriate modalities to help minimize the effects of fibrosis of the hands in patients with scleroderma.

3. Adaptive equipment, assistive devices, and compensatory techniques may be offered to the patient with scleroderma to reduce hand pain and improve function.

REFERENCE

Melvin JL. Scleroderma (systemic sclerosis): Treatment of the hand. In Hunter JM, Mackin EJ, Callahan AD (eds): Rehabilitation of the Hand: Surgery and Therapy, 4th ed. St. Louis, Mosby, 1995, pp 1385–1397.

PATIENT 2

A 37-year-old woman with longstanding "bent fingers"

A 37-year-old woman presents with the complaint that the small finger is bent on each of her hands, and she desires correction. She states that her fingers have always had this deviation, and the amount of curvature has not significantly changed since she was a child. She denies any other medical problems. The patient is employed as a computer programmer. She has two sisters: the older one does not have any finger abnormalities, but the younger sister and their mother both had similar-appearing hands. She denies any functional difficulty, and can perform all of her activities (e.g., typing, writing) without limitation.

Physical Examination: Vital signs: normal. General: no abnormalities. Hands: 5th fingers deviated radially at level of middle phalanx (see figures); normal range of motion at MCP, PIP, and DIP joints of these fingers. Radiograph (see figure): delta phalanx.

Question: What is the diagnosis?

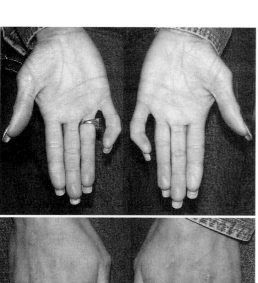

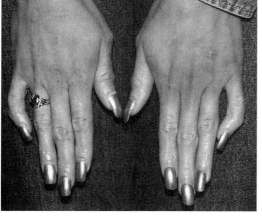

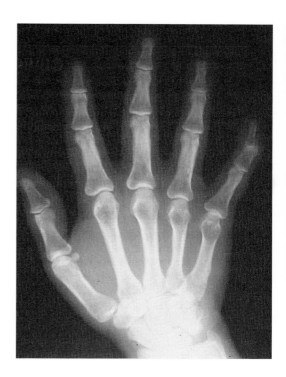

Diagnosis: Clinodactyly

Discussion: Clinodactyly is an inherited condition in which the finger deviates in the radial-ulnar plane. The condition is most often bilateral, and most commonly affects the 5th fingers, with a radial deviation toward the ring fingers. This deviation is usually caused by a **delta phalanx** (of the middle phalanx)—the asymmetrical growth of this bone causes the resultant radial deviation (see x-ray). The delta phalanx is so named because the triangular shape of the bone is reminiscent of the Greek delta symbol (Δ). The growth plate is curved (C-shaped) and therefore the bone grows more on one side than the other, producing an angulation deformity. Because this deformity is caused by abnormal growth, it usually is not as readily apparent at birth, and becomes more evident as the child grows.

This is an inherited condition (typically autosomal dominant) with variable penetrance. There is a high association with mental retardation, although certainly these patients can have normal intelligence. There are over 30 different syndromes that have clinodactyly as a component: perhaps the most valuable thing a hand surgeon can do for these patients when they present is to identify any associated anomalies.

Surgical correction is usually not medically indicated to correct any *functional* deficits. As this patient illustrates, complete and normal function of the hand and digits is the rule. Nevertheless, patients (or the patient's parents) may strongly desire surgical correction for aesthetic reasons. The angular deformity can usually be corrected with a wedge osteotomy of the middle phalanx.

Clinical Pearls

1. This is typically an autosomal-dominant, inherited condition that does not impair hand function.
2. There is a high association with mental retardation.
3. Surgical correction (for a cosmetic improvement) involves a wedge osteotomy of the affected middle phalanx to straighten the bone.

REFERENCES

1. Burke F, Flatt AE: Clinodactyly: A review of a series of cases. Hand 3:269–280, 1979.
2. Dobyns JH, Wood VE, Bayne LG: Congenital hand deformities. In Green DP, Hotchkiss RN, Pederson WC (eds): Green's Operative Hand Surgery, 4th ed. New York, Churchill Livingstone, 1999.
3. Flatt AE: The care of congenital hand anomalies. St. Louis, CV Mosby, 1977, pp 146–155.
4. Poznanski AK, Pratt GB, Manson G, Weiss L: Clinodactyly, camptodactyly, Kirner's deformity, and other crooked fingers. Radiology 93:573–582, 1969.
5. Wood VE: Clinodactyly. In Green DP, Hotchkiss RN, Pederson WC (eds): Green's Operative Hand Surgery, 4th ed. New York, Churchill Livingstone, 1999.

PATIENT 3

A 43-year-old man with finger numbness and hand clumsiness

A right hand–dominant man who is an avid golfer presents with numbness on the ulnar aspect of his right hand. He also complains of increasing clumsiness of the hand. He feels that this hand is weaker and that he cannot make as tight a fist as he used to. He denies any history of trauma to the hand or arm.

Physical Examination: General: wasting of dorsal 1st web space (see figure, *arrow*), particularly when compared to other hand. Neurologic: decreased sensation on volar ring and fifth fingers; normal sensation on index and long fingers and thumb; dorsal ulnar hand also numb. Musculoskeletal: decreased grip strength on right; patient can weakly cross fingers on right hand; strong thumb opposition, but weak finger abduction.

Laboratory Findings: Normal.

Questions: What is the affected anatomic structure? What is the location of the pathology?

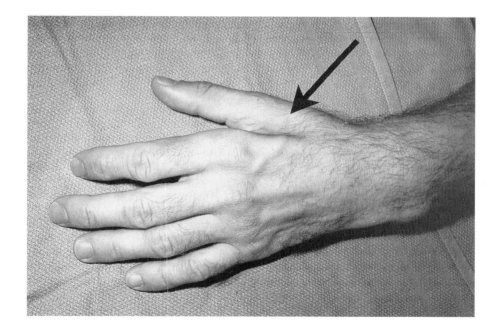

Diagnosis: Compression of the ulnar nerve at the elbow (cubital tunnel syndrome)

Discussion: Cubital tunnel syndrome (ulnar nerve compression) is the second most common nerve compression syndrome of the upper extremity, behind carpal tunnel syndrome. The two most common locations of compression of the ulnar nerve are at the elbow (cubital tunnel syndrome), and within Guyon's canal at the wrist. The former is approximately 20 times more typical than the latter.

An effective method to determine the level of the compression is to assess the sensation at the dorsal aspect of the ring and 5th fingers. The sensory branch to the dorsal hand arises at the distal forearm, *proximal* to Guyon's canal. If the compression is at the elbow (proximal to the sensory nerve origin), the dorsal hand will be symptomatic; if the compression occurs within Guyon's canal, dorsal ulnar hand sensation will be normal.

Diagnosis is usually straightforward, although electrodiagnostic studies may be helpful to document the severity of the injury to the nerve. The presence of muscle wasting (usually most evident at the dorsal 1st web space, the location of the 1st dorsal interosseous muscle) is a late sign.

At or around the elbow, the compression of the nerve can be caused by several different anatomic structures, including:

- The arcade of Struthers (a fascial band above the elbow)
- Compression by overlying muscles (such as the anconeus epitrochlearis, or the medial head of the triceps)
- The arcuate ligament (the fascial arcade of the flexor carpi ulnaris)
- Local mass effect (and compression) by osteophytes, ganglions, or other tumors.

During surgical exploration, each of these possibilities must be specifically searched for—and released if necessary.

There is no consensus on the best surgical treatment plan for cubital tunnel syndrome. Options include medial epicondylectomy, simple cubital tunnel release, and techniques that decompress the nerve and transpose it anteriorly (to reduce tension and place the nerve within a well-vascularized bed).

Clinical Pearls

1. Surgical decompression is nearly always indicated for these patients.

2. When using electrodiagnostic studies to evaluate the patient, significant conduction delays correlate with severe and possibly permanent nerve injury. Therefore, delay of surgical release until significant conduction delays exist is contraindicated.

3. If there are significant findings on electrodiagnostic testing and muscle wasting on physical exam, surgical decompression and transposition are still indicated, to prevent progressive nerve damage (although complete resolution of symptoms is less likely than in patients diagnosed earlier).

4. The location of the nerve compression can be determined by evaluating the sensation at the dorsal ulnar hand.

5. A quick assessment of ulnar nerve motor function can be evaluated by testing forceful finger abduction (fingers spread apart) and adduction against resistance.

REFERENCES
1. Concannon MJ: Common hand problems in primary care. Philadelphia, Hanley & Belfus, 1999, pp 137–139.
2. Dellon L: Techniques for successful management of ulnar nerve entrapment at the elbow. Neurosurg Clin North Am 2:57–73, 1991.
3. Dellon L: Review of treatment results for ulnar nerve entrapment at the elbow. J Hand Surg 14A:688–700, 1989.
4. Denman EE: The anatomy of the space of Guyon. Hand 10:69–76, 1978.
5. Eversmann Jr WW: Entrapment and compression neuropathies. In Green DP, Hotchkiss RN, Pederson WC (eds): Green's Operative Hand Surgery, 4th ed. Philadelphia, Churchill Livingstone, 1999.

Perspectives For Therapy

Standard evaluations performed by the hand therapist may be used to confirm the diagnosis of cubital tunnel syndrome. Visual appraisal of hand contours and mechanical faults such as clawing of the ring and small fingers with an associated Froment's sign are indicative of loss of motor units. Semmes Weinstein monofilament testing, in the ulnar nerve distribution, is valuable for staging sensory thresholds. Grip and pinch strength assessment, the manner in which the dynamometers are held to compensate for muscle weakness, and manual muscle testing help confirm the patient's subjective complaints of weakness, clumsiness, and loss of coordination. Provocative maneuvers include neural tension and Tinel's tests.

The cumulative effects of external compressive and tensile forces acting on the ulnar nerve are well understood—they cause ischemia and inflammation resulting in sensorimotor dysfunction. The goal of conservative treatment is to reduce nerve inflammation and restore vascular perfusion. Conservative treatment for cubital tunnel syndrome is therefore premised on educating the patient to avoid postures that result in ulnar nerve compression and traction. Postural and activity modification to limit forceful end-range elbow flexion and wrist extension is beneficial.

A homemade elbow pad, created from a small dish sponge and secured with a tube sock that has had the toe removed, provides an inexpensive and well-tolerated means of protecting the patient's ulnar nerve. Such pads are also commercially available.

Should the patient require a more rigid modality to protect the ulnar nerve and optimize recovery of neural function, a custom long-arm splint may be fabricated from perforated thermoplastic such as Orthoplast. The patient's elbow is positioned at approximately 30° flexion with the forearm in neutral. If based posteriorly, the medial and lateral epicondyles and olecranon process are prepadded. The splint material is then molded around the patient's elbow, upper arm, and forearm using a 4-inch ace bandage. Prepadding material, used to protect the bony prominences, is then transferred directly to the splint base. The splint is secured with wide strapping to minimize force concentration, and cotton stockinette is used as a splint interface.

Splint wear is matched to the patient's subjective complaints of pain and paresthesia. Thus, the splint may be worn at all times to protect and rest the ulnar nerve, or only at bedtime for 1–6 months. From a practical standpoint, it may be rather difficult for the patient to comply with static splinting during waking hours because of the invariant posture of elbow extension. A hinged-elbow orthosis, or dropout splint, permitting 0–45° of elbow flexion, may meet with improved patient acceptance, compliance, and nerve relief.

With early intervention, mild cases of ulnar nerve compression at the elbow are responsive, over time, to conservative care. However, moderate or severe symptoms and conditions that are recalcitrant to conservative treatment require surgical intervention to decompress the ulnar nerve.

Surgical procedures fall into one of two categories, and postoperative therapy is determined by the procedure. Either the ulnar nerve is decompressed in situ, thereby maintaining its normal anatomic position, or the nerve is relocated to a new environment anterior to the elbow joint complex. In theory, this is intended to decrease tensile and compressive forces acting on the nerve. In either case, the goal of surgery is to restore a favorable environment for the ulnar nerve. Accordingly, postoperative treatment is designed to optimize the surgical results.

Staging of postoperative therapy involves protection of the patient's surgical site, edema management, and wound care, with progression to range of motion and strengthening exercises. In general, when the surgeon must disrupt the flexor-pronator muscle attachments to decompress the ulnar nerve, the duration of protection is prolonged and motion is delayed.

Protection of the patient's surgical site is provided by a "sugar-tong" or posterior long arm splint with a wrist component, applied 24–72 hours after surgery. The patient's elbow is immobilized in as much as 90° flexion, with the forearm in neutral rotation. Bony prominences are well padded as previously described.

Range of motion of uninvolved joints, shoulder and hand, is encouraged. If the flexor-pronator muscle attachment has *not* been disrupted/repaired, active elbow and forearm motion, within the patient's pain-free range, may be initiated at the initial evaluation. When the flexor-pronator muscles *have* been operated, the patient may begin active-assist elbow flexion to end-range, followed by active extension to the limit of the splint at the first postoperative visit. At 2–3 weeks after nerve relocation surgery, active wrist and forearm motion may be initiated outside of the splint, and the patient may also actively extend his or her elbow through the full available range.

For patients having undergone in situ ulnar nerve decompression, protective splinting is discontinued at the end of the third postoperative week. Patients who have had ulnar nerve transposition will continue splint use for an additional 3 weeks (total of 6 weeks of splint protection).

Once splint use is discontinued, the emphasis in therapy should be on full active motion at the elbow, forearm, and wrist. Multiple angle isometric strengthening is safe and reproducible for the patient (for example, at 0°, 45°, 90°, and end-range elbow flexion). At 5–7 weeks after surgery, the patient may begin general strengthening and conditioning isotonic exercises. It may also be advisable for the patient to wear an elbow pad with transition to more vigorous ADLs, and the hand therapist will have discussed postural and activity modification with the patient to minimize the risk of recurrence.

Hand Therapy Pearls

1. Early recognition of ulnar nerve compression improves the likelihood that the use of conservative modalities will relieve symptoms.

2. Conservative care is premised on patient education regarding activity modification and splinting to protect the ulnar nerve.

3. Choice of surgical procedure guides the choice of postoperative therapy regimen. When the origin of the flexor-pronator muscles is disrupted to transpose the ulnar nerve, mobilization and strengthening exercises are delayed for 2–3 weeks.

REFERENCES

1. Blackmore SM, Hotchkiss RN: Therapist's management of ulnar neuropathy at the elbow. In Hunter JM, Mackin EJ, Callahan AD (eds): Rehabilitation of the Hand: Surgery and Therapy, 4th ed. St. Louis, Mosby, 1995, pp 665–677.
2. Harper BD: The drop-out splint: An alternative to the conservative management of ulnar nerve entrapment at the elbow. J Hand Ther 3:199–201, 1990.
3. Sailer SM: The role of splinting and rehabilitation in the treatment of carpal and cubital tunnel syndromes. Hand Clinics 12:223–241, 1996.
4. Tetro AM, Pichora DR: Cubital tunnel syndrome and the painful upper extremity. Hand Clinics 12:665–677, 1996.

PATIENT 4

A 30-year-old man with a distal forearm laceration from a motor vehicle crash

You are called to the emergency department to evaluate a man who was ejected from a motor vehicle in a crash. He is currently intubated and sedated; he is unable to respond to questions or follow directions. No other history is currently available, but the trauma surgeon informs you that his diagnoses at this time include closed head injury, pneumothorax, several rib fractures, and a small subcapsular liver laceration.

Physical Examination: General: dried blood on arm and hand, but no active bleeding currently. Arm: deep, obliquely oriented laceration on volar ulnar aspect of distal forearm (see figure); single, cut tendon visible at base of wound (on distal aspect); gentle traction on this tendon flexes and ulnarly deviates wrist. Hand: all fingers pink and well perfused, with strong Doppler signals; with compression of radial artery, Doppler signal at digits is lost. Finger positions: see figure; with gentle wrist extension, thumb, index, and long fingers flex, but not ring and small fingers.

Laboratory Findings: Blood alcohol level 0.17%. Radiographs: no fractures or dislocations identified.

Question: Identify the injured structures.

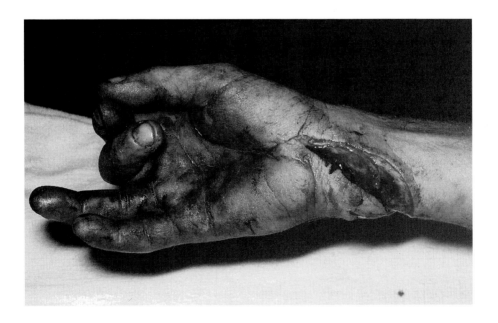

Answer: Complete transection of the ulnar artery; the flexor digitorum superficialis (FDS) and flexor digitorum profundus (FDP) to the ring and small fingers; the flexor carpi ulnaris (FCU) tendon; and the ulnar nerve (probable).

Discussion: Occasionally, the evaluation of a patient with hand trauma has to be performed without full cooperation of the patient, as in this case. Even though the patient cannot assist in the evaluation process, you must assess the injuries as much as possible prior to surgical consultation or repair.

On initial examination of this patient, there is no active bleeding noted, and all fingers are pink and well perfused. However, with compression of the radial artery, the hand becomes ischemic (as noted by the loss of Doppler signal). In this situation, the entire hand is being perfused by the radial artery, due to connections between the distal ulnar and radial arteries in the hand. Since there is no active bleeding, the ulnar artery at the laceration must be in severe vasospasm, with perhaps thrombosis of the cut vessel ends as well. This is not uncommon with complete transections of either the radial or ulnar arteries at this level, and therefore the absence of active bleeding does not rule out an occult arterial injury. (Vasospasm does not stop bleeding of *partial* arterial lacerations, which represent one of the few life-threatening injuries of the upper extremity.)

The hand posture at rest gives clues to the status of the tendon integrity. Normally, the fingers curl at rest in a characteristic cascade due to the resting tension of the flexor tendons. In this case, the ring and small fingers are extended, indicating disruption of these tendons. This is confirmed by the maneuver of gently extending the wrist: the **tenodesis effect** of the flexor tendons will cause the fingers to move and flex even more with wrist extension. In this patient, both the FDS and FDP tendons were cut, giving a complete loss of resting cascade. If a patient has lost only the FDS tendon, the resting finger cascade may not be altered at all (due to the remaining tone of the FDP tendon).

The distal transected FCU tendon is visible at the base of the wound, and its identity is confirmed by gently pulling on it to confirm its function.

In this nonresponsive patient, ulnar nerve function could not be assessed. However, since the ulnar artery and FCU have been transected, it is highly likely that the nerve has been transected as well, due to its very close association with these structures.

Clinical Pearls

1. Visual inspection of the resting cascade of the fingers, combined with testing for the tenodesis effect of these flexor tendons, can provide insight into the status of the tendons in a nonresponsive or uncooperative patient.

2. The absence of active bleeding and the presence of strong distal perfusion do not rule out vascular injury.

3. In the absence of arterial injury, tendon and nerve injuries can be repaired in a delayed setting following preliminary closure in the emergency room.

REFERENCES

1. Brown PW: Open injuries of the hand. In Green DP, Hotchkiss RN, Pederson WC (eds): Green's Operative Hand Surgery, 4th ed. New York, Churchill Livingstone, 1999.
2. Concannon MJ. Common Hand Problems in Primary Care. Philadelphia, Hanley & Belfus, 1999, pp 27–55.

PATIENT 5

A 35-year-old man with radial hand pain after a fall

The patient fell approximately 15 feet off a ladder. He now complains of pain throughout the radial aspect of his hand. He has no other medical conditions, and no other complaints related to the fall.

Physical Examination: Circulation: excellent perfusion, with brisk capillary refill. Musculoskeletal: decreased range of motion of thumb (patient is limited by pain); full passive range of motion after local anesthetic infiltration. Neurologic (prior to local infiltration): sensation intact throughout thumb and hand (no sensory defects).

Laboratory Findings: Radiograph: see below.

Questions: What is the name of this injury? What is the recommended treatment?

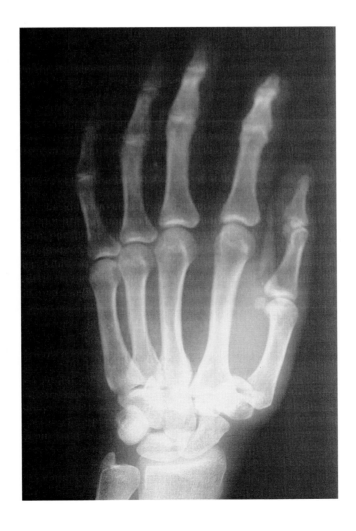

Answers: Bennett's fracture. The recommended treatment is surgical reduction and fixation (although the precise best method for accomplishing the reduction and fixation remains controversial).

Discussion: This fracture of the base of the 1st metacarpal was first described by Bennett in 1882 to the Dublin Pathological Society. The salient features of this fracture today are that it is an intra-articular fracture of the first (thumb) metacarpal: the distal metacarpal tends to be pulled radially and sometimes proximally by the attachment of the abductor pollicis longus. It is this deformational pull that must be addressed when treating these fractures, and surgical intervention is necessary to maintain the reduction.

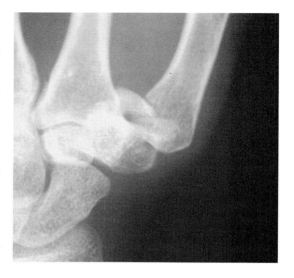

Bennett's fractures are a *single* bony fracture of the base of the thumb metacarpal. Fractures in the same location but with more bony fragments of the base are termed Rolando's fractures (see figure, *right*). They have a Y- or T-shaped intra-articular component, unlike Bennett's fractures. Another possible permutation is the reversed Bennett's fracture, which is a fracture of the base of the *fifth* metacarpal (see figure, *bottom*). While the fifth metacarpal is not subjected to as many degrees of freedom in regards to mobility when compared to the thumb, treatment options remain similar due to the ulnar pull of the attached musculature.

Recommended treatment options remain controversial, ranging from conservative management in a splint, to open reduction and internal fixation. Some authors advocate tailoring treatment options depending on the amount of articular surface involved in the fracture. In practice, it is often difficult to accurately determine the amount of articular involve-

ment radiographically, and patients tend to do quite nicely with simple reduction of the distal metacarpal (usually anchored to the index metacarpal) and fixation using percutaneous K-wire placement. Stabilizing the distal bony fragment (overcoming the radially displacing forces of the abductor pollicis longus and extensor pollicis brevis) appears to be more than adequate in maintaining ultimate hand function with a minimum amount of morbidity. Stabilization is easily achieved with percutaneous K-wire fixation under fluoroscopic guidance.

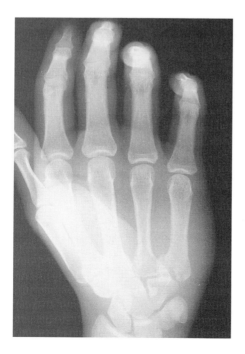

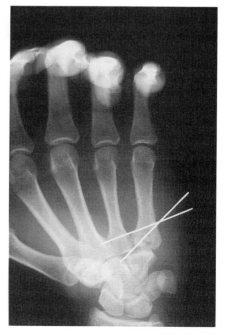

Clinical Pearls

1. The most efficacious way to treat Bennett's fractures is with percutaneous fixation of the distal/middle thumb metacarpal to the index metacarpal. Immobilizing in a splint for 4 weeks further protects this reduction.

2. A single fracture fragment at the base of the thumb metacarpal (intra-articular) is termed a Bennett's fracture; if there are multiple bony fragments it is called a Rolando's fracture; and if the fracture occurs on the proximal 5th metacarpal it is called a reversed Bennett's fracture.

3. The radial displacement so characteristic of these fractures is due to pull from the APL and EPB muscles (contained within the 1rst extensor compartment).

REFERENCES

1. Bennett EH: Fractures of the metacarpal bones. Dublin J Med Sci 73:72–75, 1882.
2. Charnley J: The Closed Treatment of Common Fractures, 3rd ed. Edinburgh, Churchill Livingstone, 1974, pp 143–149.
3. van Niekerk JLM, Ouwens R: Fractures of the base of the first metacarpal bone: Results of surgical treatment. Injury 20:359–362, 1989.

Perspectives For Therapy

Following removal of Kirschner wires and transarticular pins, and discontinuation of a thumb spica cast, the patient can be returned to a removable thumb spica splint. The duration of splint use is empirical and depends upon the degree of osteosynthesis, compression tenderness of the fracture site, and the patient's functional demands. A prefabricated or custom-fabricated, forearm-based, thermoplastic splint that is volar in design with a radial gutter component, and permitting freedom of the thumb IP joint, provides adequate stability for the trapeziometacarpal joint. The splint is applied when the patient performs vigorous activities. Splint use at rest and at bedtime are typically not necessary.

The trapeziometacarpal articulation is a saddle-shaped joint with 3° of freedom permitting abduction, adduction, extension, flexion, and rotation about a long axis. Postoperative care therefore includes active exercise to regain physiologic motion, in addition to joint mobilization. Gliding the base of the thumb metacarpal on the fixed trapezium, in the plane of the hand in radial and ulnar directions, helps restore extension and flexion, respectively, and follows the "concave on convex rule" of joint mobilization. Gliding the base of the thumb metacarpal on the fixed trapezium in dorsal and palmar directions helps restore abduction and adduction, respectively, and follows the "convex on concave" rule of joint mobilization. Treatment progression includes grip- and pinch-strengthening exercises using therapy putty, and general upper extremity strengthening and conditioning exercises using graded rubber bands.

Hand Therapy Pearl

Joint mobilization is indicated for restoring motion to the trapeziometacarpal articulation. Because it is saddle-shaped, the thumb CMC joint is mobilized radially and ulnarly, in the plane of the palm, to restore extension and flexion, respectively. Dorsal and palmar glides restore abduction and adduction, respectively.

REFERENCES

1. Kisner C, Colby LA: Peripheral joint mobilization. In Therapeutic Exercise Foundations and Techniques, 2nd ed. Philadelphia, FA Davis, 1990, p 186.
2. Wilson RL, Hazen J: Management of joint injuries and intraarticular fractures of the hand. In Hunter JM, Mackin EJ, Callahan AD (eds): Rehabilitation of the Hand: Surgery and Therapy, 4th ed. St. Louis, Mosby, 1995, pp 377–394.

PATIENT 6

A 23-year-old man who cannot extend his index finger

A 23-year-old man presents with an index finger that he cannot fully extend. He states that he "jammed" it nearly 3 weeks ago trying to catch a softball. At that time, he did not suffer any lacerations, and had full active extension and flexion of the finger. However, the finger was mildly swollen and painful (particularly at the PIP joint) for several days after the injury.

Physical Examination: Musculoskeletal: slightly tender around PIP joint of affected index finger; patient cannot actively extend PIP joint (see figure); DIP joint flexion difficult; PIP joint passively extended nearly −20°, but further extension limited by pain. Neurologic: finger sensation intact.

Laboratory Findings: Radiograph: no bony defects of the digit; no fractures or dislocations.

Questions: What is the diagnosis? How would you treat this patient?

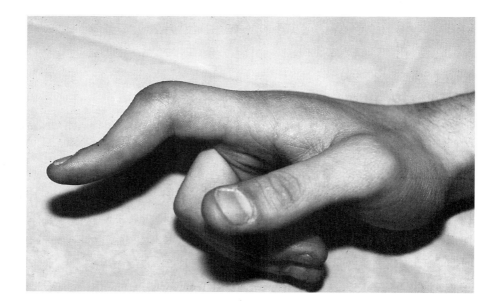

Answer: Boutonnière deformity. Treatment should include extended splinting of the finger.

Discussion: The boutonnière deformity is defined by specific joint positioning: flexion of the PIP joint and hyperextension of the DIP joint. It is caused by a derangement of the extensor mechanism of the finger; typically the central slip insertion (at the base of the middle phalanx) is disrupted. With time, the lateral bands migrate volarly to their usual position (this **volar displacement** typically does not occur acutely, and therefore the characteristic posture is not demonstrated until several weeks after the original injury). Ultimately, contracture of the oblique retinacular ligament of Landsmeer further adds to the characteristic positioning of the joints.

It is not uncommon for these injuries to become manifest some weeks after the original injury. The finger deformity does not occur until the lateral bands of the extensor mechanism migrate to their pathologic position. Early recognition of the injury and initiation of therapy is important in the treatment of this potentially difficult problem.

When the central slip has been cut sharply (i.e., an open injury), immediate surgical repair is indicated. In closed injuries, however, early surgical intervention is not nearly as successful. In this avulsive type of injury, there usually is inadequate tendon substance to repair (much like the situation of a closed mallet finger injury, another injury to the extensor mechanism of the finger). The best early treatment of these injuries is splinting of the PIP joint in full extension, leaving the DIP joint free to actively flex and extend. When constructing these splints, the MCP joint is also left free; only the PIP joint is immobilized. Patients need to be warned that this treatment is not a "quick fix": splinting will be required for 8 to 12 weeks, or even longer. Noncompliance with splinting is perhaps the greatest obstacle to a successful outcome. It is important for the patient to know that late surgical treatments are often disappointing to both patient and surgeon.

Obtain radiographs of these injured fingers when initially evaluating them, to rule out a volar PIP joint dislocation as the cause of the deformity (which would involve an entirely different treatment approach) and to look for a dorsal bony chip at the proximal middle phalanx. If there is a dorsal bony chip, this may represent the avulsion of the central slip (still attached to this bony fragment). Consider open reduction and internal fixation of the fracture in this situation. Another diagnosis to consider when evaluating patients with these symptoms is the "pseudo-boutonnière" deformity: flexion contracture of the PIP joint without DIP hyperextension. This can be caused by direct injury to the PIP joint and volar plate, resulting in a late, fixed flexion deformity of the PIP joint.

Other pathologic processes besides direct trauma may cause the boutonnière deformity, including post-burn deformity (due to injury to both the dorsal skin and underlying extensor tendon) and rheumatoid arthritis. Treatment options for these conditions are different than those for traumatic boutonnière deformities, and should be taken into account when planning treatment options. If conservative management is not successful, surgical intervention *may* be indicated. As mentioned above, surgical reconstruction of the extensor mechanism is often disappointing, and fusion of the PIP joint may be the best method for providing the most functional finger for these patients.

Clinical Pearls

1. For closed injuries, the best treatment option is splinting of the PIP joint in extension, allowing motion of the DIP joint. Patients should be warned that splinting might be required for 3 months or more.

2. This deformity is caused by volar subluxation of the lateral bands of the finger: by acting **volar** to the axis of the PIP joint, the lateral bands function as flexors of the joint, rather than extensors. With prolonged subluxation, contraction of the oblique retinacular ligament of Landsmeer will prevent even passive reduction of the deformity.

3. Surgical options are typically disappointing in the late treatment of this injury.

4. Prolonged splinting is also the best option for a closed mallet finger—another injury of the extensor mechanism.

REFERENCES

1. Caroli A, Zanasi S, Squarzina PB, Guerra M, Pancaldi G: Operative treatment of the post-traumatic boutonnière deformity: A modification of the direct anatomical repair technique. Year Book of Hand Surgery, 1992:Article 6–10.
2. Concannon MJ: Common Hand Problems in Primary Care. Philadelphia, Hanley & Belfus, 1999, pp 151–152.
3. Tubiana R, Grossman JA: The management of chronic posttraumatic boutonnière deformity. Bull Hosp Jt Dis Orthop Inst 44(2):542–51, 1984.
4. Urbaniak JR, Hayes MG: Chronic boutonnière deformity—An anatomic reconstruction. J Hand Surg 6(4):379–383, 1981.

Like their zone I and II counterparts, it is preferable to treat acute, closed, extensor tendon injuries in zone III with continuous extension splinting. For acute, closed injuries, it is critical that the splint position the PIP joint at absolute 0° and be worn at all times. In the present patient, static splinting should immobilize the PIP joint at the maximum passive extension possible of −20°. Follow-up hand therapy can then address splint revisions to achieve PIP joint extension as close to 0° as the patient will permit. Due to the amount of time elapsed between injury onset and clinical presentation, the extensor tendon will probably have healed in an elongated position resulting in an extension lag at the PIP joint.

Immobilization of the PIP joint is obtained using a custom-fabricated, volar finger–based splint. The splint is designed with high sides to help immobilize the PIP joint, and it clears the MCP and DIP joints of the finger. Dorsal pressure is applied using elasticized Velcro loop, which is preferable to regular Velcro for maintaining the joint in maximum extension (see figure, *below*).

Because of the duration of immobilization, hand therapist and patient must be vigilant for skin maceration and breakdown. The immobilization splint is lined with moleskin and the patient is instructed to change the lining as needed. The patient's PIP joint must be maintained in full extension during lining changes and performance of hygiene. It may be preferable for the patient to have two splints: one unlined for hygiene, and a second that is lined to help absorb moisture. Use of baby-powder, talcum, or corn-starch is also de-sirable. Both the splint base and moleskin lining can be windowed to promote air circulation.

Active MCP joint and DIP joint flexion are encouraged while wearing the splint. Active DIP joint flexion will promote elongation of the ORL and permit the PIP joint to be passively extended. Both PIP joint position in the splint and skin condition need to be checked at regular intervals, and the splint revised to accommodate increased PIP joint extension.

After 8–12 weeks of continuous extension splinting, gentle active PIP joint flexion is initiated using an exercise template. During the first week of mobilization, no more than 30° of active PIP joint flexion is permitted, with up to 10 repetitions every other waking hour. The MCP joint should be maintained in extension by the patient while he or she performs active PIP joint flexion. The patient is encouraged to "meet" the exercise template with the involved finger, rather than try to push beyond the template.

If no extension lag develops, the patient may perform 40° of active PIP joint flexion during the second week, adding 10°/week during successive weeks. Each week the exercise template is modified to permit the augmented range of motion at the PIP joint. The patient should splint between exercise sessions for an additional 2 weeks (that is, during the 30° and 40° weeks) and at bedtime for an additional 4 weeks after discontinuation of splint use during waking hours. Any recurrence of PIP joint extension lag requires prompt resumption of continuous extension splinting for 2 weeks. Range of motion exercises may then be carefully reinitiated; however, the patient should be encouraged to back-up by 10° the PIP joint flexion exercise.

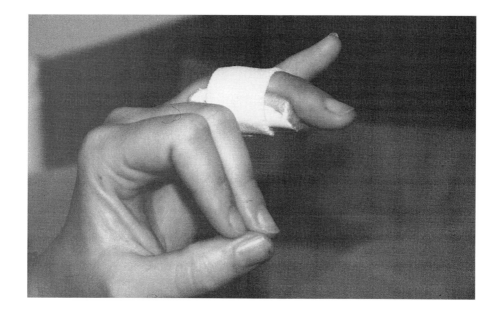

Hand Therapy Pearls

1. With managed care limiting the number of hand therapy visits and duration of care, additional consideration needs to be given to the management of closed, extensor tendon injuries. For example, beyond 8–12 weeks of continuous splint use, the patient may be ready to initiate active motion with supervision, only to learn that insurance benefits for hand therapy have been exhausted.

2. When treating patients with closed extensor tendon injuries in zone III, vigilance regarding skin condition is essential due to the prolonged interval of immobilization.

3. It is preferable to manage the closed extensor tendon injury in the acute stage; custom splints should immobilize the joint of interest at 0°. Immobilization with the joint flexed can lead to elongation of the tendon callus and formation of an extensor lag.

REFERENCE

Evans RB. An update on extensor tendon management. In Hunter JM, Mackin EJ, Callahan AD (eds): Rehabilitation of the Hand: Surgery and Therapy, 4th ed. St. Louis, Mosby, 1995, pp 565–606.

PATIENT 7

A 50-year-old man with progressive finger flexion contractures

A 50-year-old man presents with flexion contractures of his left ring finger and, to a lesser degree, small finger. The contractures have been increasing in severity over the past year and a half. He denies any prior injury to the hand.

Physical Examination: General: hard "cord" beneath skin along distal ulnar palm and extending to ring finger. Skin: appears tethered to deep tissue in several places; pits at base of palmar skin. Musculoskeletal (see figure): MCP joint of ring finger cannot be fully extended; slight flexion contracture of PIP joints of both ring and fifth fingers (approximately 10°). Neurologic: sensation normal and intact throughout hand.

Question: What is your diagnosis? Suggest a treatment protocol.

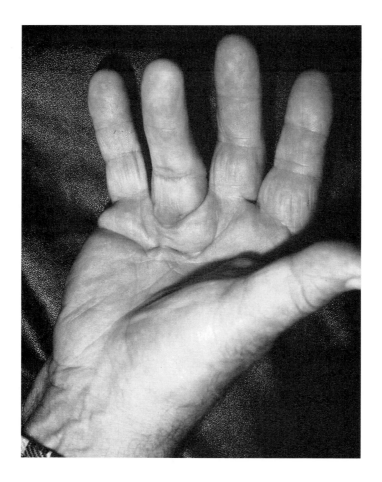

Answer: Dupuytren's contracture. Recommended treatment is resection of the underlying diseased palmar fascia (regional fasciectomy).

Discussion: Dupuytren's contracture is a progressive disease of the palmar fascia. It typically starts with a palmar nodule, and then progresses to form cords which may progressively limit extension of both the MCP and PIP joints of the affected digits. The ring and fifth rays are the most commonly involved; the thumb is affected least often. There is a higher incidence of Dupuytrens's among people of Celtic origin, epileptics, and alcoholics. A cause-and-effect relationship between these pre-existing conditions and development of this disease has never been established.

Knuckle pads (on the dorsal aspect of the MCP joints) occur in nearly one-fifth of patients. They are typically of little consequence and do not need to be addressed surgically.

Previously, it was believed that surgical correction with regional fasciectomy was indicated when MCP contracture was at 20°, or when any flexion contracture of the PIP joint was present. The logic behind this was that MCP extension is usually easily recovered, while PIP contracture is much more difficult to recapture. Recently, however, a large study by McFarlane's group has shown that when PIP joint contracture is less than 30° preoperatively, it tends to get worse postoperatively; the fifth finger is the most problematic in this regard. For this reason, McFarlane et al now recommend nonoperative management of PIP joint contractures of less than 30°.

Clinical Pearls

1. Dupuytren's diathesis comprises early onset, positive family history, knuckle pads, and plantar fibromatosis. Such patients are more likely to experience progression of their disease despite surgical treatment.

2. The spiral cord is an anatomic structure that is "formed" by the Dupuytren's process. This cord is composed of fibers from the pretendinous band, the spiral band, the lateral digital sheet, and Grayson's ligament. As it contracts, it pulls the digital neurovascular bundle superficially and centrally on the digit, making it much more vulnerable to inadvertent injury during surgical resection.

3. Incidence of recurrent disease after surgical resection is higher in patients with Northern European ancestry, bilateral disease, or multiple digit involvement.

REFERENCES
1. Armstrong JR, Hurren JS, Logan AM: Dermofasciectomy in the management of Dupuytren's disease. J Bone Joint Surg [Br] 82-B:90–94, 2000.
2. McFarlane RM: Dupuytren's contracture. In Green DP, Hotchkiss R, Pederson WC (eds): Green's Operative Hand Surgery, 4th ed. New York, Churchill Livingstone, Inc, 1999.
3. Lubahn JD, Lister GD, Wolfe T: Fasciectomy and Dupuytren's disease: A comparison between the open-palm technique and wound closure. J Hand Surg 9A:53–58, 1984.

Perspectives For Therapy

The natural history of Dupuytren's disease, from the standpoint of impairment of hand function, is fairly well understood. Gradually increasing flexion contractures involving the MCP and IP joints persuade the patient to seek treatment. The contracting tissues are incised or excised in a corrective effort. Palmar wounds may be sutured, left to close by secondary intention, or skin grafted.

The role of the hand therapist in treating the patient who has undergone a Dupuytren's contracture release is three-fold: first, to maintain the augmented range of joint extension restored in the OR;

second, to ensure optimal wound healing after an operation that may have been quite extensive, depending upon the severity of disease and the surgeon's preferred method of treatment; and third, to promote finger flexion with progression to strengthening. These roles are not mutually exclusive.

If feasible, perform a preoperative assessment of the patient's hand function. These data provide the hand therapist with important background against which to set therapeutic goals, judge efficacy of treatment and progress, and alter or discontinue treatment.

The cornerstones of postoperative therapy are hand splinting, wound care, and early active motion. At initial evaluation, 48–72 hours after surgery, the postoperative dressings are removed. Surgical wounds, edema, and range of motion are documented. A sensory evaluation may also be conducted. Wounds are redressed with a nonadherent material such as Xeroform or Adaptic, to which a small amount of topical antibiotic ointment has been applied. A light dressing of 2-inch Kling is then applied to the patient's hand in a circumferential manner.

At the initial therapy visit, a hand-based, volar, static splint is fabricated from perforated thermoplastic material and applied to position the operated fingers, and thumb if necessary, in composite IP joint extension. The splinting material should conform to the postoperative dressing and may permit a slight flexion cascade at the MCP joints; the splint can be modified into further extension during the second postoperative week. Gradually accomodating MCP joint extension does not compromise the surgical result and is preferable to instantaneous application of an excess extensor force to the operated hand. Excessive wound site tension can cause ischemic skin necrosis at the tips of the triangular flaps of the Z-plasty, increased inflammation, and decreased nutritional flow. Accordingly, the splint is adjusted gradually at follow-up therapy visits to ensure proper positioning on the patient's hand, with regard given to soft tissue healing, circulatory adaptation to finger extension after a prolonged interval of flexion, and fluctuant edema. The splint is strapped dorsally through the first webspace and over the operated fingers to maintain PIP joint extension. Velstretch is an ideal strapping material for applying dorsal pressure to the PIP joints.

Instruct the patient in wound care, including hand cleansing with a mild soap such as Ivory. Soap is applied to the periwound area only and rinsed with running water, and the skin is thoroughly dried. Wound coverings only need to be changed when serosanguinous discharge has seeped through. If adherent, dressings can be safely removed with a saline solution prepared by the patient at home. This solution consists of one tablespoon of salt dissolved in one quart of water. The solution is allowed to cool, and small amounts are drizzled over the adherent dressing until it can be removed easily; dressings do not require soaking prior to removal. The remaining saline solution can be stored at room temperature until needed at a future time. The patient should be instructed to avoid mechanical trauma—for example, caused by over-exuberant removal of dressings—as it may damage new granulation tissue. Similarly, chemical trauma of healing wounds caused by the use of cytotoxic solutions such as rubbing alcohol, hydrogen peroxide, or peroxide-saline is also to be avoided.

The patient is directed to wear the splint at all times, except during wound care and exercise. Continuous splint use during early treatment lasts *approximately* 3 weeks; note that this interval is determined empirically by the completion of soft tissue healing. Tendon gliding and thumb opposition exercises are initiated at the first therapy visit and are performed with up to ten repetitions every other waking hour. The patient is reminded to perform the exercises gently, and to come to each position without exerting excessive effort. The patient is also instructed in edema control, consisting of elevation of the operated hand and application of compressive dressings such as CoFlex in distal-to-proximal fashion, without tension. CoFlex is preferable to Coban and CoWrap because it is breathable and promotes air circulation.

The duration of wound healing depends upon the size of the surgical defect. When surgical

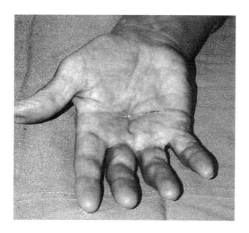 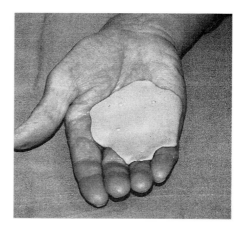

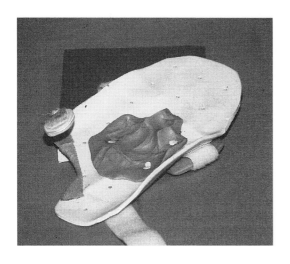
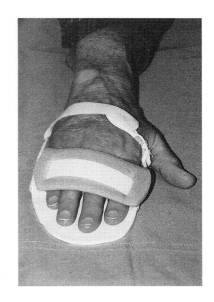

wounds are well-healed and sutures removed, an elastomer putty appliance is custom-molded to the patient's palm and operated fingers (see figures, *previous page*). While curing, the patient's splint is applied directly over the elastomer appliance. When fully cured, the appliance and splint are removed as one unit from the patient's hand, and the elastomer is galvanized to the splint base using thermoplastic rivets (see figures, *above*). In this manner, the elastomer appliance may be re-seated on the patient's hand, exactly molding with the scar and applying even compression each time the splint is applied. At this time, splint wear for scar remodeling is decreased to bedtime use only for a minimum of 12 more weeks, and the patient is instructed in scar massage, performed every other waking hour for 5 minutes each session. In addition to tendon gliding, the patient may also begin gentle grip-strengthening exercises using therapy putty; this material is an excellent adjunct to scar massage and desensitization exercises.

Clinic activities such as the use of thermal modalities, joint mobilization techniques, IP-blocking exercises, passive extension, and functional activities are components of a therapeutic program that can be adjusted to suit the demands of each patient. Periodic reassessment of the patient's hand motion is important to determine if intermittent extension splinting is indicated during waking hours.

The use of a skin graft to close the surgical site may delay active motion for 5–7 days during postoperative rehabilitation. However, the need for static splinting to promote composite MCP and IP extension, and to minimize graft contraction, is nonetheless indicated. Active motion must be initiated gently because healing grafts, while well-vascularized, have little tensile strength and are prone to shear injury and epidermolysis. Graft recipient sites can be covered with a nonadherent dressing such as Adaptic. The donor sites, when sutured closed, require monitoring until sutures are removed; then scar management can be initiated. Postoperative dressings used to protect split-thickness graft donor sites will typically fall away from the donor site without assistance from the hand therapist.

Hand Therapy Pearls

1. When surgery is anticipated for the patient with Dupuytren's disease, *preoperative* assessment of the patient's hand function is highly desirable to help judge the efficacy of surgical intervention and postoperative hand therapy.

2. A custom-fabricated, static, hand-based splint that is placed on the palmar surface should achieve composite IP joint extension. However, the splint may accomodate slight flexion of the MCP joints during the first 2 postoperative weeks.

3. Early stages of wound care are directed at protection of the wound environment, hygiene, and avoidance of mechanical and chemical irritants that interfere with wound granulation. Later stages of wound care emphasize scar remodeling and scar massage.

4. Early, active motion is indicated for patients who have had contracture release, but the hand therapist should emphasize that exercises are to be performed *gently*.

REFERENCES

1. Evans RB. The source of our strength. J Hand Ther 10:14–23, 1997.
2. Evans RB. Wound classification and management. In Hunter JM, Mackin EJ, Callahan AD (eds): Rehabilitation of the Hand: Surgery and Therapy, 4th ed. St. Louis, Mosby, 1995, pp 217–235.
3. Fietti VG, Mackin EJ. Open-palm technique in Dupuytren's disease. In Hunter JM, Mackin EJ, Callahan AD (eds): Rehabilitation of the Hand: Surgery and Therapy, 4th ed. St. Louis, Mosby, 1995, pp 995–1006.
4. McFarlane RM, MacDermid JC. Dupuytren's disease. In Hunter JM, Mackin EJ, Callahan AD (eds): Rehabilitation of the Hand: Surgery and Therapy, 4th ed. St. Louis, Mosby, 1995, pp 981–994.
5. Mullins PA. Postsurgical rehabilitation of Dupuytren's disease. Hand Clin 15:167–174, 1999.
6. Singer DI, Moore JH, Byron PM. Management of skin grafts and flaps. In Hunter JM, Mackin EJ, Callahan AD (eds): Rehabilitation of the Hand: Surgery and Therapy, 4th ed. St. Louis, Mosby, 1995, pp 277–290.

PATIENT 8

A 24-year-old woman with thumb pain and weak grip after a fall

A 24-year-old woman presents to your office complaining of ulnar-sided thumb pain (at the base of her thumb) for the past 4 days. She remembers falling while at a bar, but is uncertain of other details of the accident. She did complain of swelling and some bruising along the dorsal aspect of her hand. Besides pain, she has noticed that she cannot grip tightly with that hand without causing a significant amount of pain.

Physical Examination: General: tenderness over entire thumb MCP joint; subtle swelling. Musculoskeletal: full active extension and flexion of thumb; patient can actively oppose thumb tip to other digits, but with pain; significant pain on passive radial deviation, but little resistance after local anesthesia (see figure); injured thumb has about 30° more laxity in this direction than uninjured thumb.

Laboratory Findings: Radiograph: no fractures or dislocations.

Questions: What is your diagnosis? What is the recommended treatment?

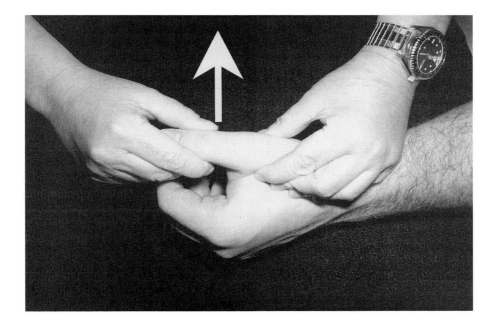

Answer: Gamekeeper's thumb (also known as skier's thumb). Operative exploration and repair are warranted due to the strong possibility of a Stener lesion.

Discussion: Gamekeeper's thumb is the partial or complete rupture of the ulnar collateral ligament (UCL) of the thumb MCP joint. It is typically caused by forceful abduction of the thumb (in skiers, this commonly occurs when the thumb is trapped in the strap of the ski pole during a fall). X-rays of the thumb may be normal (as in the present patient), or they may show a chip/avulsion fracture of the base of the proximal phalanx. In the latter case, the UCL remains attached to the bony chip, which is then a reliable indicator on x-ray as to whether the UCL is significantly displaced (this will have some impact on treatment options).

Typically the UCL is torn from the proximal phalanx and remains attached to the superior aspect of the distal metacarpal. The UCL can move as a "hinged flap," and can easily be held out of position by the adductor aponeurosis: this is called a Stener lesion, named after the physician who described this anatomical derangement. The presence of a Stener lesion is an absolute indication for surgical repair, because the UCL can never heal while held out of anatomic position. Patients who do not undergo repair experience chronic pain and weak grip.

Diagnosis of a Stener lesion is not necessarily straightforward. It is easy in patients with an avulsion fracture of the proximal phalanx: since the bone marks the distal end of the UCL, significant displacement confirms a Stener lesion (see figure;

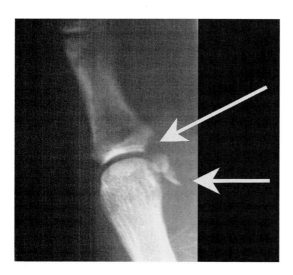

upper arrow is point of avulsion). The bony chip (*lower arrow*) remains attached to the UCL. Both the chip and the UCL are blocked from returning to their anatomic positions by the adductor aponeurosis, and surgical correction is required. In those patients without an avulsion fracture, a Stener lesion cannot be ruled out without surgical exploration.

Diagnosis of gamekeeper's thumb is usually made clinically, by tenderness over the ulnar aspect of the thumb MCP, combined with increased laxity of the MCP joint to radial deviation *when compared to the other side*. Comparison to the contralateral hand is important, because every patient has a different amount of baseline laxity. A patient that has 30 degrees or more laxity of the MCP joint when compared to the other hand most likely has a complete tear of the UCL; those with 20 degrees or less who still complain of tenderness and pain over the ulnar aspect of the MCP joint probably have a partial tear of the ligament.

During evaluation it is helpful to anesthetize the area, so that evaluation of the joint laxity can be done without severe patient pain. Both the median and radial nerves should be blocked at the wrist. Note that in patients with a complete tear, aggressive radial deviation of the thumb may actually *create* a Stener lesion, by flipping the distal end of the UCL up over the adductor aponeurosis.

In partial tears of the UCL, immobilization usually is all that is required. The thumb MCP joint should be held in a slightly adducted position (as opposed to more traditional thumb splint positions, in which abduction is necessary to preserve web space). In complete tears (whether a Stener lesion is confirmed or not), operative exploration and repair are required. In equivocal cases, this author (MC) prefers to explore the joint, because early intervention is much more efficacious than attempted late repair of the UCL. Repair of the UCL can be done with nonabsorbable suture if enough remains at the proximal phalanx to hold the suture. If there is not enough ligament substance at the proximal phalanx, the UCL can be repaired using an anchor suture placed at the base.

In the present patient, the significant degree of laxity represented a complete UCL tear. It was repaired using a suture anchored to the base of the proximal phalanx.

Clinical Pearls

1. Diagnosis of gamekeeper's thumb is made clinically by tenderness at the ulnar aspect of the MCP joint, and laxity to radial deviation of the MCP joint (when compared to the contralateral hand). In complete tears of the UCL, there is usually more than 30° of laxity when compared to the uninjured hand.

2. A Stener lesion occurs when the UCL is held out of its normal anatomic position by the fibers of the adductor pollicis. Since the ligament will not heal while held in this position, the presence of a Stener lesion is an absolute indication for surgery.

3. If a patient has an incomplete tear of the UCL (i.e., less than 30° of laxity of the MCP joint), immobilization in a thumb spica cast is appropriate treatment. Be careful to adduct the thumb at the MCP joint to minimize stretch at the healing ligament.

REFERENCES

1. Dray GJ, Eaton RG: Dislocations and ligament injuries in the digits. In Green DP, Hotchkiss, R, Pederson WC (eds): Green's Operative Hand Surgery, 4th ed. New York, Churchill Livingstone, Inc, 1999.
2. Frank WE, Dobyns JH: Surgical pathology of collateral ligamentous injuries of the thumb. Clin Orthop 83:102–114, 1972.
3. Stener B: Displacement of the ruptured ulnar collateral ligament of the metacarpophalangeal joint of the thumb. A clinical and anatomical study. J Bone Joint Surg 44B:869–879, 1962.

Perspectives For Therapy

Following interval immobilization in a thumb spica cast for conservative management of **Grades I and II** UCL sprains, patients are returned to a custom-fabricated, removable, hand-based thumb spica splint that permits freedom of the IP joint. Perforated thermoplastic is selected to promote air circulation and, rather than sealing the spica portion of the splint, the two ends are secured with a small Velcro strap; this allows adjustment for edema. The CMC joint may be positioned in abduction; however, to minimize stresses acting on the UCL, the MCP joint should be positioned in 10° flexion and in neutral, relative to the mediolateral plane. Normally, the UCL is maximally lengthened when the MCP joint is in extension, and this represents the close-pack position of the joint. Thus, positioning the MCP joint in flexion minimizes tension on the UCL.

The patient wears the splint at all times for 2–4 weeks, except during hygiene activities and exercise. Every other waking hour, the patient removes the splint and performs up to 20 repetitions of active composite thumb flexion and extension, and gentle opposition to the medial four fingers. Thermal modalities and joint mobilization may be employed in the clinic; however, care must be taken to stabilize the MCP joint mediolaterally when performing oscillations. The patient is also encouraged to perform active motion exercises for the uninvolved upper extremity joints.

The patient is re-evaluated following 2–4 weeks of interval splinting. If painfree, they may decrease splint use during activity, with the exception of vigorous ADLs and participation in sports. A playing cast is recommended for football; taping for volleyball and basketball; and use of a splint or reinforced glove for skiing. Grip-strengthening exercises for the fingers, while protecting the thumb in extension and adduction, and isolated lateral pinch for the thumb may also be initiated at this time.

Following surgery and interval immobilization to manage **Grade III** injuries of the UCL, the patient is returned to a hand-based thumb spica splint for 4 weeks. Splint design is identical to that used for conservative management. The patient is instructed in active motion exercises for the thumb, including extension, flexion, and gentle opposition. Exercise frequency and duration are also identical to conservative management guidelines. Postoperative care also involves edema management through elevation of the upper extremity in addition to retrograde massage, as needed. It is particularly important to address range of motion of the uninvolved joints of the patient's upper extremity. The patient may gradually resume ADLs such as handwriting, eating, grooming, and dressing without the splint. Once sutures are removed and the wound well healed, scar massage may be initiated, and thermal modalities used in the clinic. Joint mobilization may also be performed with care given to stabilizing the MCP joint as previously described.

At 4–6 weeks postoperatively, the patient decreases splint use during activity, with the exception of vigorous ADLs and participation in sports. At this time, the patient also begins passive range-of-motion exercises for thumb flexion, and dy-

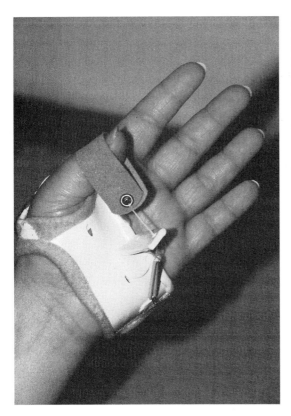

namic splinting may be initiated at this time, if indicated (see figure; the thumb hole of this custom, hand-based splint clears the MCP joint, and the finger loop is secured to the IP joint to promote composite MCP and IP flexion. The line of pull is perpendicular to the distal phalanx, and the rubber-band traction is adjusted, bringing the thumb into end-range flexion at both joints.)

At 8 weeks postoperatively, the patient is instructed in progressive, resisted exercises for general upper extremity strengthening and conditioning using graded rubber bands or tubes. Exercise putty may be used for increasing grip and pinch strength.

At 12 weeks, the patient may return to his or her preinjury level of activity. However, it is advisable to continue some type of protective splinting when engaged in vigorous ADLs and sports.

Hand Therapy Pearl

The primary consideration for the hand therapist, whether treating ulnar collateral ligament injury of the thumb MCP joint conservatively or postoperatively, is to protect the MCP joint and UCL from valgus stresses during interval healing.

REFERENCES
1. Cannon NM. Ligamentous/soft tissue injuries and reconstruction. In Diagnosis and Treatment Manual for Physicians and Therapists 3rd ed. Indianapolis, Hand Rehabilitation Center of Indianapolis, 1991, pp 130–131.
2. Wilson RL, Hazen J. Management of joint injuries and intraarticular fractures of the hand. In Hunter JM, Mackin EJ, Callahan AD (eds): Rehabilitation of the Hand: Surgery and Therapy, 4th ed. St. Louis, Mosby, 1995, pp 377–394.
3. Wright HH. Hand therapists set the pace in sports medicine. J Hand Ther 4:37–41, 1991.

PATIENT 9

A 45-year-old woman who cannot actively extend her small finger

A 45-year-old woman was playing softball at her company picnic when she "jammed" her right 5th finger attempting to field a fly ball. She presents now (2 days after the injury) with persistent swelling of the finger, pain over the entire digit, and an inability to actively extend the distal phalanx of that finger. She denies any other injuries to the hand. She smokes approximately 10 cigarettes per day, and is employed as a transcriptionist.

Physical Examination: Skin: no lesions or lacerations on finger. Musculoskeletal: full (passive) extension and flexion at MCP, PIP, and DIP joints; moderate tenderness with movement; patient can strongly flex finger into a fist, but cannot extend the distal phalanx (see figure).

Laboratory Findings: Radiograph: no fractures or dislocations.

Questions: What is your diagnosis? Describe the recommended treatment.

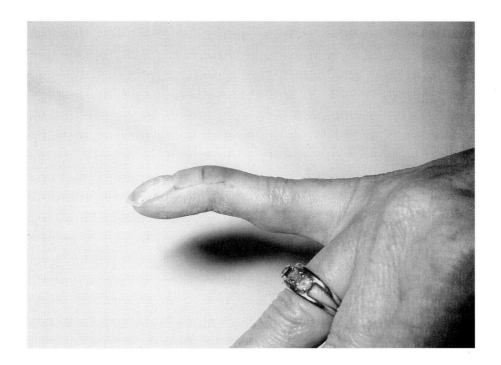

Answer: Mallet finger (closed). Immobilization is the recommended treatment.

Discussion: Mallet finger represents a disruption of the terminal extensor mechanism as it inserts at the distal phalanx. The injury is classified based on whether it is closed or open (i.e., a laceration) and whether there is an associated avulsion fracture of the distal phalanx. Treatment options depend on these factors.

Open injuries (such as a cut on the distal dorsal finger) are best treated with operative direct repair of the tendon. These injuries differ very little from extensor tendon lacerations located more proximally on the finger. Closed injuries, in which the tendon has been avulsed from its insertion at the distal phalanx, are a bit more problematic. There is rarely enough tendon substance available to hold a suture in this situation. Therefore, in closed mallet finger injuries (without an associated fracture), operative intervention is not indicated. These digits should be splinted in neutral or slight hyperextension for a minimum of 12 weeks. There are several types of splints available that will maintain this immobilization while still allowing PIP motion, such as the Link or Stack splints (see figure, *below*). These are easy for the patient to use.

It is important that the patient understand that splinting must be maintained 24 hours a day, 7 days a week. After 8 weeks (if the patient can maintain the distal phalanx in extension without the splint), he or she can wear the splint only at night for an additional 4 weeks, after which splinting is stopped altogether. Let the patient know that if extension lag recurs, splinting will have to be resumed immediately. If a patient is unable to comply with external splinting, percutaneous K-wire placement maintaining full extension is occasionally helpful (see figure).

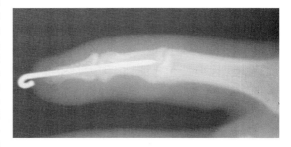

Lateral x-rays should be obtained in these injuries, because they occasionally occur with a small, dorsal, bony chip fracture (see *A, next page*). The bony chip is still attached to the distal tendon. If the bone fragment is large enough, open reduction and internal fixation can be accomplished relatively early (see *B, next page*). Because the bone-to-bone interface heals faster and more strongly than the tendon, patients who undergo this procedure may be able to resume normal activity as quickly as 5–6 weeks after surgical repair. If the injury is not large enough to accommodate a small screw or pin, the treatment remains the same as for a closed mallet finger without a fracture.

Patients sometimes present several months after their original injury. The initial treatment plan for these individuals still involves splinting, although it has a higher risk of not being successful.

If a patient has failed conservative management, operative repair is indicated. At 3 months after the original injury, operative repair involves resecting the dorsal scar, incorporating and replacing the extensor tendon, repairing the shortened tendon with several nonabsorbable sutures, and extensive immobilization. Left untreated, the mallet finger deformity can progress to a swan neck deformity. If late operative repair is not successful, a final alternative for these patients is fusion of the DIP joint in a functional position (i.e., 0–10 degrees of flexion)

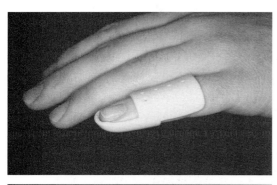

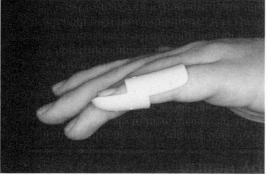

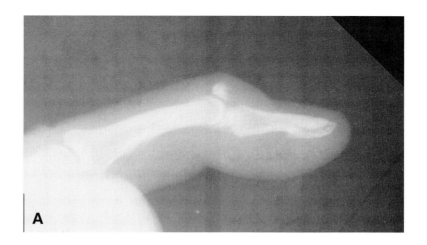

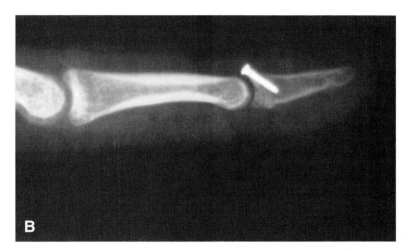

Clinical Pearls

1. Closed mallet finger injuries (i.e., the extensor tendon was not sharply cut) are best treated with prolonged splinting of the DIP in extension. Patients should be warned that splinting may last 12 weeks or longer.

2. If a patient presents with a chronic mallet finger, operative repair involving imbrication of the extensor tendon and protection of this repair with a percutaneous K-wire (maintaining the DIP in full extension) may be required.

3. For patients who may be less compliant with splinting, consider placement of a percutaneous K-wire across the DIP to maintain the digit in proper position during the tendon healing phase.

REFERENCES

1. Patel MR, Desai SS, Bassini-Lipson L: Conservative management of chronic mallet finger. J Hand Surg 11(4):570–573, 1986.
2. Shankar NS, Goring CC: Mallet finger: Long-term review of 100 cases. J R Coll Surg Edinb 37(3):196–198, 1992.
3. Stern PJ, Kastrup JJ: Complications and prognosis of treatment of mallet finger. J Hand Surg 13(3):329–334, 1988.

Custom-fabricated splints, based on the Stack design, may be indicated in the event that adequate fit in a prefabricated Link or Stack splint is not possible. An effective custom splint can be made from a piece of ⅛-inch-thick Aquaplast of sufficient size to encircle approximately 80% of the circumference of the middle and distal phalanges, with the distal edges finished parallel to the lateral and medial borders of the nail-fold. A hole is punched in the splint material while cold, using a leather-punch tool. The splint material is molded by sliding it over the patient's fingertip through the hole created in the material.

The splint material that projects below the plane of the finger is used to create the distal component of the splint, volar to the distal phalanx and DIP joint, and supporting the distal joint in 5–10° of hyperextension. The splint material projecting above the plane of the finger is used to create the proximal component of the splint, dorsal to the middle phalanx. This is secured with Velcro and permits PIP joint motion.

The edges of the hole are finished by pressing them into the splint base, and the distal component of the splint, supporting the distal phalanx in hyperextension, is windowed with the leather-punch to promote air circulation. It has been suggested that two splints be fabricated for the patient; one is specifically for wear during performance of hygiene.

Due to the length of time required for continuous splinting during extensor tendon healing, skin breakdown due to perspiration, inadequate drying technique after hygiene, or neglect is a potential complication. The patient should be instructed in monitoring skin condition and in proper splint application, ensuring that the DIP joint of the involved finger remains in full extension. Absorbent materials such as moleskin can be used to line the splint, and must be changed when soiled. Splint revisions to provide a precise fit will be necessary with decreased edema.

After 8 weeks of splinting, provided there is no extension lag, the patient is instructed in gentle, active flexion of the DIP joint. Exercise templates that permit 20–25° of isolated DIP flexion during the first week and 35° isolated flexion during the second week are useful. Up to 10 repetitions are performed every other waking hour, and the patient should return to the immobilization splint between exercise sessions during this 2-week interval. Splinting at bedtime should be continued for an additional 4 weeks, once intermittent daytime splinting is discontinued. If an extension lag emerges, exercises should be halted and extension splinting resumed on a continuous basis for 2 weeks. Gentle, active DIP motion should be reattempted only after that interval.

As mentioned, if left untreated, mallet finger can evolve into a swan-neck mechanical fault. The extensor digitorum and hand intrinsics concentrate their extensor forces at the base of the middle phalanx, resulting in PIP joint extension while the unopposed FDP flexes the DIP joint. Hyperextension of the PIP joint is initially resisted by the accessory collateral ligaments and volar plate; however, as these structures yield, PIP joint hyperextension results. PIP joint hyperextension increases as the released oblique retinacular ligament migrates to a position *dorsal* to the PIP joint, with resultant adaptive shortening.

Hand Therapy Pearl

Vigilance regarding skin condition and revisions of custom splints are essential when treating patients with zone I and II extensor tendon injuries due to the prolonged interval of immobilization.

REFERENCES

1. Evans RB. An update on extensor tendon management. In Hunter JM, Mackin EJ, Callahan AD (eds): Rehabilitation of the Hand: Surgery and Therapy, 4th ed. St. Louis, Mosby, 1995, pp 565–606.
2. Rosenthal EA. The extensor tendons: Anatomy and management. In Hunter JM, Mackin EJ, Callahan AD (eds). Rehabilitation of the Hand: Surgery and Therapy, 4th ed. St. Louis, Mosby, 1995, pp 519–564.

PATIENT 10

A 60-year-old man with a 2-year history of a nail deformity

A 60-year-old man presents with a nail deformity that first arose 2 years ago. He cannot recall any specific trauma to the nail itself, but he did "break a hand bone" in a car accident 3 years ago (those records are unavailable, but he relates that the only treatment was cast immobilization).

Physical Examination: General: all systems normal. Musculoskeletal: excellent range of motion and strength. Neurologic: sensation intact. Skin: nail thickened and discolored; rough and irregular surface.

Questions: What is your diagnosis? What treatment options (if any) can you suggest?

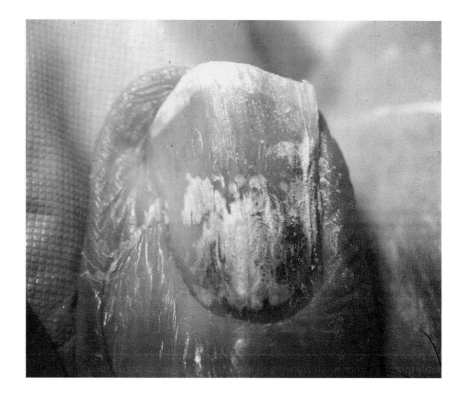

Answers: Onychomycosis. Recommend medical management with Lamisil (terbinafine) or Sporonox (itraconazole).

Discussion: About 50% of patients who present with dystrophic nails have a nail bed fungal infection, or onychomycosis. The diagnosis is confirmed by microscopic visualization of hyphae present on nail scrapings using a 20% KOH preparation. Causes for the disorder in the other 50% are multiple, including psoriasis, lichen planus, and trauma. Fungal infections of the nail are much more common in the foot than the hand. In either location, they can result in a highly annoying aesthetic and functional deformity.

In the past, medical treatment was problematic, requiring long-term administration of systemic (oral) antifungal agents, with significant toxicity. In addition, recurrence was the rule rather than the exception. Recently, several agents have been developed that appear to be more effective in the treatment of onychomycosis, require a much shorter treatment period, and have less potential toxicity.

Lamisil (terbinafine) is an antifungal agent that is effective in the treatment of onychomycosis. The dosing schedule is 250 mg PO once a day for a total of 6 weeks. This short treatment period removes the necessity for liver function tests (LFTs) prior to treatment, if your patient is otherwise healthy. If he or she has a history of hepatitis, liver disease, or heavy alcohol abuse, it may be prudent to obtain LFTs prior to initiating treatment. Remember that the treatment of *fingernail* onychomycosis is not the same as the treatment in the foot (toe infections require longer therapy). If your patient has affected toes as well, refer to the dosing information to adjust the treatment. Even though this agent is markedly more effective than older antifungal agents for this problem, approximately 30% of patients will have a recurrence.

An alternative agent for this problem is Sporanox (itraconazole), which can be given 200 mg PO once a day for 6 weeks. An alternative method of administering this drug is "pulsed" therapy, in which the patient takes 200 mg twice a day for 1 week, then no drug for 3 weeks; this is repeated for a total of 3 months. Although this type of dosing is much more convenient for the patients (easier to maintain compliance), preliminary reports indicate that Lamisil is more effective and is associated with less recurrence than Sporonox.

Clinical Pearls

1. Toenail onychomycosis is more prevalent than fingernail infections and requires longer medical therapy.

2. Onychomycosis is the leading cause of dystrophic nails (approximately 50% of all cases).

3. Current medicinal options have fewer side effects and less impact on the overall health of your patient than previous options.

REFERENCES

1. Baran R: Onychia and paronychia of mycotic, microbial and parasite origin. In Pierre M (ed): The Nail. New York, Churchill Livingstone, Inc, 1981.
2. Lawry MA, Haneke E, Strobeck K, et al: Methods for diagnosing onychomycosis: A comparative study and review of the literature. Arch Dermatol 136(9):1112–1116, 2000.
3. Sigurgeirsson B, Billstein S, Rantanen T, et al: L.I.ON. study: Efficacy and tolerability of continuous terbinafine (Lamisil) compared to intermittent itraconazole in the treatment of toenail onychomycosis. Br J Dermatol 56 (Suppl 141):5–14, 1999.
4. Zaias N: The Nail in Health and Disease. Robert B. Luce Incorporated, New York, McGraw-Hill, 1980.
5. Zook EG, Brown RE: The perionychium. In Green DP, Hotchkiss R, Pederson WC (eds): Green's Operative Hand Surgery, 4th ed. New York, Churchill Livingstone, Inc, 1999.

PATIENT 11

A newborn infant with a thumb deformity

You have been called to the nursery to consult on a newborn baby boy. His thumb appears normal distally, but is attached to the hand by only a small skin bridge. There is no family history of a similar newborn deformity. This is the parents' first child (no sibling data).

Physical Examination: Musculoskeletal: no bone in skin bridge between thumb and hand; thumb completely viable, but voluntary movement of digit by patient not discernible.

Laboratory Findings: Radiograph of right hand: see below.

Questions: What is the diagnosis? What is the recommended treatment?

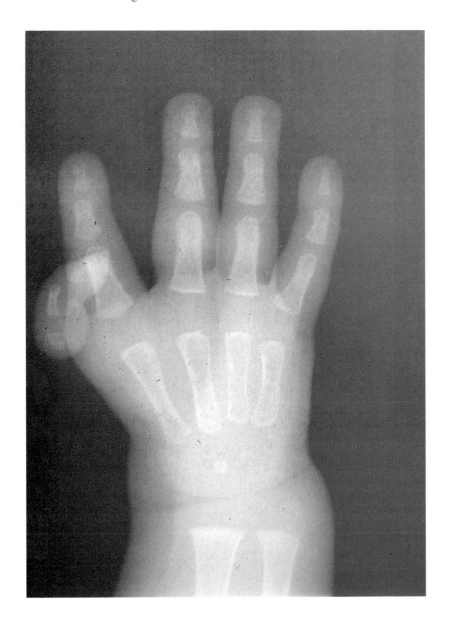

Answer: Hypoplastic thumb (*pouce flottant* variant)

Discussion: Hypoplastic thumb is defined as rudimentary thumb with no (or very little) metacarpal and no thumb musculature. The pouce flottant variant, also called "floating thumb," is one of the more severe forms of thumb hypoplasia. It can range in severity from a digit that is slightly smaller than the unaffected side, to complete thumb absence. Interestingly, the distal aspect of the thumb may appear relatively normal. However, there is often only one rudimentary neurovascular bundle supplying the digit, and little or no skeletal support.

The distal thumb's relatively normal appearance often misleads parents into being overly optimistic about the functional future of the digit. Despite appearances, any attempt to salvage the original segment is destined to failure, as the thumb will have very little function.

The best functional outcome is achieved by re-section of the floating segment in the neonatal period (see figure, *left;* appearance at 15 months of age) and later pollicization.

Pollicization provides these individuals with a functional opposable digit and a relatively normal hand (see figure, *right;* hand 4 weeks after pollicization). The principles of this relatively complex procedure include shortening of the index metacarpal, with repositioning of the index finger to act as the new thumb. The technical details have evolved; currently, the technique put forth by Buck-Gramcko has a reliable track record, as well as good aesthetic and functional results. The timing of surgery remains somewhat controversial, with most doctors advocating elective pollicization between 12 and 24 months of age.

Initial postoperative care involves primarily protection of the digit with long arm casting. After adequate healing has occurred, hand therapy is very helpful in recovering mobility of the digit.

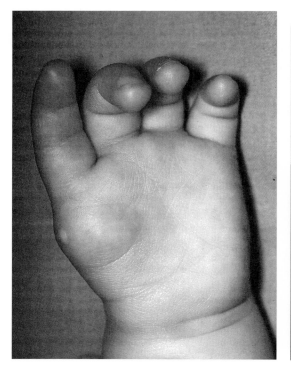

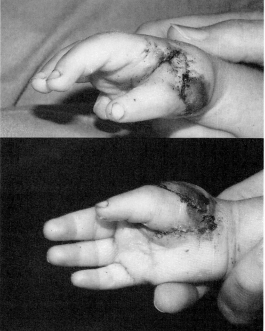

Clinical Pearls

1. Despite a relatively normal-appearing distal thumb, individuals with the *pouce flottant* deformity will not be able to achieve reasonable function of that digit, despite heroic attempts to salvage it.

2. Timing of pollicization is not "set in stone": surgery should be delayed until the structures (neurovascular bundles, tendons) are large enough to be safely dissected and mobilized. Most authors advocate pollicization between 1 and 2 years of age.

3. Patients with hypoplastic thumbs have been associated with the following: ring D chromosome abnormalities, Holt-Oram syndrome, trisomy-18 syndrome, Rothmund-Thompson syndrome, and thalidomide exposure.

4. A completely absent thumb is almost always associated with an absent radius (radial club hand)—except in thrombocytopenia radial aplasia (Fanconi's syndrome), where the thumb is present even though the radius is absent.

REFERENCES

1. Buck-Gramcko D: Pollicization of the index finger. J Bone Joint Surg 53A:1605–1617, 1971.
2. Flatt AE: The Care of Congenital Hand Anomolies. St. Louis, CV Mosby, 1977.
3. Kleinman WB: Management of thumb hypoplasia. Hand Clin 6(4):617–641, 1990.
4. Manske PR, Rotman MB, Dailey LA: Long-term functional results after pollicization for the congenitally deficient thumb. J Hand Surg [Am] 17(6):1064–72, 1992.

Perspectives For Therapy

Perhaps the most important aspect of pediatric therapeutic management is parental education regarding their active involvement in the rehabilitative process. In the current managed healthcare climate, the progress of the pediatric patient simply cannot be followed by the hand therapist with the frequency and duration required for skeletal-motor maturation. Accordingly, the hand therapist must be capable of communicating to the parents all aspects of postoperative care. Additionally, he or she should ameliorate the emotional uncertainty of the parents regarding their child's integration into society. The hand therapist may even play a role in educating the child's teacher regarding the patient's functional status.

It is critical for the hand therapist to perform a preoperative assessment of the pediatric patient. Patterns of established hand use, motion, strength, and sensation are key elements of the preoperative evaluation. The pediatric patient's success in using the pollicized index finger for prehensile activities will depend, in part, upon the manner in which they have learned to achieve functional grasping. For example, if the patient functioned effectively using the long and ring, or ring and small fingers for small object manipulation, these established prehensile patterns will probably be retained postoperatively. The patient will then rely on their thumb and long finger for grasping large objects, due simply to the amplified first web-space.

Wound care, splinting, range-of-motion exercises, sensation monitoring, and play and functional activities all have a place during the postoperative interval. The parents are instructed in wound and skin care, range-of-motion exercises, and motor activities for the operated hand, as these become incorporated into a home program. Meticulous wound care, scar massage, and monitoring of skin condition will complement the hand surgeon's skills and help improve the appearance of the operated hand. The more normal the hand appears, the higher the likelihood of parental, patient, and social acceptance, and chances are improved that the pediatric patient will use his or her pollicized digit.

The goals of hand splinting are twofold: first, position the thumb for function, and second, prevent development of deformity. To optimize the surgical result and prevent adduction contracture of the pollicized digit, hand splinting consists of fabricating a thermoplastic C-web spacer to maintain thumb opposition/abduction. A splint interface, such as light cotton or similar thin, absorbent material is indicated for skin protection. If available, brightly colored, $\frac{1}{16}$-inch, perforated thermoplastics are desirable for splint fabrication, as they are lightweight and promote air circulation. Custom thermoplastic splints are secured with a cohesive bandage and worn between exercise sessions and at bedtime.

Soft straps, to promote thumb opposition/abduction, offer an alternative to thermoplastics. A simple abduction strap, based low on the thumb, is led across the palm and secured on the wrist in circumferential fashion. This may be worn at all times, except during wound care and hygiene performance. Securing splints with adhesive tape is relatively contraindicated due to concerns about skin condition, and even paper tape should be used judiciously.

Parents are instructed in splint application and removal and are encouraged to practice in the clinic with therapist supervision to ensure carryover at home. They also receive information about splint care and skin precautions. As active motion develops in the thumb, splint use normally decreases.

Therapeutic intervention must be matched with the cognitive status and motor development skills of the pediatric patient. Developmentally appropriate motor tasks emphasize reaching, grasping, and pinching using thumb opposition, and these activities are incorporated into play behavior.

Patient age does not seem to be a critical determinant of functional outcome following pollicization. Pollicization may be performed prior to the first birthday through the mid-teens. Patients readily initiate developmentally appropriate activity of the pollicized index finger, and recognize the transposed index finger as a thumb. Total active motion is approximately 50% of the normal thumb, and pinch strength averages 25% when compared to age- and sex-matched controls. The pollicized index finger is used for manipulation of small objects 60% of the time, and for large objects 90% of the time. Patients having undergone pollicization require 40% longer than controls to perform similar tasks.

Hand Therapy Pearls

1. Parent education is the most important aspect of pediatric patient management. If the parents readily accept the appearance of their child's hand, successful (re)integration into society is likely.

2. A preoperative assessment of hand function should be performed. Established prehensile patterns are generally retained postoperatively.

3. Postoperative treatment includes wound care, splinting, range-of-motion exercises, sensation monitoring, and play and functional activities.

4. Therapeutic intervention must be matched with the cognitive status and motor development skills of the pediatric patient.

REFERENCES

1. Byron PM: Splinting the hand of a child. In Hunter JM, Mackin EJ, Callahan AD (eds): Rehabilitation of the Hand: Surgery and Therapy, 4th ed. St. Louis, Mosby, 1995, pp 1443–1449.
2. Candish S. Zimmer P: Post-op pollicization: The paediatric challenge. J Hand Ther 9:267, 1996.
3. Fuller M: Treatment of congenital differences of the upper extremity: Therapist's commentary. J Hand Ther 12:174–177, 1999.
4. Manske PR, McCarroll HR: Reconstruction of the congenitally deficient thumb. Hand Clin 8:177–196, 1992.

PATIENT 12

A 45-year-old man with progressive hand weakness and clumsiness

A 45-year-old man complains of weakness and clumsiness of his dominant (right) hand. He denies any injury or trauma to this hand. The symptoms have been slowly progressive over the past 8 months. He does not experience pain or numbness in the hand, but does suffer cramping and pain in his forearm with exertional activity.

Physical Examination: Neurologic: sensation intact throughout volar and dorsal hand; moving two-point discrimination < 5 mm on all fingers. Musculoskeletal: full passive range of motion of fingers and thumb, with no limitations; negative Phalen's and Tinel's tests at volar wrist; no detectable muscular atrophy; slightly weaker right grip compared to left (despite right-handedness). Patient cannot actively flex distal phalanx of thumb nor index finger, but denies any pain during attempt; also is unable to pinch thumb *fingertip* to index *fingertip* (see figure).

Questions: What is the diagnosis? What is your treatment recommendation?

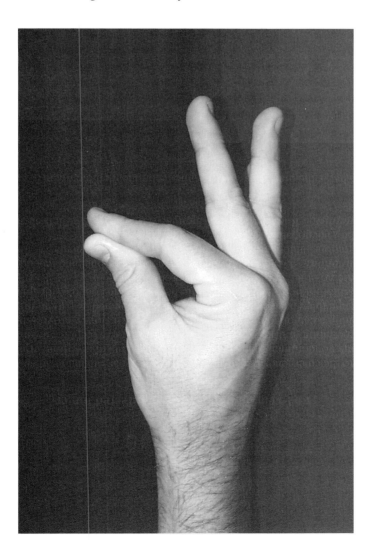

Answer: Anterior interosseous nerve compression. Treatment requires surgical decompression.

Discussion: The anterior interosseous nerve is a branch of the median nerve that arises in the mid-forearm. It innervates three muscles:

- Flexor pollicis longus (thumb distal phalanx flexion)
- Flexor digitorum profundus to the index and long fingers (distal phalanx flexion)
- Pronator quadratus (forearm pronation).

Since forearm pronation is reproduced by other muscles (pronator teres), weakness of pronation is a rare presenting complaint. The anterior interosseous nerve is a motor branch of the median nerve and has no sensory branches; therefore, patients with compression or injury to this nerve have no complaints of anesthesia or other sensory alterations.

The loss of active flexion of both the distal phalanges of the index and thumb fingers results in a very characteristic pinch conformation, as shown in this patient. Patients with this condition compensate for the loss of function by using the key pinch provided by the ulnar-innervated musculature (adductor pollicis and first dorsal interosseous muscles). This compensation should not be confused with the classic **Froment's sign,** which shows evidence of *ulnar nerve pathology.* Froment's sign is seen when patients with an ulnar nerve lesion are asked to demonstrate key pinch (forcefully holding the thumb against the index, such as when using a key to open a door (see figure, *A*). In these patients, because of the loss of both the adductor pollicis and the first dorsal interosseous muscles, compensation is via the FDP and FPL, producing the characteristic posture called Froment's sign (see figure, *B*).

Diagnosis of compression/entrapment of the anterior interosseous nerve is first made clinically, and confirmed with electrodiagnostic studies. If these studies are negative, consider a more proximal lesion of the median nerve (such as pronator syndrome). If a lesion cannot be positively identified, hold surgical exploration and repeat the studies in 4 to 6 weeks. If the repeat studies are still nonconfirmatory, and the patient remains symptomatic, surgical exploration is warranted to definitively exclude the possibility of nerve entrapment.

Compression of the nerve by the deep head of the pronator teres is the most common cause of this syndrome. Other causes include compression by an enlarged bicipital tendon bursa, or by a fascial band at the origin of the flexor digitorum su-

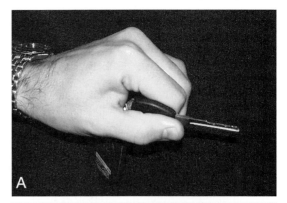

A

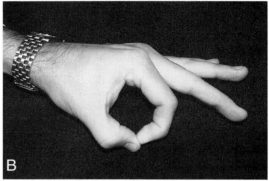

B

perficialis. If the decision is made to proceed with exploration, the entire length of the median nerve from 8 cm above the elbow to the mid-forearm should be examined (see figure below) to definitely exclude all possible sites of compression.

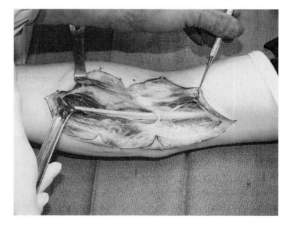

See color panel.

Clinical Pearls

1. Entrapment/compression of the anterior interosseous nerve—a purely motor nerve—is one of the few nerve compression symptoms without sensory derangements.

2. The clinical diagnosis is confirmed by the classic, compensatory, pinch posture using the "key-pinch" muscles (adductor pollicis and 1st dorsal interosseous) when the patient is trying to pinch the tip of the index finger to the tip of the thumb.

3. Electrodiagnostic studies can help confirm and locate the lesion. However, even if studies are negative, surgical exploration and decompression are still indicated in the face of persistent symptoms within this nerve distribution.

REFERENCES
1. Bucher TPJ: Anterior interosseous nerve syndrome. J Bone Joint Surg 54B:555, 1972.
2. Eversmann Jr WW: Entrapment and compression neuropathies. In Green DP, Hotchkiss R, Pederson WC (eds): Green's Operative Hand Surgery, 4th ed. New York, Churchill Livingstone, 1999.
3. Farber JS, Bryan RS: Anterior interosseous nerve palsy. J Bone Joint Surg 47B:91–93, 1968.
4. Maeda K, Miura T, Komada T, Chiba A: Anterior interosseous nerve paralysis. Report of 13 cases and review of Japanese literatures. Hand 9:165–171, 1977.

Perspectives For Therapy

Compression of the median nerve at elbow level, or within the proximal forearm, is regarded as high median nerve entrapment. Commonly described locations of median nerve compression are the pronator teres muscle, lacertus fibrosus of the biceps brachii, and the arcuate proximal origin of the FDS in the forearm. The hand therapist can provide objective results of manual muscle testing and sensory threshold data on light touch, through the use of Semmes-Weinstein monofilaments, to aid the hand surgeon in making a diagnosis. Anterior interosseous nerve syndrome is characterized by median nerve compression resulting in weakness of FPL, FDP II and III, and pronator quadratus. Absence of paresthesia is useful for differential diagnosis. In pronator syndrome, median nerve compression results in mixed motor (weakness) and sensory (paresthesia in the median nerve distribution of the hand and pain) disturbances.

Provocative testing to implicate the pronator teres muscle consists of active forearm pronation against manual resistance and passive elbow extension with overpressure. To implicate the lacertus fibrosus of the biceps brachii muscle, the patient's elbow is placed in 120° flexion, and manual resistance is applied. Resisted forearm supination, with the elbow positioned at 90° flexion, is also assessed because the biceps is a powerful supinator of the forearm. Resisted PIP joint flexion of the long finger may implicate the FDS where its humeroulnar and radial heads converge upon the arcuate proximal tendon of origin.

Conservative treatment for anterior interosseous nerve syndrome and pronator syndrome consists of immobilizing the affected extremity with a sugartong splint with wrist component; this splint design positions the elbow at 90° flexion, forearm in neutral rotation, and wrist at 0°. A posterior long-arm splint with wrist component can be fabricated if additional stability is desirable. With conservative treatment, the patient should anticipate 8–12 weeks of continuous splint use, to provide an interval of relative rest for the median nerve. However, if symptoms are responsive, the patient may be permitted to decrease splint use.

Any surgical procedure with the goal of releasing all constricting structures may potentially lead to scar formation consistent with extensive exposure. Scar tissue may result in motion restriction where it crosses flexion creases, and adherent scar may limit soft tissue gliding along connective tissue planes. Postoperative management of scar is therefore prioritized once adequate wound healing has occurred and skin staples or sutures have been removed. Scar tissue is mobilized by deep massage. Silicone gel sheeting or custom-made elastomer appliances secured with elastic stockinette are used for scar compression. As edema decreases, stockinette of decreasing diameter should be issued to the patient to ensure adequate scar compression.

Exercises combining elbow extension, forearm supination, and wrist extension are used to mobilize the median nerve, and these can be initiated as early as 48–72 hours following surgery. Early exercise also contributes to scar remodeling and helps set the stage for progression to general upper extremity strengthening and conditioning exercises at 3 weeks postoperatively.

Hand Therapy Pearls

1. The hand therapist can provide the hand surgeon with objective information about high median nerve entrapment through clinical, provocative testing of muscle performance and sensory thresholds.

2. Conservative treatment of median nerve compression requires a period of relative rest for the nerve; this is provided by static splinting.

3. In cases of surgical management of median nerve entrapment, the hand therapist plays an important role during postoperative treatment. Scar management and nerve gliding exercises are critical.

REFERENCE
Tetro AM, Pichora DR. High median nerve entrapments: An obscure cause of upper-extremity pain. Hand Clin 12:691–703, 1996.

PATIENT 13

A 15-year-old boy unable to extend his thumb after a wrist fracture

The patient broke his wrist while skateboarding nearly 6 weeks prior to presentation. He had been diagnosed as having a "Colles fracture" according to his mother (the records are not available for review). He was treated with cast immobilization by an orthopedic surgeon, and last week the cast was removed. He states that he has been unable to extend his thumb since that time.

Physical Examination: Neurologic: no tenderness over dorsal and volar wrist; intact sensation throughout hand. Musculoskeletal: wrist stiff; reduced flexion and extension compared to other (non-injured) side; full active flexion and extension of index, long, ring, and 5th fingers; can fully flex thumb into palm, but cannot actively extend distal phalanx. When thumb is fully extended by examiner, patient cannot maintain extension upon release (see figure).

Laboratory Findings: Radiographs: original films (provided by patient)—distal radius fracture. Recent films—good anatomic position of the distal radius and anatomic reduction; early bony healing of fracture.

Questions: What is the diagnosis? What surgical treatment is advisable?

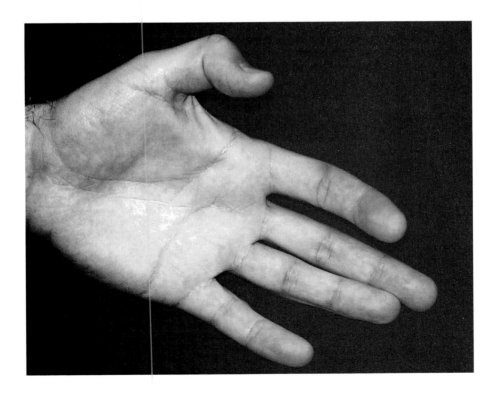

Answers: Rupture of the extensor pollicis longus (EPL) tendon. The best treatment option is tendon transfer using the extensor indicis proprius as the proximal motor.

Discussion: The EPL tendon lies within the 3rd extensor compartment and functions to extend the distal phalanx of the thumb. Injury to this tendon is a known complication of distal radius fractures, regardless of which method of fracture fixation is employed (i.e., closed vs. open technique). This injury often is an attenuation-type rupture, making success of direct repair unlikely.

Two treatment options remain for restoration of active thumb distal phalanx extension: repair using a tendon graft, or repair using a tendon transfer. Because of a high incidence of tendinous adhesions after tendon repair using a tendon graft, and the close proximity of an excellent donor muscle whose harvest leaves little donor morbidity, we greatly favor the use of the extensor indicis proprius (EIP) as a tendon transfer for reconstruction.

The EIP duplicates the action of the extensor digitorum communis at the index finger. At the MCP joint, the EIP typically lies ulnar to the extensor digitorum communis tendon. Harvest of the tendon is relatively straightforward, with transection at the level of the MCP joint through a small 1.5 cm incision. The tendon is then pulled back through a separate incision at the level of the dorsal radial wrist (see figure, *below*) and sutured to the distal end of the EPL using nonabsorbable suture. The wrist, fingers, and thumb are splinted in extension to minimize tension on the healing tendon in the postoperative period.

The similar action of the EIP and EPL (finger extension) makes rehabilitation training fairly easy for the patient. Using the tendon transfer is relatively straightforward and quickly relearned. Patients are instructed to "shoot the gun," a motion that simultaneously extends the index and thumb distal phalanges (see figure).

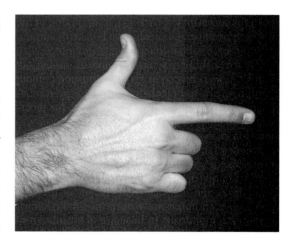

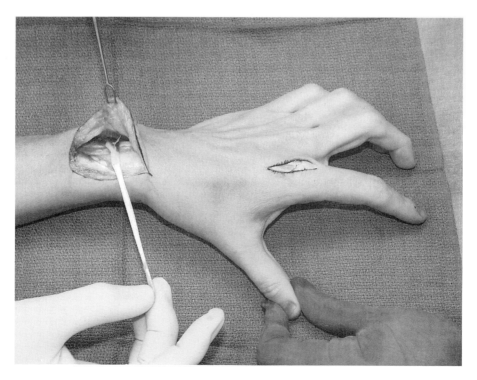

Clinical Pearls

1. Rupture of the EPL is a known complication of distal radius fractures, regardless of the treatment used for fracture reduction or fixation.
2. EPL rupture is also a common complication of rheumatoid arthritis; treatment options in these patients are similar to those with rupture due to acute trauma.

REFERENCES

1. Chapman DR, Bennett JB, Bryan WJ, Tullos HS: Complications of distal radius fractures: Pins and plaster treatment. J Hand Surg 7:509–512, 1982.
2. Cooney III WP, Dobyns JH, Linscheid RL: Complications of Colles' fractures. J Bone Joint Surg 62A:613–619, 1980.
3. Dobyns JH, Linscheid RL: Complications of treatment of fractures and dislocations of the wrist. In Epps Jr CH (ed): Complications in Orthopaedic Surgery. Philadelphia, JB Lippincott, 1978, pp 271–352.
4. Feldon P, Millander LH, Nalebuff EA: Rheumatoid arthritis in the hand and wrist. In Green DP, Hotchkiss R, Pederson WC (eds): Green's Operative Hand Surgery, 4th ed. New York, Churchill Livingstone, 1999.

Perspectives For Therapy

At 4 weeks postoperatively, patients are placed in a custom-fabricated, thermoplastic splint that positions the wrist in 20° extension and the thumb in composite extension at the CMC, MCP, and IP joints. The fingers are permitted freedom of motion. The splint is worn for protection at bedtime and between exercise sessions.

Each waking hour, the patient removes the splint and performs 20 repetitions of the following exercises:

- Active thumb IP joint extension performed simultaneously with extension of the index finger. The patient maintains the wrist in neutral; medial three fingers and thumb CMC in flexion; and thumb MCP joint at 0°. In this manner, the tension of the transferred EIP is transmitted primarily to the thumb IP joint.
- Active wrist exercises in all planes with the fingers and thumb relaxed
- Thumb opposition and composite flexion with the wrist positioned in radial deviation and extension to minimize tension on the transferred EIP.

Electrical stimulation of the transferred EIP may also be initiated at this time. Instrument settings should accord with the goal of facilitating muscle *recruitment,* rather than muscle strengthening.

At this postoperative stage, it is also important to instruct the patient in scar massage to minimize the risk of tendon adherence to underlying soft tissues, which can result in diminution of extensor power transmitted to the thumb IP joint. The use of elastomer putty or silicone gel sheeting is useful for scar compression, and these modalities may be employed at bedtime, either galvanized directly to the splint base or secured over the scar with elastic stockinette.

At 6 weeks postoperatively (providing the patient can consistently achieve and sustain at least 0° active IP extension of the thumb), passive composite flexion of the thumb, performed with the wrist flexed, may be initiated. Joint mobilization and dynamic splinting may also be indicated to manage flexion limitations.

If the patient is unable to consistently achieve and sustain active IP extension to 0°, the static extension splint may be revised to include only the IP, which is positioned in 10° hyperextension. The patient continues those exercises initiated at 4 weeks postoperatively, and electrical stimulation to re-educate the transferred EIP is also indicated.

Splinting may be discontinued at 8 weeks postoperatively, providing the patient is able to actively achieve and sustain 0° IP extension. Otherwise, intermittent extension splinting of the IP joint may be continued during waking hours, one hour on:one hour off, and at bedtime. Resistive exercises, using light resistance therapy putty and rubber bands/tubes, may also be initiated at this time.

Hand Therapy Pearls

1. Following transfer of EIP to substitute for EPL, the patient performs active IP joint extension of the thumb, simultaneously with extension of the index finger. Tension is transmitted preferentially to the thumb IP joint by maintaining the CMC joint in flexion and the MCP joint in neutral.

2. Scar massage is important to minimize soft tissue adherence to the transferred EIP tendon and resultant diminution of extensor power to the thumb IP joint.

3. When using electrical stimulation to re-educate the transferred EIP, instrument settings should be consistent with muscle recruitment rather than muscle strengthening.

REFERENCE

Cannon NM: Tendon transfers for extension of the thumb. In Diagnosis and Treatment Manual for Physicians and Therapists 3rd ed. Indianapolis, Hand Rehabilitation Center of Indianapolis, 1991, pp 181–182.

PATIENT 14

A 60-year-old woman with progressive thumb swelling and deformity

A 60-year-old woman presents with a 2-month history of slowly increasing thumb swelling and pain. She relates that the symptoms started when she hit the thumb with a hammer. She denies any cuts to the thumb, but did relate that after the hammer injury the thumb nail turned black (although this has since resolved). She has not sought medical attention up to this point, but recent changes to her thumbnail have caused concern. She is a nonsmoker, and is otherwise in good health.

Physical Examination: General: distal phalanx of thumb markedly swollen and tender; fingernail grossly deformed (see figures). Musculoskeletal: thumb flexion somewhat limited, largely due to swelling of volar digit; range of motion, sensation, and motor strength normal in other digits. Neurologic: no tenderness proximal to distal phalanx.

Laboratory Findings: Radiograph (distal phalanx): see figure, *next page*. WBC 9400/µl with a left shift. ESR 94 mm/hr.

Questions: What is your diagnosis? Name the nail deformity. What treatment option would you recommend?

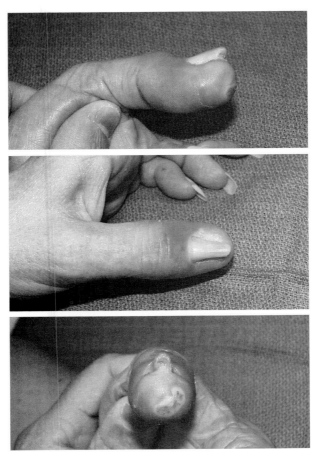

See color panels.

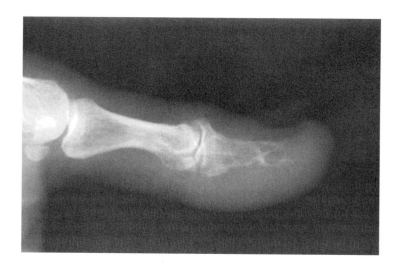

Answers: Osteomyelitis of the distal phalanx. The nail lesion is called the "pincer" deformity. Treatment involves irrigation and debridement of the involved thumb and distal phalanx, antibiotics, and nail removal.

Discussion: In the pincer deformity, the lateral edges of the nail fold inward, producing a tube or pincer shape. Although this patient did not have a classic history of penetrating trauma, the presentation is very suspicious for an infectious etiology (swelling, erythema, tenderness). The radiographs demonstrate bone involvement, with erosion of the bone (the lytic areas of the phalanx) indicative of osteomyelitis. Treatment of an infectious process like this requires debridement and drainage (especially if there is any purulence present within the deep tissue) and directed antibiotic coverage. Antibiotics are typically selected based on culture results, but in the initial treatment phase (before the culture results are finalized) gram-positive coverage is a reasonable place to start.

In this patient, the purulence was drained from an incision on the lateral border of the thumb, and the involved bone of the distal phalanx was resected. The incision was left open (i.e., not sutured) to facilitate dressing changes and to provide egress of any residual purulence. In addition, the nail was removed; the pincer deformity was secondary to the underlying infectious process. After correcting the underlying infection, the nail regrew normally. If it had not, the deformity could potentially be corrected with dermal grafting as described by Brown et al.

In evaluating patients that have suspected osteomyelitis, laboratory tests that may be helpful include a CBC. The WBC may be elevated, but is often normal; a more frequent finding is a left shift, with increased polymorphonuclear leukocytes. The ESR may be elevated in over 90% of these patients, but this is a nonspecific test. Approximately 40–50% focal bone loss is necessary to detect lucency on plain films (as in this case). A much more sensitive test is the MRI scan, which can detect osteomyelitis at a much earlier stage. Although MRI is relatively more expensive than other testing modalities, several studies have shown its superiority over plain films, CT, and radionuclide scanning in the early diagnosis of osteomyelitis.

Clinical Pearls

1. The most sensitive test for detecting osteomyelitis at this point remains the MRI scan. Plain films will show characteristic changes later in the course of the disease, when a significant amount of bone has been involved.

2. The mainstays of treatment for hand infections of this type are adequate drainage and debridement of devitalized tissue, in conjunction with directed antibiotic coverage. The use of either of these modalities without the other is likely to fail.

3. Nail deformities that are secondary to other pathologic processes (as in this case, or like the grooving seen in nails adjacent to mucous cysts) usually resolve spontaneously with successful treatment of the underlying pathologic problem.

REFERENCES

1. Boutin RD, Brossmann J, Sartoris DJ: Update on imaging of orthopedic infections. Orthop Clin North Am 29(1):41–66, 1998.
2. Brown RE, Zook EG, Williams J: Correction of pincer-nail deformity using dermal grafting. Plast Reconstr Surg 105(5):1658–1661, 2000.
3. Sammak B, Abd El Bagi M, Al Shahed M: Osteomyelitis: A review of currently used imaging techniques. Eur Radiol 9(5):894–900, 1999.
4. Tsukayama DT: Pathophysiology of posttraumatic osteomyelitis. Clin Orthop 360:22–29, 1999.

PATIENT 15

A 64-year-old man with an infected finger

You are called to the emergency department to treat a 64-year-old man with an infection of the distal index finger on his nondominant hand. The patient complains of swelling, erythema, and pain. He cannot recall any penetrating injuries or cuts to the hand or finger, except for a "minor" cut he suffered 2 weeks earlier opening a can of soup. His symptoms have been slowly progressive over the past few days. He is afebrile, and there has been no drainage from the finger. The patient is a heavy smoker, and he suffered a myocardial infarction 2 years ago. He has a chronic cough, with sputum production and hemoptysis. There are no other significant medical problems.

Physical Examination: General: significant erythema, swelling, and tenderness of distal left index finger; no lacerations, fluctuance, or drainage visible. No erythema of forearm; no palpable epitrochlear or axillary adenopathy.

Laboratory Findings: Radiographs: see figures. WBC normal; no left shift of polymorphonuclear leukocytes.

Questions: What is the diagnosis? What is the recommended treatment?

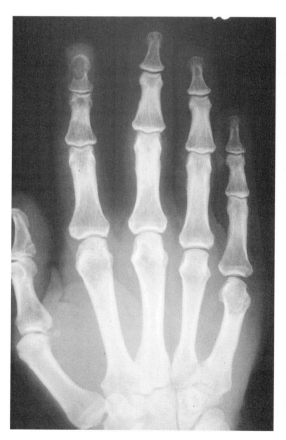
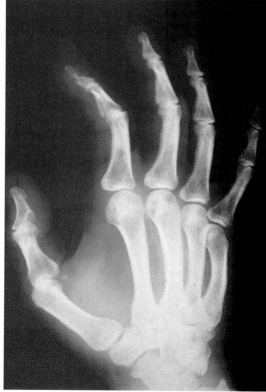

Answers: Metastatic tumor to the distal phalanx. Recommended treatment is palliative amputation.

Discussion: Metastatic cancer does not commonly affect the hands. When it does, it frequently mimics the situation of an infection, with the finger becoming tender and erythematous. The diagnosis may be missed or delayed if radiographic examination is not performed.

Most metastatic tumors of the hand involve the distal phalanx (see x-rays), and the primary tumor is most commonly lung cancer or renal cell cancer. Other tumors that may metastasize to the hand include head and neck malignancies, or chondrosarcoma (from the long bones).

Amadio and Lombardi published a review of the Mayo Clinic experience with metastatic hand lesions. During 1940–1983, a total of 18 patients with these lesions were identified; five had a lung cancer primary, and five had kidney cancer. These diseases were the two most commonly occurring in this group. Since the incidence of lung cancer is much higher than renal cell cancer, and the absolute numbers of occurrence of metastasis to the hand are similar, on a case-by-case basis it appears that renal cell cancer is *more likely* to metastasize to the hand. In regards to location, approximately 55% of all metastases occurred within the distal phalanx. Other locations were soft tissues of the hand (18%), carpal bones (13%), and proximal phalanx (9%). The overall incidence of metastatic lesions to the hand in the population identified with any malignancy was 9/75,000 (.012%).

This diagnosis has a grim prognosis, and treatment is based on providing palliation. Ray amputation is perhaps the most efficacious way to maintain the maximum amount of function with minimal discomfort to the patient. Despite the poor prognosis, long-term survival has been noted in some patients, and therefore complete surgical resection is indicated.

Clinical Pearls

1. The two most common primary tumors to metastasize to the hand are lung cancer and renal cell cancer.

2. The most common location for metastases to the hand is within the distal phalanx. Radiographically, the lesions have a lytic appearance.

3. Initial presentation of these lesions can often be confused with an infectious etiology. Erythema, swelling, and pain are often the initial complaints.

REFERENCES

1. Amadio PC, Lombardi RM: Metastatic tumors of the hand. J Hand Surg 12A:311–316, 1987.
2. Bryan RS, Soule EH, Dobyns JH, et al: Metastatic lesions of the hand and forearm. Clin Orthop 101:167–170, 1974.
3. Rose BA, Wood FM: Metastatic bronchogenic carcinoma masquerading as a felon. J Hand Surg 8:325–328, 1983.

PATIENT 16

A 35-year-old man with a proximal phalanx fracture

A 35-year-old man presents 1 day after having suffered a fracture to his index finger when he fell off a bike. The diagnosis was made at his local emergency department, where x-rays were taken after the fall; he has these films with him (see figure). He is currently employed as a claims adjustor for a local insurance company, and prefers to avoid surgery if at all possible.

Physical Examination: General: index finger edematous and somewhat ecchymotic; markedly tender over proximal phalanx; no lacerations. Musculoskeletal: mobility limited by pain. Neurologic: sensation intact at digit; perfusion adequate.

Question: What is the best treatment option for this injury?

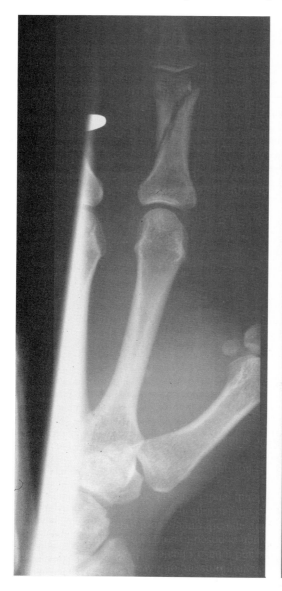 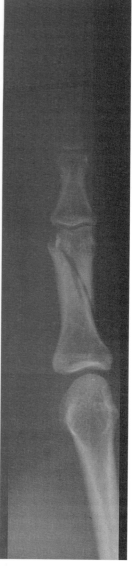

Answer: Open reduction and internal fixation of the fracture

Discussion: The main complications that can occur after a fracture of a hand bone are nonunion and malunion. A **nonunion** occurs when there is a failure of bony repair at the fracture site: the fracture site is bridged with scar tissue rather than bone. This happens most commonly when there is a large gap between the bony fragments, or excessive mobility during the early healing process. A **malunion** is when the bone heals in a poor (nonanatomic) position. Malunions are more of a concern in treating phalangeal fractures (as compared to metacarpal fractures) because there are no adjacent supporting ligaments that maintain the digit in a proper position during and after healing.

The most common type of malunion problem in phalangeal fractures is a rotational deformity. This can cause a significant functional disorder, because with flexion the rotated digit "crosses out" of its normal axis, usually impinging on the adjacent digits. Scissoring is one of the possible complications after malunion of a phalangeal fracture (see figure, *right*). As a result of the higher likelihood of scissoring in phalangeal fractures, it is recommended that the bony fragments be reduced and held in reduction with some type of bony fixation (using screws, plates, or even K-wires to temporarily maintain the reduction during healing).

Spiral and comminuted proximal phalanx fractures also benefit from this treatment (see preop-

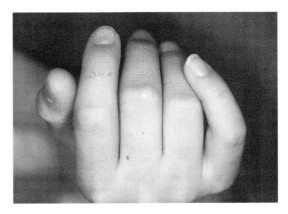

erative x-rays, *below*). The fracture is exposed and partially reduced (same patient, *A* on next page), and then fixed with either lag screws (*B* and *C*) or plates. One advantage of the precise and stable fixation afforded by plates and/or screws is early mobilization, which can greatly speed recovery and limit post-injury stiffness.

In the present patient, there is already some telescoping of the fracture fragments, with subtle finger shortening due to the oblique orientation of the fracture. Combined with the angular and possible rotational deformities, direct fixation of the fracture would provide the patient with the best ultimate outcome.

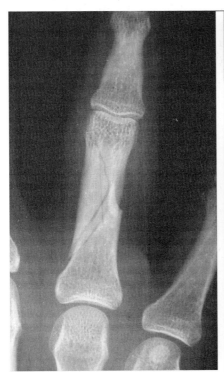

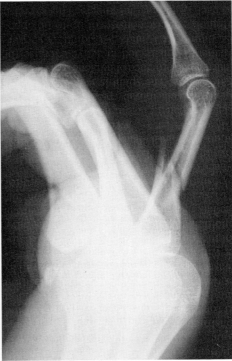

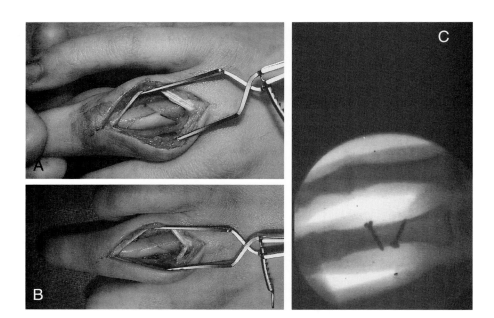

Clinical Pearls

1. If possible, internal fixation with plates and screws affords the opportunity for early range of motion of the adjacent joints. This can significantly decrease late stiffness after bony healing has occurred.

2. After the bone fragments have been reduced in the operating room (but before permanent fixation), gently flex the fingers into a fist to check for any rotational deformity and scissoring. You want to avoid fixation in a position that will guarantee a malunioun.

3. Some fractures of the digits occur too close to the adjacent joint to allow adequate purchase with plates and screws. In these patients, temporary fixation with a K-wire to maintain the bony alignment is an acceptable option.

4. Obliquely oriented fractures are particularly unstable, as they are prone to "telescope," sliding the finger proximally as the bone fragments override each other.

REFERENCES

1. Agee J: Treatment principles for proximal and middle phalangeal fractures. Orthop Clin North Am 23:35–40, 1992.
2. Green DP: Complications of phalangeal and metacarpal fractures. Hand Clin 2:307–328, 1986.
3. Stern PJ: Fractures of the metacarpals and phalanges. In Green DP, Hotchkiss R, Pederson WC (eds): Green's Operative Hand Surgery, 4th ed. New York, Churchill Livingstone, 1999.
4. Widgerow AD, Edinburg M, Biddulph SL: An analysis of proximal phalangeal fractures. J Hand Surg [Am] 12(1):134–139, 1987.

Perspectives For Therapy

Fifteen to 20% of all hand fractures involve the proximal phalanx. Proximal phalanx fractures occur in the workplace and also result from motor vehicle accidents, sports and recreational activities, and household mishaps.

One of the advantages of managing proximal phalanx fractures using open reduction and internal fixation (ORIF) is the ability to begin active motion within 24–72 hours postoperatively. Early active motion, in conjunction with extremity elevation and cohesive dressings, controls edema formation and induration associated with the increased soft-tissue dissection required for ORIF. Because soft tissues heal more quickly than bone, and are therefore liable to form dense adherent scar, early controlled mobilization is ideal for managing proximal phalanx fractures. Early active motion results in decreased edema and fibrosis, improved tendon excursion, and diminished likelihood of PIP flexion contracture.

As a general rule, passive motion is not indicated at this early stage of hand rehabilitation. Mini- and microplate fixation systems may be prone to deformation or outright breakage through injudicious, but well-intentioned application of passive force by the hand therapist or patient.

Tendon gliding and DIP blocking exercises are also indicated during early postoperative rehabilitation. The intrinsic minus-to-full flexion maneuver is particularly useful for increasing active IP flexion, while joint blocking improves PIP extension by stretching the oblique retinacular ligaments, periarticular soft tissues, and joint capsule. Despite the fact that composite flexion is the more functional hand position, every effort should be made to regain full active PIP extension, also.

The hand therapist can fabricate a custom, hand-based, thermoplastic splint to rest the patient's hand and fingers between exercise sessions and at bedtime. Alternatively, a volar finger gutter that maintains the IP joints in extension may be satisfactory. Choice of splint design is based on the patient's plan to return to work and/or avocational activities, with consideration given to the type of protection required.

Wound care, consisting of scar massage, is indicated after suture removal. This is an excellent modality to help minimize soft tissue sensitivity and enhance skin/tendon mobility. The patient may begin weaning from the splint at 3 weeks postoperatively, with discontinuation of splint use at 6–8 weeks postoperatively. At this latter time, progressive resistance exercises are initiated gradually. Passive motion and/or dynamic splinting may also be used.

Under no circumstances are finger injuries to be treated in the field by a well-intentioned athlete, player, coach, or trainer by relocating a seemingly minor injury ("jammed" finger). Such action can produce an unstable, displaced fracture from one that was formerly stable. Instead, the patient's finger should be immobilized in its injured posture and cold pack(s) applied. Play should obviously be discontinued and the patient transported to hospital for evaluation and definitive management by a hand surgeon.

Hand Therapy Pearls

1. When ORIF is used to manage proximal phalanx fractures, hand therapy consisting of active motion may be initiated between 24 and 72 hours postoperatively.

2. Passive motion is *not* indicated during early hand rehabilitation efforts, as it can damage hardware used for ORIF.

3. On-field management of finger injuries consists of discontinuing play, immobilizing the patient's finger in the posture of injury, applying cold pack(s), and transporting the patient to the hospital for evaluation and treatment by a hand surgeon. Relocating a "jammed' finger in the field is to be condemned.

REFERENCES

1. Cannon NM: Proximal phalanx fracture. In Diagnosis and Treatment Manual for Physicians and Therapists 3rd. ed. Indianapolis, Hand Rehabilitation Center of Indianapolis, 1991, pp 103–104.
2. Lee S-G, Jupiter JB: Phalangeal and metacarpal fractures of the hand. Hand Clin 16:323–332, 2000.
3. Meyer FN, Wilson RL: Management of nonarticular fractures of the hand. In Hunter JM, Mackin EJ, Callahan AD (eds): Rehabilitation of the Hand: Surgery and Therapy, 4th ed. St. Louis, Mosby, 1995, pp 353–375.
4. Stern PJ: Management of fractures of the hand over the last 25 years. J Hand Surg 25A:817–823, 2000.

PATIENT 17

A 47-year-old woman with a painful volar wrist mass

A 47-year-old woman presents complaining of a volar wrist mass of 3-year duration. Approximately 5 years ago, she fell and suffered a laceration on the volar aspect of her wrist; according to the patient, it only involved the skin (no deeper structures) and was sutured in the emergency department. Since the mass first appeared, she has noticed progressive swelling.

Physical Examination: General (see figure): swelling at volar wrist, consistent with a mass of some kind (although not well defined). Skin: well-healed, irregular incision in same location. Neurologic: area quite soft (easily compressible) and extremely sensitive; light tapping over mass causes significant pain, which patient describes as an "electrical shock" into her hand; poor sensation on volar thumb, index, and long fingers. Musculoskeletal: full active and passive range of motion of all fingers and wrist, with confirmed function of FDS, FDP, and volar and dorsal interossei muscles; patient can actively oppose thumb to ring and 5th digits without difficulty.

Questions: What is your diagnosis? What is your treatment recommendation?

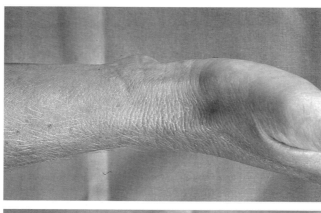

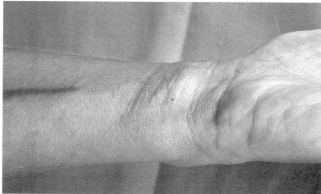

See color panels.

Answers: Median nerve laceration with neuroma formation. Recommend exploration, excision of neuroma, and reconstruction with nerve graft.

Discussion: Despite the patient's belief, and evidently her previous doctor's belief as well, that no deep-structure injury occurred during the accident 5 years ago, her symptoms—exquisite tenderness, a positive Tinel's sign over the injured nerve ("electrical shocks"), and soft tissue swelling—are classic for nerve transection with subsequent neuroma formation. Traumatic neuromas are usually due to penetrating trauma, and arise from the proximal end of nonrepaired nerve lacerations. The regenerating axons grow beyond the borders of the nerve in an attempt to rejoin the distal nerve. If the nerve ends are not immediately adjacent or coapted surgically, they form a jumble of highly sensitive nerve fibers.

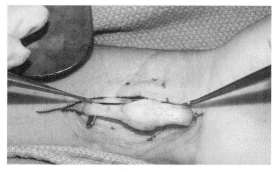

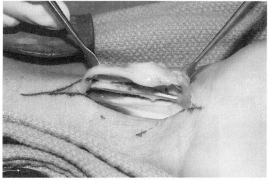

The present patient's symptomatic neuroma was evident upon initial surgical exposure (see figure *next page, A;* note the flexor carpi radialis tendon just radial and superficial to the mass). Further surgical exploration demonstrated that the mass was in fact a neuroma-in-continuity of the median nerve (see figure, *right*), as suggested by the physical examination.

In the present patient, a confounding physical finding was active opposition of the thumb, a function that is supplied by the intrinsic thenar muscles (abductor pollicis brevis, opponens pollicis, flexor pollicis brevis [FPB]; innervated primarily by the median nerve). In fact, loss of the median nerve frequently requires a tendon transfer (opponensplasty) to recover this lost function. The presence of active opposition in this patient could be due to one of two possibilities:

- The original nerve injury was not a complete transection, and the motor fibers to the thumb intrinsic muscles remained intact.
- Remember that half of the FPB is innervated by the ulnar nerve. A significant number of people, even with complete median nerve transection, will be able to oppose the thumb using the FPB.

Treatment involves resection of the neuroma (protecting intact nerve fascicles, if possible) and reconstruction of the nerve using nerve grafts, if necessary. Nerve grafting is almost always required after resection of the neuroma and scar in the treatment of these late injuries, or there would be too much tension on the nerve repair (see figure *next page, B*). In this patient, there is a risk of damaging fibers that remained intact (if any) during the neuroma resection. Resection of the neuroma with preservation of intact neural fibers might be facilitated by intraoperative electrodiagnostic studies, using either nerve action potentials or evoked responses. In the present patient, the nerve was reconstructed with multiple cables of sural nerve graft.

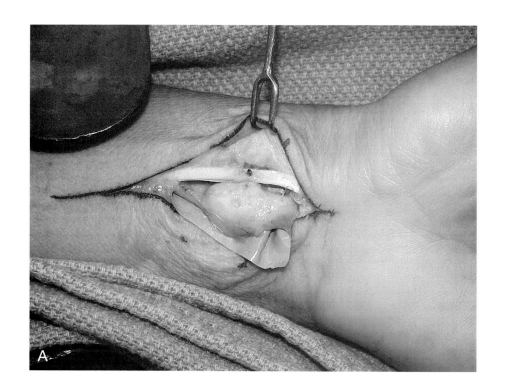

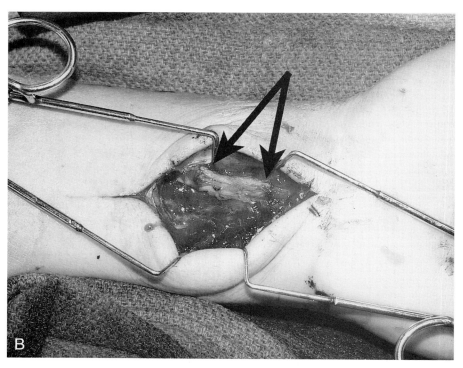

Clinical Pearls

1. Quite commonly, the nerve is not completely transected in traumatic neuromas. Patients should be warned that in the course of neuroma resection, intact fibers may be disrupted. Even with nerve graft reconstruction, recovery of any function lost during neuroma resection is not assured. Typically, these neuromas are so painful that most patients are willing to accept this risk.

2. Painful neuromas only occur in nerves containing sensory fibers; cut motor nerves do not form these exquisitely symptomatic lesions.

3. Opposition of the thumb is possible in some individuals via the ulnarly innervated FPB in the situation of complete median nerve transection.

REFERENCES

1. Kline DG: Evaluation of the neuroma in continuity. In Omer G, Spinner M (eds): Management of Peripheral Nerve Problems, Philadelphia, WB Saunders, 1980.
2. Kline DG, Nulsen FE: The neuroma in continuity: Its preoperative and operative management. Surg Clin North Am 52:1189–1209, 1972.
3. Sunderland S: The anatomy and physiology of nerve injury. Muscle Nerve 13:771–784, 1990.
4. Wilgis EF, Brushart TM: Nerve repair and grafting. In Green DP, Hotchkiss R, Pederson WC (eds): Green's Operative Hand Surgery, 4th ed. New York, Churchill Livingstone, 1999.

Perspectives For Therapy

The most important consideration for the hand therapist is protection of the nerve graft during: (1) vascularization from the host capillary bed, and (2) axonal regeneration into the distal nerve segment. The hand surgeon therefore guides post-operative therapy by performing controlled motion intra-operatively to determine the optimal position of the wrist that will minimize tension on the nerve graft. In this patient, a dorsal block splint, immobilizing the wrist in 30° flexion for up to 3 weeks, would be appropriate, and unless contraindicated, the patient is permitted to perform active motion of her fingers and thumb. The splint is revised 10°/week into extension for 3 weeks until a neutral position is achieved during the sixth postoperative week. At the conclusion of 6 weeks of protection, the dorsal block splint is discontinued with initiation of progressive wrist motion.

Nerves traumatized by injury, fibrosis, neuroma formation, and surgical intervention may experience varying degrees of hypersensitivity during regeneration. Desensitization of the volar wrist may be initiated following removal of skin sutures. Patients undergo a three-phase hand sensitivity test which includes Downey textured dowels, contact/immersion particles, and vibration at 30 and 256 cycles/second. Scar massage, texture, and percussion techniques are then selected to match to the patient's level of hyperesthesia.

There are two groups of patients appropriate for sensory re-education following peripheral nerve repair:

1. Those in whom protective sensation is lacking or severely impaired, as judged by Semmes-Weinstein thresholds $\geq$ the 4.31 monofilament (2.04 gmf). These patients are at increased risk for soft tissue injury due to thermal extremes, laceration, and shear stress, and will benefit from protective sensation re-education.

2. Those with protective sensation, as demonstrated by Semmes-Weinstein thresholds $\leq$ the 4.17 monofilament (1.48 gmf), but who lack discriminative sensation. These patients are unable to localize a brief sensory stimulus; cannot tell whether two sensory stimuli are the same or different; and cannot determine what kind of object they may be manipulating, when challenged without visual guidance. These patients will benefit from discriminative sensory reeducation.

Certainly there will be variation within that group of patients regarded as having diminished or absence of protective sensation, in terms of their Semmes-Weinstein thresholds. The operational criterion for placement of a specific patient into one of the two above groups will be their risk of soft tissue damage due to thermal injury, laceration, and shear stress.

Compensatory techniques for lack of protective sensation may be initiated as soon as the patient is allowed to use the hand for activities of daily living (ADLs). Patients are educated about: (1) minimizing skin contact pressure—for example, increasing total contact surface by building-up the handles of work implements, (2) lessening repetitive motion through task mix, and (3) maintaining soft, pliant skin with frequent applications of skin moisturizers. In addition to general vigilance for conditions (e.g., thermal extremes and contact with sharps) that could subject their soft tissues to increased risk of injury, the patient must be taught the early warning signs of skin breakdown, such as erythema and ecchymosis, and be encouraged to perform frequent skin checks.

Success in discriminative sensory re-education depends upon, at a minimum, axonal regeneration into the distal nerve segment and contact made with an appropriate target end-organ. Under the most optimal conditions, rates of axonal regeneration are 1–4 mm/day. Thus, it will be extremely challenging for both the hand therapist and motivated patient to accomplish discriminative sensory re-education, given current insurance constraints on the duration of postoperative hand therapy.

Training in localization and discrimination of sensory stimuli involves integrating visual and sensory modalities over gradually smaller skin surface areas. Appreciation of texture, shape, and object identification requires timed tasks with vision occluded, and helps integrate sensory and motor functions. From a practical standpoint, the success of discriminatory sensory re-education can be measured in accuracy of patient response, duration of timed tasks, and increased amounts of time spent using the hand for performance of ADLs.

Unfortunately, no one can determine *a priori* the specificity of nerve regeneration following injury and repair—this can only be determined empirically by challenging the system. Fortunately, the nervous system demonstrates sufficient plasticity to compensate for fragmentary and mismatched primary somatosensory cortical representations caused by misdirected axons and receptor degeneration. Given sufficient time to complete, the motivated patient can relearn and interpret sensory stimuli. This sensory re-education process relies on higher-order secondary and tertiary association areas that are superordinate to the primary cortical areas.

Hand Therapy Pearls

1. The most important consideration for the hand therapist is protection of the nerve graft during vascularization from the host capillary bed and axonal regeneration into the distal nerve segment.

2. There are two groups of patients appropriate for sensory re-education following peripheral nerve repair: those in whom protective sensation is lacking or severely impaired, and those with protective sensation, but who lack discriminative sensation, localization, and object identification.

3. The central premise of sensory re-education is plasticity of the nervous system. Under optimal conditions, higher order secondary and tertiary cortical association areas can compensate for fragmentary and mismatched primary somatosensory cortical representations caused by misdirected axons and receptor degeneration.

REFERENCES

1. Dagum AB: Peripheral nerve regeneration, repair, and grafting. J Hand Ther 11:111–117, 1998.
2. Waylett-Rendall J: Desensitization of the traumatized hand. In Hunter JM, Mackin EJ, Callahan AD (eds): Rehabilitation of the Hand: Surgery and Therapy, 4th ed. St. Louis, Mosby, 1995, pp 693–700.
3. Callahan AD: Methods of compensation and reeducation for sensory dysfunction. In Hunter JM, Mackin EJ, Callahan AD (eds): Rehabilitation of the Hand: Surgery and Therapy, 4th ed. St. Louis, Mosby, 1995, pp 701–714.
4. Anatomy and physiology of the peripheral nerve. In MacKinnon SE, Dellon AL (eds): Surgery of the Peripheral Nerve. New York, Thieme, 1988, pp 1–33.
5. Lundborg G: Peripheral nerve injuries: Pathophysiology and strategies for treatment. J Hand Ther 6:179–188, 1993.

PATIENT 18

A 53-year-old woman with longstanding left thumb pain and grip weakness

A 53-year-old woman is referred to your office for evaluation of right thumb pain of 1-year duration. She cannot recall any injury to the hand or thumb, either recently or in the remote past. She complains of discomfort mostly when grasping objects, such as gripping a doorknob and turning it, or holding a carton of milk. Her past medical history is significant for hypothyroidism; she is on thyroid replacement therapy. Otherwise, she has no other medical problems.

Physical Examination: General: right hand and thumb appear atraumatic. Musculoskeletal: full active range of motion of all fingers; slight discomfort with extreme abduction of thumb; more significant pain localized at volar proximal thenar eminence when pinching thumb to index finger; no tenderness over A1 pulley; no mobile masses at volar thumb; no thumb triggering with thumb flexion and extension; significant pain upon axial compression of thumb (see figure); Finkelstein's test negative. Wrist flexion with radial deviation against resistance does not reproduce her symptoms.

Laboratory Findings: Radiographs: see figure.

Questions: What is the diagnosis? What is your recommended treatment option?

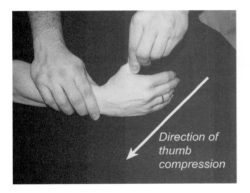

Direction of
thumb
compression

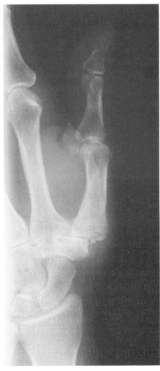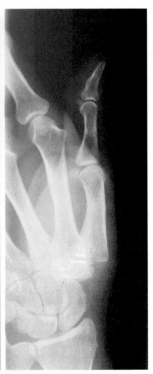

Answer: Basilar joint arthritis (thumb CMC joint). Best option for relief of pain at this advanced stage is trapeziectomy with ligamentous reconstruction.

Discussion: The carpometacarpal (CMC) joint of the thumb is saddle shaped, which allows for the circumduction mobility of the thumb. This joint and the DIP joints of the fingers are the more commonly affected joints of the hand in degenerative arthrititis. CMC joint arthritis typically affects postmenopausal women.

The differential diagnosis in patients that present with pain at the base of the thumb includes de Quervains's tenosynovitis, flexor carpi radialis (FCR) tendonitis, and stenosing tenosynovitis of the flexor pollicis longus (FPL).

In the present patient, de Quervain's tenosynovitis is less likely because she has a negative Finkelstein's test. She is not tender over the FCR, nor upon wrist flexion and radial deviation—both of which are symptoms of FCR tendonitis. She is not tender over the thumb A1 pulley and shows no triggering with thumb flexion and extension—both of which are symptoms of stenosing tenosynovitis of the FPL tendon. The symptom that sheds most light on the diagnosis of CMC arthritis is the **positive grind test,** which reproduces the patient's symptoms. This is performed by placing axial compression on the metacarpal onto the trapezium.

In nearly one-third of individuals with this disorder, carpal tunnel syndrome coexists. Therefore, symptoms of median nerve compression should be specifically searched for.

There are four stages to the pathologic process of CMC arthritis (proposed by Dell):

Stage 1 is characterized by mild joint narrowing or subchondral sclerosis. There may be minimal joint effusion or ligament laxity. In this stage there is no subluxation, nor osteophyte formation.

Treatment in this early stage is conservative, involving NSAIDs and immobilization of the thumb in an abducted position.

Stage 2 involves narrowing of the CMC joint and sclerotic changes of the subchondral bone. There may be osteophyte formation at the distal trapezium. There may be mild to moderate subluxation (the base of the first metacarpal subluxes radially and dorsally). Treatment for this and the more severe stages of CMC arthritis entails trapeziectomy and ligament reconstruction.

Stage 3 is characterized by more severe joint space narrowing; there may be cystic changes and sclerotic bone. Osteophyte formation is usually evident at the distal trapezium. There is moderate to severe subluxation of the base of the first metacarpal radially and dorsally (which may not be reducible).

Stage 4 radiographs are almost identical to those in stage 3, but there is evidence of scaphotrapezial joint involvement. At this advanced stage, the CMC joint is typically not mobile, and patients have little pain.

The thinking behind trapeziectomy and ligament reconstruction (see figures, *next page*) is that stabilization of the proximal metacarpal with ligamentous reconstruction can prevent late adduction contractures of the thumb. The FCR tendon is split proximally and left intact to its insertion distally (*top*). A hole is drilled into the proximal 1st metacarpal (*arrow*). The tendon is then passed through this hole and sutured, such that it supports the proximal metacarpal and prevents radial subluxation (*bottom*). The remaining (extra) tendon is then tucked into the space left by the trapezium, to be used as a joint "spacer."

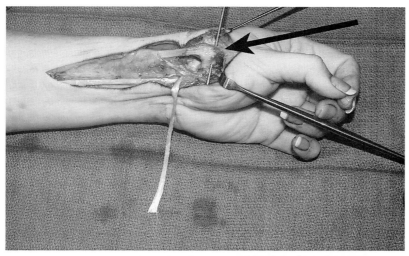

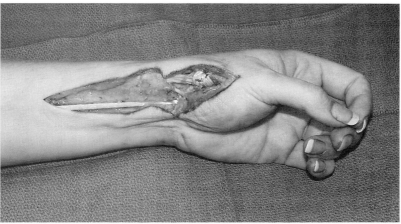

See color panels.

Clinical Pearls

1. One-third of patients with basilar joint arthritis have coexisting carpal tunnel syndrome. This needs to be searched for, so that the median nerve can be released at the time of surgical management of the CMC arthritis.

2. Treatment in the early stages involves immobilization and NSAIDs to decrease discomfort. As the process progresses, trapeziectomy with beak ligament repair reconstruction is required.

REFERENCES

1. Damen A, van der Lei B, Robinson PH: Carpometacarpal arthritis of the thumb. J Hand Surg Am 21(5):807–812, 1996.
2. Dell PC, Brushart TM, Smith RJ: Treatment of trapeziometacarpal arthritis: Results of resection arthroplasty. J Hand Surg 3:243–249, 1978.
3. Kleinman WB, Eckenrode JF: Tendon suspension sling arthroplasty for thumb trapeziometacarpal arthritis. J Hand Surg Am 16(6):983–991, 1991.
4. Tomaino MM, Pellegrini Jr VD, Burton RI: Arthroplasty of the basal joint of the thumb. Long-term follow-up after ligament reconstruction with tendon interposition. J Bone Joint Surg Am 77(3):346–355, 1995.

Degenerative change involving the first CMC joint, the trapeziometacarpal joint, is virtually a hallmark of osteoarthritis. Thumb pain is particularly debilitating for the patient, influencing all aspects of upper extremity function, including use of the involved hand for overhead activities. Screening of shoulder motion should, therefore, be included in the hand therapist's initial evaluation of patients with reconstruction of their thumb CMC joint.

Reconstruction of the first CMC joint, recommended for this patient, involves excision of the trapezium, ligament reconstruction, and tendon interposition arthroplasty. Tendon interposition arthroplasty refers to using a rolled tendon graft as a spacer within the first CMC joint, following excision of the trapezium. Historically, the FCR, abductor pollicis longus, and palmaris longus have been used as interpositional spacers. A K-wire is placed to seat the thumb metacarpal in an abducted position, thereby maintaining the arthroplasty space occupied by the tendon graft.

Following surgery, the patient is placed in a short arm thumb spica cast that permits motion of the thumb IP joint. After 4–5 weeks, the K-wire is removed and the patient is returned to a custom-fabricated, hand-based, thumb spica splint, also permitting IP motion. The splint is worn at all times, except during performance of hygiene and exercise.

The patient is instructed in active exercise for the wrist, thumb MCP, and CMC joints. A very effective thumb exercise consists of tip-to-tip opposition to each of the medial fingers. This exercise combines thumb flexion, abduction, and rotation. Blocking exercises may also be initiated for the MCP, to assist with flexion. Scar massage for the tendon donor and recipient sites is also indicated.

The patient may begin using the operated hand for ADLs such as handwriting, eating, dressing, and grooming/selfcare activities. When out of the splint, the patient is discouraged from using the index and long fingers for grasping and prehension. This "scissor pinch" is a common substitution pattern following thumb surgery, and is a difficult habit to correct. String tying, threading beads, opening/closing safety pins, and Purdue peg board can be used in the clinic to help normalize radial hand function, and verbal cues from the hand therapist serve as helpful reminders. Thermal modalities, joint mobilization, and dynamic splinting should also be considered to increase IP and MCP motion.

At 7–8 weeks postoperatively—providing the CMC joint is stable—the patient begins weaning off the spica splint, and is instructed in progressive resistive exercises. The patient can use therapy putty while performing composite flexion of the fingers and of the thumb, in isolation, and pinch strengthening. Putty is also an excellent adjunct to help increase end-range active motion.

Patients may anticipate resuming their pre-injury level of activity by 12 weeks postoperatively, regaining 50–55% grip and pinch strength, relative to the uninvolved hand. Splint use can be encouraged for the most vigorous ADLs, and on an as-needed basis for rest and support.

Hand Therapy Pearls

1. Thumb pain affects all aspects of upper extremity use. Thus, shoulder motion should be evaluated following CMC joint reconstruction, and appropriate modalities offered if shoulder motion is limited.

2. Use of the index and long fingers in a "scissor pinch" to substitute for thumb function should be discouraged. Radial hand function requires incorporation of the thumb into ADLs.

3. Treatment guidelines following thumb CMC joint arthroplasty are first directed at protection of the repair and increasing motion and functional use of the thumb. Thumb strengthening is a secondary priority and is not added until 7–8 weeks postoperatively (or even delayed up to 10 weeks, depending on the patient's symptoms).

REFERENCES

1. Berger RA, Beckenbaugh RD, Linscheid RL: Arthroplasty in the hand and wrist. In Green DP, Hotchkiss RN, Pederson WC (eds): Green's Operative Hand Surgery, 4th ed. New York, Churchill Livingstone, 1999, pp 167–168.
2. Jeter E, Degman GG, Lichtman DM: Postoperative wrist rehabilitation. In Lichtman DM, Alexander AH (eds): The Wrist and its Disorders, 2nd ed. Philadelphia, WB Saunders, 1997, pp 709–714.

PATIENT 19

A 29-year-old man with ring and fifth finger pain

A 29-year-old construction worker presents complaining of numbness and paresthesias over the ring and 5th fingers of his right hand. The symptoms are of 2-week duration. He suffered a cut on the volar aspect of his ring finger 10 days ago, and it hasn't healed. He complains of significant pain when he holds a cold drink with that hand, or when exposed to cold temperatures outside.

Physical Examination: General: ring and 5th fingers cool to touch, when compared to adjacent digits. Skin: pale; good capillary refill; recent laceration on distal aspect of ring finger, with no evidence of healing or infection. Musculoskeletal: tender mass (1.5 cm) (see figure, *arrow*) at ulnar aspect of mid-palm, just barely palpable.

Laboratory Findings: Radiographs: normal.

Questions: Which further diagnostic studies would you recommend? What is your presumptive diagnosis?

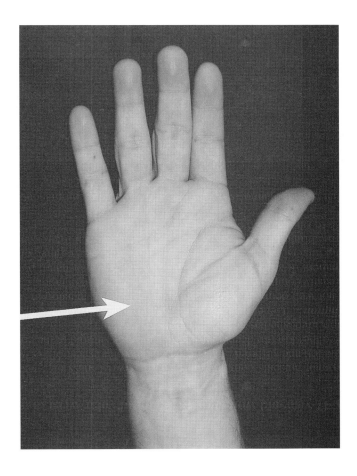

Answers: Angiography is recommended. Hypothenar hammer syndrome is the presumptive diagnosis.

Discussion: Thrombosis and/or aneurysm formation of the ulnar artery at the hand secondary to repetitive trauma (e.g., when using the hand as a hammer) can occur from direct trauma to the artery and its intima against the hook of the hamate. In women, this entity is rare, but not unheard of. Interestingly, a study of workers in an auto shop showed that 14% of the men that admitted using their hands as hammers had overt evidence of ulnar artery occlusion (they were all symptomatic). The diagnosis of hypothenar hammer syndrome is strongly suggested by any combination of the following signs and symptoms:

- A tender mass within the hypothenar area of the volar palm
- Symptoms of ulnar nerve compression (anesthesia/paresthesias within the ulnar nerve distribution)
- Ischemic symptoms of the distal fingertips, particularly of the ring and fifth fingers.

Angiography is typically not necessary for diagnosis, but is quite helpful prior to surgical repair and reconstruction (see figures). In patients with hypothenar hammer syndrome, the angiogram may demonstrate occlusion of the ulnar artery at the palm (*A*). In this particular individual, sufficient collateral flow from the radial artery allowed perfusion of the ulnar digits. Approximately 10–15% of the population does not have this crossover perfusion. Compare this image with the normal arterial anatomy of an adult forearm and hand (*B*).

Several nonoperative treatment options have been described for this entity, but surgical management remains the mainstay of definitive treatment. Suggestions for medical solutions have included vasodilators, stellate ganglion block, and lytic agents such as streptokinase or urokinase. None of these modalities have a role in the long-term treatment of this disease.

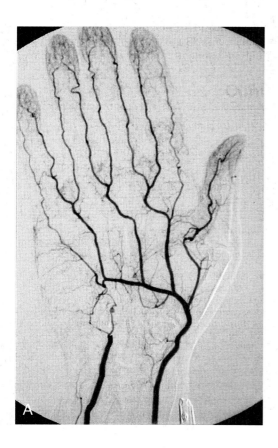

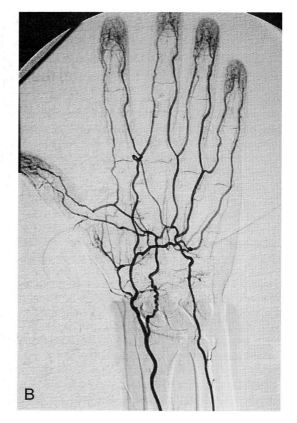

Clinical Pearls

1. Hypothenar hammer syndrome is suggested by any combination of: a tender volar hypothenar mass, ulnar nerve compression, and ischemic symptoms of distal fingertips, particularly of ring and 5th fingers.

2. Since the dorsal innervation to the ring and 5th fingers arises proximal to Guyon's canal (and presumably proximal to compression from an ulnar artery aneurysm within Guyon's canal), symptoms on the dorsal aspect of these digits in conjunction with volar symptoms imply a more proximal lesion, such as at the cubital tunnel.

3. Resection of the affected arterial segment appears to be a significant component of successful treatment. It is controversial whether this improvement is due to resection of the sympathetic nerve fibers (allowing distal vascular dilatation) or removal of a source of possible emboli.

4. Approximately 15% of people who use their hands as a hammer have symptomatic hypothenar hammer syndrome.

REFERENCES

1. Fowler IC, Workman CE: Aneurysm of the ulnar artery due to blunt trauma to the hand. MO Med 61:927–929, 1964.
2. Given KS, Puckett CL, Kleinert HE: Ulnar artery thrombosis. Plast Reconstr Surg 61:405–411, 1978.
3. Koman LA, Urbaniak JR: Ulnar artery insufficiency: A guide to treatment. J Hand Surg 6:16–24, 1981.
4. Little JM, Ferguson DA: The incidence of hypothenar hammer syndrome. Arch Surg 105:684–685, 1972.

Perspectives For Therapy

The most important role for the hand therapist, when treating patients with hypothenar hammer syndrome, is that of patient educator. Accordingly, the patient must learn to avoid using the heel of their hand as a hammer. It is also critical, in cases where sensory function of the ulnar nerve is either recovering or frankly compromised secondary to longstanding compression, that the patient be instructed in visual monitoring of his or her skin, to minimize the risk of thermal injury and related soft tissue trauma to the involved hand. This is particularly important if the patient is planning to return to work in an environment where sharp and blunt hand tools and power machinery are the mainstays of work-related activities. The use of Semmes-Weinstein monofilaments can provide objective information about light-touch thresholds.

Additional intervention may be offered in the form of a prefabricated, circumferential wrist strap. Made of neoprene, these straps serve two purposes: they support the ulnar aspect of the wrist, and they provide a thermal effect. Commercially available heated gloves are particularly beneficial in patients who complain of cold intolerance. For patients who anticipate returning to work using vibrating and high-impact tools, cyclist gloves with Viscolas inserts provide padding for the palm and good shock absorption characteristics.

Postoperatively, patients are instructed in active range-of-motion exercises and edema management using circumferential compression dressings that neither restrict blood flow nor compromise the sensation of the hand. Wound care, including scar massage and desensitization exercises, is beneficial following suture removal. The use of silicone gel sheeting or a custom-fabricated elastomer appliance is desirable for scar compression and improves skin compliance. Either material, when applied directly to the scar and secured with elasticized stockinette, can also help manage hyperesthesia.

Hand Therapy Pearls

1. The most significant role of the hand therapist in treating patients with hypothenar hammer syndrome is that of educator. Avoiding use of the hand as a hammer and visual monitoring when paresthesia is present will minimize the risks of recurrent ulnar artery and soft tissue injuries.

2. Neoprene wrist supports, heated gloves, and padded-palm gloves may be offered to support the ulnar wrist, provide a thermal effect in patients with cold intolerance, and provide shock absorption in patients who anticipate returning to employment that places high physical and environmental demands on their hands.

REFERENCES

1. Levin LS, Moore RS: Vascular disorders of the hand: Surgeons' perspective. J Hand Ther 12:152–159, 1999.
2. Talley M: Vascular disorders of the hand: Therapist's commentary. J Hand Ther 12:160–163, 1999.
3. Taras JS, Lemel MS, Nathan R: Vascular disorders of the upper extremity. In Hunter JM, Mackin EJ, Callahan AD (eds): Rehabilitation of the Hand: Surgery and Therapy, 4th ed. St. Louis, Mosby, 1995, pp 959–978.

PATIENT 20

A 45-year-old man with loss of volar finger coverage

The 45-year-old athletic director of the local university suffered loss of the entire volar aspect of his nondominant fifth finger, from the PIP crease to the distal nail, when the digit was caught in a log splitter. He presented emergently to the emergency department, where examination confirmed loss of the skin, but no exposed deep structures. X-rays revealed no underlying bony dislocations or fractures. He was taken to the operating room, and a full-thickness skin graft was applied to the volar aspect of the digit. Ten days following this procedure, examination revealed that the skin graft over the distal finger (involving the distal phalanx and the distal aspect of the middle phalanx) did not survive (see figure). The underlying soft tissue (particularly at the most distal aspect of the digit) was also felt to be nonviable (the likely cause of skin graft failure), leaving very little coverage over the volar distal phalanx. This gentleman is an avid golfer and desires surgical reconstruction that would not negatively impact this avocation.

Question: What is the best method of digit reconstruction allowing restoration of skin and padding with maximal function?

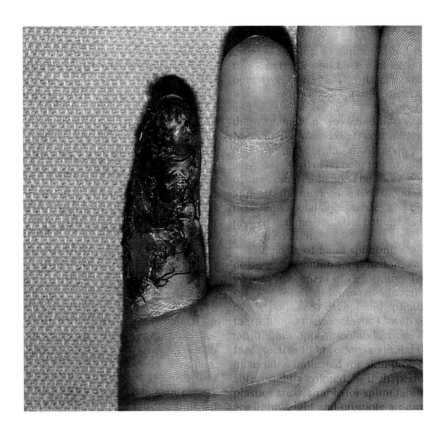

Answer: Crossfinger flap from the dorsal ring finger

Discussion: In the situation of loss of skin and soft tissue of the volar finger, numerous flaps for reconstructing the digit have been described. Local advancement flaps would not be appropriate in this case due to the proximal loss of volar tissue that had already been reconstructed with the skin grafts. Reconstruction with a palmar flap is subject to trouble with long-term joint flexion contracture and stiffness. A Littler neurovascular island flap may be possible; this option is attractive because in addition to restoring skin and soft tissue, sensation can be regained as well. However, when the adjacent ring finger is not injured, a crossfinger flap is a relatively easy and efficacious way to restore soft tissue in reconstruction of volar defects of the distal 5th finger.

The crossfinger flap is not immune to difficulties (such as joint stiffness) in the postoperative period, due to prolonged immobilization (particularly of the donor finger PIP joint in flexion). After division and inset of the flap, fastidious attention must be paid to regaining full active and passive range of motion (ROM) of not only the recipient finger, but also the donor. Another potential drawback of the crossfinger flap is persistently decreased sensation on the volar finger. While some sensation can be expected to ultimately recover, this is a potential disadvantage to any noninnervated flap coverage of the volar finger—the crossfinger flap is no exception.

Execution of this type of coverage is relatively straightforward. After completely debriding the recipient bed, the crossfinger flap is designed over the adjacent (donor) finger overlying the middle phalanx. The flap can be harvested as far as the mid-lateral line away from the injured finger. This can add length, which is particularly useful in coverage of large defects. Care must be taken during flap elevation to preserve the paratenon over the extensor mechanism. The paratenon is required for the full-thickness skin graft (covering the donor defect) to reliably take and for preventing donor digit problems. After the flap is inset, the fingers are carefully immobilized to prevent motion during the postoperative period. Some physicians advocate placement of K-wires between the donor and recipient digits to further immobilize and prevent motion.

The flap is left in place for at least 3 weeks, during which time neovascularization is occurring between the flap and its recipient bed. After this time, the patient is brought back to the operating room for flap division; it can now survive completely on the new blood supply formed. Elaborate insetting maneuvers at this point typically are not indicated, and if too enthusiastic can cause vascular embarrassment and some flap loss. It is best to leave the raw edges of the flap open to heal by secondary intention.

In the present patient, a crossfinger flap was transferred from the dorsal aspect of the ring finger to provide coverage of the distal fifth finger (see figure, *below*). A full-thickness skin graft was placed over the donor defect to provide skin coverage over the extensor mechanism. Long-term results, 3 years after reconstruction using a crossfinger flap, were excellent (see figure, *next page*).

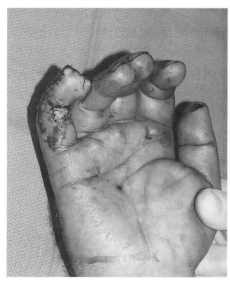 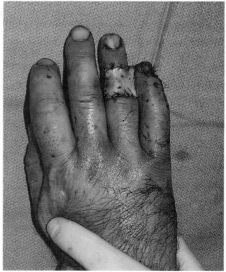

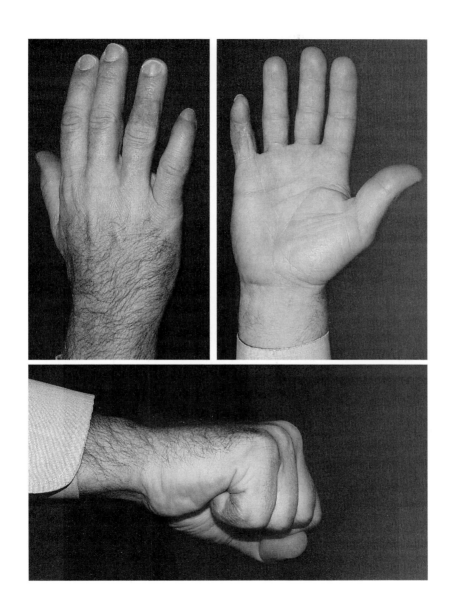

Clinical Pearls

1. The level of dissection of the crossfinger flap is important: preservation of the peritenon over the extensor mechanism of the donor finger is critical to allow survival of the full-thickness skin graft over the donor defect.

2. Careful immobilization between the donor and recipient fingers is vital in the establishment of the new blood supply to the flap. Some physicians advocate placement of K-wires between the digits.

3. Crossfinger flaps can be designed as far across the finger as the midlateral line. This added length is helpful when insetting the flap to the recipient digit.

4. Fastidious attention to ROM exercises in the post division and inset period is critical to avoid flexion contractures of the PIP joint, particularly at the donor digit.

5. At division, careful insetting of the flap is usually not required. Aggressive defatting and trimming of the flap can compromise its vascular supply, as can sutures that are placed too tightly. A few strategically placed sutures will suffice in maintaining the edge position of the flap; the raw edge will heal by secondary intention within a few weeks.

REFERENCES

1. Atasoy E: Reversed cross-finger subcutaneous flap. J Hand Surg 7:481–483, 1982.
2. Cohen BE, Cronin ED: An innervated cross-finger flap for fingertip reconstruction. Plast Reconstr Surg 72:688-
3. Concannon MJ: Common Hand Problems in Primary Care. Philadelphia, Hanley & Belfus, Inc, 1999, pp 93–95.
4. Kappel DA, Burech JG: The cross-finger flap: An established reconstructive procedure. Hand Clin 1:677–684, 1985.

Perspectives For Therapy

This patient is an ideal candidate for a custom-fabricated, thermoplastic splint designed to support, protect, and contribute to immobilizing the operated ring and small fingers. The splint may be hand-based, molded to conform to the flexed postures of the operated fingers and position the MCP joints in flexion. The period of immobilization during neovascularization may be 3 to 3½ weeks, and an opportunity to exercise the uninvolved joints is desirable. Thus, the splint should permit freedom of motion of the lateral three digits and the wrist. Such exercise should place minimal stress on the operated fingers, particularly if K-wire fixation has been employed, and the splint will protect any exposed hardware, also.

Upper extremity elevation, to the level of the patient's heart, is mandatory, and attention to wound care during immobilization may be indicated. The hand therapist should consult with the hand surgeon to determine the manner in which dressing changes are to be performed, the frequency, and the type(s) of dressings to be used.

Following flap division, and depending upon the condition of the soft tissues, the patient will require fairly aggressive ROM exercise for the operated fingers. Continued attention to wound care and edema management are required during soft tissue healing by secondary intention. A light cotton, cohesive dressing, placed over a nonadherent dressing, addresses both needs, and atraumatic dressing changes can be performed by the patient at home.

Regaining PIP joint extension, particularly of the donor finger, may require joint mobilization and use of a dynamic PIP extension splint. This splint is worn intermittently during waking hours, and a static volar gutter splint is used at bedtime. The static splint should be revised to reflect extension gains. Splint use must be accompanied by active exercise to reinforce the motion gained by dynamic splinting. Broad finger loops, supporting the middle and distal phalanges, will minimize contact pressure on new skin. Plaster-of-Paris serial static splints are another extremely useful modality for correcting recalcitrant PIP flexion contractures; however, the patient must return to the clinic every 2 days or so, to have a new splint applied.

When all soft tissues are adequately healed, the hand therapist can issue silicone gel sleeves to the patient for digital scar compression and desensitization. These are worn at bedtime and between splinting and exercise sessions. The patient may also be a candidate for progression to protective and discriminative sensory re-education.

Hand Therapy Pearls

1. Consider early active motion for the patient's uninvolved joints during interval immobilization of the operated fingers.

2. Discuss with the hand surgeon any dressing changes that are required during neovascularization of the crossfinger flap.

3. Splinting modalities used to regain motion of the operated fingers must be augmented by active exercises.

4. The patient should be educated about the potential need for sensory re-education secondary to diminished protective sensation in the operated fingers.

REFERENCES

1. Callahan AD: Methods of compensation and reeducation for sensory dysfunction. In Hunter JM, Mackin EJ, Callahan AD (eds): Rehabilitation of the Hand: Surgery and Therapy, 4th ed. St. Louis, Mosby, 1995, pp 701–714.
2. Colditz JC: Modification of the digital serial plaster casting technique. J Hand Ther 8:215–216, 1995.
3. Singer DI, Moore JH, Byron PM: Management of skin grafts and flaps. In Hunter JM, Mackin EJ, Callahan AD (eds): Rehabilitation of the Hand: Surgery and Therapy, 4th ed. St. Louis, Mosby, 1995, pp 277–290.
4. Waylett-Rendall J: Desensitization of the traumatized hand. In Hunter JM, Mackin EJ, Callahan AD (eds): Rehabilitation of the Hand: Surgery and Therapy, 4th ed. St. Louis, Mosby, 1995, pp 693–700.

PATIENT 21

A 36-year-old man with wrist pain for the past 3 months

A 36-year-old musician fell onto his nondominant hand while loading musical equipment onto his band's truck. He originally sought medical attention at a local emergency department; x-rays were read as "normal, no bony injury noted" (see figure, *left*). The diagnosis at that time was "wrist sprain," and he was treated with a prefabricated wrist cock-up splint and given a prescription for ibuprofen 800 mg TID. While immobilized, his symptoms subsided considerably. Nevertheless, the symptoms of wrist pain with activity recurred once the splinting was discontinued.

Physical Examination: Skin of hand: atraumatic. Musculoskeletal: full active and passive range of motion (ROM) of digits, without pain or limitation; vague wrist pain with motion, particularly flexion. With your thumb pressed against his volar radial wrist, radial movement of the wrist (from an ulnar deviated position) causes pain, and you can feel a "clunk" or popping of the wrist.

Laboratory Findings: Second radiograph (with fingers clenched in a tight fist): see figure, *right*.

Questions: What is your diagnosis? Is any therapy or surgical treatment necessary?

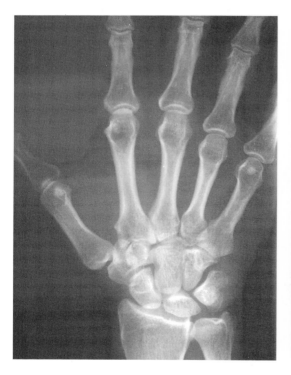 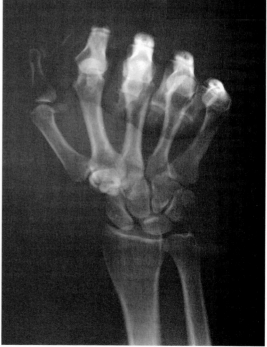

Answers: Dynamic (reducible) scapholunate dissociation. The best treatment option is dorsal (Blatt) capsulodesis, with scapholunate ligament repair if possible.

Discussion: The diagnosis was hinted at in the physical examination, when pressure on the volar scaphoid by the examiner's thumb caused pain and a "clunk" with radial deviation of the wrist: this is **Watson's shift test**. As the wrist moves from a position of ulnar deviation to radial deviation, the scaphoid volar-flexes, and with scapholunate dissociation this becomes painful. This test has been criticized for having low specificity: one study showed that up to 36% of normal individuals may have a positive test.

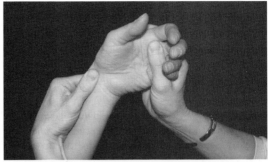

Watson's shift test is performed by grasping the patient's hand at the ulnar aspect of the fifth metacarpal, with the examiner's thumb on the palmar surface of the distal pole of the scaphoid (see figure). It is important for the examiner's thumb to apply pressure to the distal pole of the scaphoid, to prevent it from flexing. The patient's wrist is then slowly moved from ulnar to radial deviation (*arrow*), and the distal tuberosity is compressed by the examiner's thumb. With this radial deviation, the scaphoid flexes to a more vertical orientation, and the tuberosity compression forces proximal pole subluxation dorsal to the lip of radius. As the examiner's thumb pressure is released, the subluxed scaphoid reduces, often producing a palpable "clunk" and dorsal wrist pain (indicating instability of the scapholunate ligament).

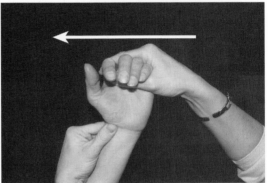

The reason this patient's condition remained undiagnosed is that the scapholunate injury is still early (and reducible). Static x-rays may not (and did not, in this case) show the characteristic widening between the scaphoid and the lunate (the **Terry Thomas sign**). This sign is more easily seen when the hand forms a tight fist.

This injury is early, and the scaphoid remains reducible; therefore, good results may be achieved with Blatt dorsal capsulodesis. Scapholunate ligament repair may be performed simultaneously, if there is sufficient substance of the ligament to repair. The Blatt approach has the advantage of maintaining a very reasonable amount of wrist motion, which would be particularly important to this gentleman, as he is a musician.

Furthermore, if the capsulodesis is not successful at maintaining reduction or minimizing pain, other options (such as scaphotrapeziotrapezoid [STT] fusion, or scaphocapitate fusion) would remain available as salvage procedures. The objectives with the STT or scaphocapitate fusion are:

- Reduction of the malrotated, vertically displaced scaphoid
- Closure of the scapholunate interval
- Maintenance of carpal height.

Clinical Pearls

1. The Watson shift test is a sensitive maneuver to quickly ascertain both static and dynamic instabilities of the scaphoid.

2. When performing a Blatt capsulodesis, it is currently recommended to secure the dorsal wrist capsule flap to the prepared and reduced scaphoid with a pull-out suture (as opposed to a bony anchor). This appears to provide more direct contact of the ligamentous reconstruction to the cancellous bone of the scaphoid, with better ultimate healing.

3. Arthritic degenerative changes noted intraoperatively are a strong contraindication for soft tissue repair (capsulodesis); intercarpal fusion is a better alternative.

REFERENCES

1. Blatt G: Dorsal capsulodesis for rotary subluxation of the scaphoid. In Gelberman RH (ed): The Wrist. New York, Raven Press Ltd, 1994, pp 147–165.
2. Lane LB: The scaphoid shift test. J Hand Surg 18:366–368, 1993.
3. Watson HK, Ashmead D, Makhlouf MV: Examination of the scaphoid. J Hand Surg 13:657–660, 1988.
4. Wolfe SW, Gupta A, Crisco 3rd JJ: Kinematics of the scaphoid shift test. J Hand Surg 22:801–806, 1997.

Perspectives For Therapy

At 8–10 weeks postoperatively, a short-arm thumb spica cast is discontinued and the patient is returned to a removable wrist support splint with a radial gutter thumb spica component. This can either be custom-fabricated from perforated thermoplastic material or issued prefabricated. The splint is worn for protection between exercise sessions and at bedtime, and permits freedom of the thumb IP joint.

Scar and edema management techniques are initiated at the patient's first hand therapy visit. Active ROM exercises for the patient's forearm, wrist, and hand are prioritized. Shoulder and elbow motion should be screened and limitations addressed. Neither passive ROM nor strengthening exercises are indicated during this early stage of postoperative rehabilitation, as both would put the dorsal capsulodesis at risk and possibly cause significant irritation of joint and soft tissues neighboring retained hardware.

At 10–12 weeks postoperatively, retained hardware is removed by the hand surgeon, and passive ROM exercises may be initiated. However, to protect the dorsal capsulodesis, neither dynamic splinting nor weighted stretches are indicated for wrist flexion. Thermal modalities and joint mobilization may be employed in the clinic to help increase motion of the radiocarpal and ulnocarpal joints. Continued active motion of the wrist will result in gradual increases in physiologic motion of the midcarpal and intercarpal joints.

Progressive resisted exercises, using rubber bands or tubes, emphasize general upper extremity strengthening and conditioning, and the patient is also instructed in grip strengthening exercises using therapy putty. The patient returning to manual labor or sports activity must be encouraged to continue splint use for wrist protection and support. Otherwise, the splint can be discontinued at this time, also. At 24 weeks postoperatively, the patient may gradually resume his or her preinjury level of activity.

In the current patient, return to work concerns can be addressed by having him play his instrument in the clinic, if practical. Range of motion and strengthening exercises can be tailored to meet the specific postures and movements required for play.

While patients undergoing Blatt capsulodesis may regain almost full forearm rotation and wrist extension; experience a maximum deficit of 20° wrist flexion; and, on average, recover approximately 80% of grip strength, as judged by comparison to the contralateral hand, short-term results are more conservative. For example, while the forearm rotation arc may approach 160–165°, wrist extension may differ 15–30°, wrist flexion 45–50°, and grip strength by 32% when compared to the uninvolved hand.

REFERENCES

1. Blatt G. Dorsal capsulodesis for rotary subluxation of the scaphoid. In Gelberman RH (ed): The Wrist. New York, Raven Press Ltd, 1994, pp 147–165.
2. Cannon NM: Blatt Capsulodesis. In Diagnosis and Treatment Manual for Physicians and Therapists, 3rd ed. Indianapolis, Hand Rehabilitation Center of Indianapolis, 1991, pp 124–125.

PATIENT 22

A 49-year-old woman with hand numbness and weakness

A 49-year-old, right hand–dominant woman presents complaining of right hand numbness and weakness that has been troubling her for the past 8 months. She is employed as an administrative assistant at a local attorney's office. She denies any history of trauma or injury to either hand. It is difficult for her to pinpoint specifically what makes the symptoms worse: prolonged typing makes her hand numb, but the pain also awakens her at night. Her family doctor prescribed ibuprofen and gave her a wrist cock-up splint 3 months ago for these complaints. These measures helped her somewhat for a while, but she cannot discern any improvement now, despite continuing with both of these modalities.

Physical Examination: General: no evidence of trauma or injury to either hand. Musculoskeletal: full active and passive range of motion (ROM) of wrists and fingers; decreased sensation of volar thumb, index, and long fingers on right hand—tapping on volar wrist causes "sprangles" (electrical shock–type sensations) to radiate to these affected digits; finger flexion, extension, abduction, and adduction on right all strong, with no evidence of weakness or paralysis; on maximal flexion of wrist, symptoms worsen after approximately 45 seconds.

Laboratory Findings: Radiograph (right hand): normal. Electrodiagnostic studies: slowing of median sensory and motor distal latencies, with normal median motor forearm nerve conduction velocity; stimulation of median nerve distal to wrist reveals *normal* sensory latency and amplitude.

Questions: What is the diagnosis? Is any further testing required prior to definitive treatment?

Answers: Carpal tunnel syndrome. No further testing is necessary.

Discussion: Carpal tunnel syndrome (CTS) is the most common nerve compression syndrome of the upper extremity, and is a significant complaint in workers' compensation patients. The median nerve travels through the carpal tunnel at the volar wrist adjacent to nine flexor tendons. The carpal tunnel's boundaries are bone on its dorsal, radial, and ulnar borders. The volar boundary is formed by the transverse carpal ligament, a thick, fibrous (and nonyielding) structure that forms the "roof" of the carpal tunnel (see figure, *white bar*). If there is any increase in volume in the tunnel (such as can occur with edema, or inflammation of the synovium that invests the tendons within the carpal tunnel), the surrounding structures do not stretch to accommodate the increase, resulting in greater pressure within the tunnel.

This higher pressure is manifest clinically at the median nerve: it limits blood flow within that segment of nerve, leading to the local symptoms of nerve compression—numbness and paresthesias within the median nerve distribution. Long-standing compression can lead to local demyelination of the nerve and more severe nerve damage.

There are four cardinal signs and symptoms of CTS:

- Symptoms within the median nerve distribution
- Symptoms that awaken the patient at night
- A positive Tinel's sign (positive shocks or

"sprangles" that are elicited by gently tapping the volar wrist at the carpal tunnel with the wrist extended)
- A positive Phalen's test.

Phalen's test is very sensitive for CTS and is performed by having the patient maximally flex both wrists against each other and hold that position for 1–2 minutes. This test can be quantified somewhat by determining how rapidly the symptoms of paresthesias or numbness develop while holding this position.

While these are the main signs and symptoms of CTS, not all patients present with all four. If a patient presents with three of the four symptoms, CTS is probable. If only one of the four symptoms is evident, the diagnosis is less likely. In equivocal cases, electrodiagnostic testing can be performed to confirm or exclude the diagnosis. Keep in mind, however, that electrodiagnostic testing may miss up to 13% of patients with CTS (false negative error). The median to ulnar latencies are usually compared to rule out the possibility of a peripheral neuropathy, which can be another cause of slowing at the median nerve. The fact that the median study is normal *distal* to the carpal tunnel confirms that the abnormal segment is at the carpal tunnel and is neuropraxic.

CTS is associated with, and may be caused by, many different disease processes, including: pregnancy, menstruation, menopause, pyridoxine defi-

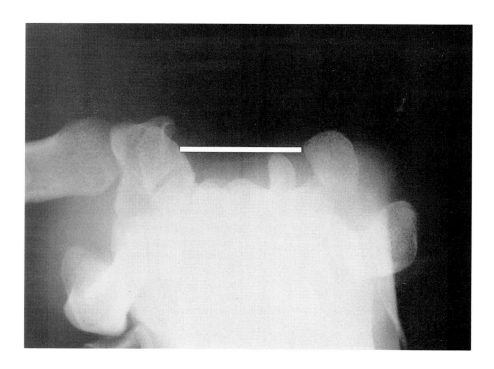

ciency, toxic shock syndrome, hemodialysis, rheumatoid arthritis, obesity, amyloidosis, mucolipidoses, chondrocalcinosis, myxedema, acromegaly, and athetoid-dystonic cerebral palsy. Processes that *add volume* into the closed space of the carpal tunnel can also cause compression of the median nerve and resultant CTS: persistent median artery with thrombosis, aneurysm, AVM, anomalous muscles, tenosynovitis, acute palmar space infections, or masses (such as neurofibroma, lipoma, ganglion cyst). Finally, CTS can be caused by any process that *decreases the volume* of the carpal tunnel: idiopathic thickening of the transverse carpal ligament, malunion or callus following distal radius fracture or carpal fracture, unreduced dislocations of the wrist or intercarpal joints (such as perilunate dislocation, in which the lunate is pushed directly into the median nerve), improper immobilization of the wrist, or incorrect positioning while placing a cast.

Since the symptoms most often arise secondary to a tenosynovitis within the carpal tunnel (crowding the median nerve and causing localized compression), early treatment has traditionally focused on reducing this swelling. This is easiest to achieve with immobilization and administration of nonsteroidal anti-inflammatory drugs (NSAIDs)—both of which must be consistently and uniformly applied. Immobilization for only part of the day (allowing wrist and finger motion at other times) will perpetuate the tenosynovitis, and the conservative management will more than likely fail.

If after a trial of conservative management the patient becomes asymptomatic, the splinting and NSAIDs can be discontinued. If the symptoms arise again (or were never completely resolved with conservative management), then operative decompression is indicated.

Clinical Pearls

1. There are four cardinal signs of carpal tunnel syndrome (CTS): symptoms within the median nerve distribution, symptoms that awaken the patient at night, a positive Tinel's sign, and a positive Phalen's test.

2. Muscular atrophy (atrophy at the thenar eminence) is a very late finding, and urgent operative decompression is indicated. The absence of thenar wasting does not rule out CTS.

3. Electrodiagnostic testing will give a false negative result in approximately 13% of patients.

4. Pillar pain, a common postoperative finding, is pain at the base of the thenar and hypothenar eminences after carpal tunnel release. It is quite variable in severity and duration of symptoms. The etiology is not well understood, but in general it does subside and resolve over time without any additional treatment or therapeutic measures needed.

REFERENCES
1. Concannon MJ: Common Hand Problems in Primary Care. Philadelphia, Hanley & Belfus, Inc, 1999, pp 133–137.
2. Concannon MJ, Brownfield ML, Puckett CL: The incidence of recurrence after endoscopic carpal tunnel release. Plast Reconstr Surg 105:1662–1665, 2000.
3. Concannon MJ, Gainor B, Petroski GF, Puckett CL: The predictive value of electrodiagnostic studies in carpal tunnel syndrome. Plast Reconstr Surg 100:1452–1458, 1997.

Perspectives For Therapy

Patients who undergo surgical decompression of the median nerve at wrist level, or carpal tunnel release, receive a postoperative bulky dressing that protects the surgical wound. This is typically a volar, forearm-based fiberglass or plaster-of-Paris splint that crosses the wrist and clears the fingers and thumb.

Patients are encouraged to initiate tendon gliding and thumb opposition exercises immediately after surgery, and they are taught to elevate their operated hand above the level of their heart to help control edema. Postoperative dressings are kept clean and dry.

Approximately 7–10 days postoperatively, the surgical dressings are discontinued, sutures are removed, and the patient is returned to a prefabricated wrist support splint. He or she is instructed in scar massage to help mobilize the palmar scar; this activity also desensitizes the scar. The patient is encouraged to continue tendon gliding exercises, and is also instructed in median nerve gliding exercises. Splint use is reviewed, and the patient gradually decreases splint wearing time over the next 2 weeks. The splint should be worn at bedtime and during the performance of work-related activities of daily living. Splint use is also indicated when the patient is in the community and at home engaged in activities requiring repetitive, sustained, or forceful use of the wrist and fingers.

Prefabricated splints that make use of a removable internal metal stay are always revised such that the stay is flattened and replaced inside the splint. This ensures that the operated wrist is immobilized in a neutral position, minimizing tensile stress and compression of the median nerve.

Grip and pinch strength and sensation may be assessed by the hand therapist, and the patient can be instructed in light, resistive exercises using therapy putty as indicated. Exercise sessions lasting up to 5 minutes and repeated six to eight times daily are sufficient, and will not irritate the patient's hand and wrist. General upper extremity strengthening and conditioning exercises, using graded rubber-bands or tubes, are well-tolerated by the patient and are preferable to isotonic extension (reverse curls) and flexion exercises (curls) that increase both the muscular and postural loads on the wrist.

A general upper-extremity exercise program often taught to these patients consists of: shoulder abduction, extension, flexion, horizontal abduction/adduction, and external/internal rotation; proprioceptive neuromuscular facilitation (diagonals D1/2E); elbow extension/flexion; and forearm rotation. This program emphasizes reconditioning of the proximal musculature, with overflow into the extrinsic and intrinsic muscles of the hand and fingers since the patient must secure the rubber band with the exercising hand.

For some patients, progression to a work-conditioning or multidisciplinary work-hardening program may be beneficial. Patients often desire, and are responsive to, suggestions made regarding worksite and home-office modifications that help minimize stresses on their hands and wrists. Handles of work implements and commonly used household items can be built up to reduce the magnitude of force application; padded-palm gloves that provide shock-absorption when handling vibrating tools can be worn; and workstations can be modified.

Hand Therapy Pearls

1. Patients who undergo carpal tunnel release surgery benefit from early active motion, including tendon and nerve gliding exercises, which help minimize adhesion formation at the surgical site.

2. Prefabricated splints that make use of a removable metal stay should be revised by flattening the metal stay, thereby promoting neutral wrist mechanics and minimizing compression and tension on the median nerve.

3. Patients may benefit from suggestions to modify tools, tasks, and work environments to lessen the risk of median nerve re-injury.

REFERENCES

1. Keir PJ, Wells RP, Ranney DA, et al: The effects of tendon load and posture on carpal tunnel pressure. J Hand Surg 22A:628–634, 1997.
2. Rozmaryn LM, Dovelle S, Rothman ER, et al: Nerve and tendon gliding exercises and the conservative management of carpal tunnel syndrome. J Hand Ther 11:171–179, 1998.
3. Sailer SM: The role of splinting and rehabilitation in the treatment of carpal and cubital tunnel syndromes. Hand Clin 12:223–241, 1996.

PATIENT 23

A 37-year-old nurse with wrist pain at work

A 37-year-old nurse presents with radial wrist pain of 8-month duration. She previously saw her primary care physician for this complaint, who prescribed ibuprofen. Her symptoms seemed to abate somewhat for a few weeks, but the medication has ceased to have an effect. She denies any prior injury to that wrist, and she does not do any strenuous labor either at work or at home.

Physical Examination: Musculoskeletal: no tenderness over volar or dorsal wrist, but mildly tender over radial aspect of distal radius; full active and passive ROM of all digits and wrist, but discomfort on extreme ulnar deviation of wrist. Watson shift test negative. The patient complains of the most pain when her thumb is clasped into her palm and the wrist is ulnarly deviated (see figure).

Laboratory Findings: Radiographs: normal, no abnormalities seen.

Questions: What is your diagnosis? What treatment options does this patient have?

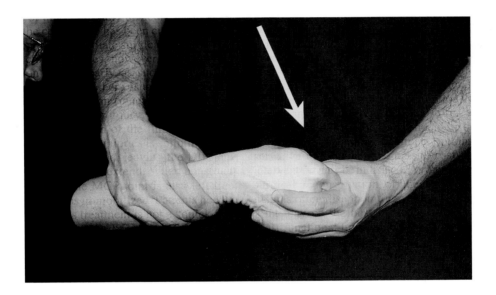

Answers: De Quervain's disease (stenosing tenosynovitis of the 1st extensor compartment). Treatment options include steroid injection within the 1st compartment, or surgical release of the 1st extensor compartment.

Discussion: The 1st extensor compartment contains the abductor pollicis longus and extensor pollicis brevis tendons: these tendons form the volar border of the anatomic snuffbox (see figure, *below*). Inflammation of these tendons within the extensor retinaculum can create a sharp tenderness over the radial styloid process. Patients with de Quervain's tenosynovitis are exquisitely tender over the 1st extensor compartment while performing **Finkelstein's test** (see figure, previous page), which confirms the diagnosis. As demonstrated in the examination of this patient, this test involves having the patient curl the thumb within his or her fist. In this position, if ulnar deviation of the wrist by the examiner causes significant pain over the 1st extensor compartment, the test is positive.

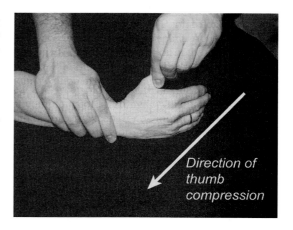

Direction of thumb compression

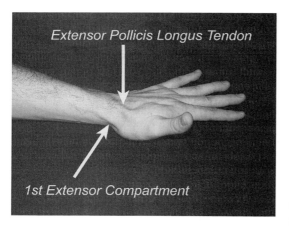

Extensor Pollicis Longus Tendon

1st Extensor Compartment

The differential diagnosis of patients who present with radial wrist pain (such as the patient in this case) includes:

- Basilar joint arthritis. CMC arthritis can be distinguished from de Quervain's syndrome by performing the **grind test,** in which axial compression is placed on the base of the thumb metacarpal (see figure, *right*) This maneuver is not painful in patients with de Quervain's tenosynovitis, but is painful if significant basilar joint arthritis is present.
- Intersection syndrome. In this syndrome, the tendons of the 1st extensor compartment (APL and EPB) cross over the tendons of the 2nd extensor compartment (ECRL and ECRB) just proximal to the extensor retinaculum. There can be irritation and tenosynovitis at this juncture, approximately 4 cm proximal to the wrist

joint. Steroid injection within the 2nd extensor compartment typically resolves the symptoms.
- Wartenberg's syndrome. This is an isolated neuritis of the superficial radial nerve at the distal forearm. This nerve is entirely sensory at this level, so there are no symptoms of weakness or motor deficit. Associated parasthesia or anesthesia in the radial nerve distribution of the hand distinguishes Wartenberg's syndrome from other diagnoses. This syndrome is most commonly caused by compression of the nerve by external forces, such as heavy wrist jewelry or watches.

De Quervain's tenosynovitis can be treated either conservatively or operatively. Conservative management involves immobilization for 4 weeks in a thumb spica splint in conjunction with steroid injection within the 1st extensor compartment. Dexamethasone (0.4–1 mg) has been advocated to reduce the risk of skin depigmentation and subcutaneous fat atrophy. It is important to inject beneath the retinaculum and not just in the subcutaneous tissue.

Surgical release is typically very straightforward. A longitudinal incision (i.e., parallel to the axis of the radius) reduces risk of iatrogenic injury to the superficial radial nerve. The extensor retinaculum is incised directly over the 1st extensor compartment. Additional slips of both the EPB and APL should be searched for and released (multiple slips of these tendons, especially the EPB, are the rule rather than the exception in these cases). In advanced cases, there may be tendonous adhesions that need to be taken down for complete release. Prior to incision closure, flex and extend the wrist to check if the released tendons sublux. If they do, *loosely* reapproximate the tendon sheath edges with a single horizontal suture to hold the tendons in place during wrist flexion. Postoperatively, the thumb should be free to move (and the patient encouraged to actively use it), but the wrist should be splinted in extension for 2 weeks to prevent volar subluxation of the APL and EPB.

Surgical complications include: injury to the superficial radial nerve, inadequate decompression (particularly likely if not all slips of the tendons are released), tendon instability (volar subluxation), and tendon scarring and adherence (prevented by allowing early range of motion of the thumb).

Clinical Pearls

1. When releasing the 1st extensor compartment, if you make the incision in the extensor retinaculum too radially (volarly), the tendons will be more likely to sublux postoperatively. If the tendons are noted to volarly sublux intraoperatively with wrist flexion, partial fixation of the tendon sheath should be performed to "splint" tendons in proper position during the early healing process.

2. A positive Finklestein's test is strongly suggestive of de Quervain's tenosynovitis. However, some patients are more sensitive to this maneuver than others, and it is a good idea to test the contralateral (unaffected) side, as well. If that is also positive, reconsider the diagnosis.

3. An increased incidence of de Quervain's disease has been found in patients with Dupuytren's disease, rheumatoid arthritis, gout, and diabetes. Approximately one-third of patients have bilateral disease.

REFERENCES

1. Albright JA: Common variations of the radial wrist extensors. J Hand Surg 3:134, 1978.
2. Jackson WT, Viegas SF, Coon TM, et al: Anatomical variations in the first extensor compartment of the wrist. J Bone Joint Surg 68(6): 923–926, 1986.
3. Lipscomb P. Tenosynovitis of the hand and the wrist: Carpal tunnel syndrome, de Quervain's disease, and trigger digit. Clin Orthop 13:164, 1959.
4. Witt J, Pess G, Gelberman RH: Treatment of de Quervain's tenosynovitis. A prospective study of the results of injection of steroids and immobilization in a splint. J Bone Joint Surg 73:219–222, 1991.

Perspectives For Therapy

Conservative management of de Quervain's tenosynovitis includes custom fabrication of a thumb spica splint that is static, forearm-based, radial, and gutter style. It should permit freedom of the thumb IP joint (see figure *A, next page*). The splint is worn at all times for 3–6 weeks, with the exception of during hygiene activities. The duration of splint use may be modified as symptoms improve.

When designing a thumb spica splint, it is important that the patient be capable of actively flexing the medial four fingers to the mid-palm, and of opposing the thumb to the tips of the medial four fingers. The wrist should be immobilized in neutral, thumb CMC joint at 40° abduction, and MCP joint in 10° flexion. Patients are cautioned against using an adduction pinch between their index and long fingers to substitute for tip pinch between the thumb and index finger while using the splint. This "scissors pinch" is a difficult habit to break, once static spinting is discontinued. The patient is also educated about activity modification, and if indicated, ergonomic adjustments can be recommended for both the patient's workplace and home to minimize stresses acting at the first extensor compartment.

Iontophoresis using dexamethasone in the active electrode may also be employed over the first extensor compartment. Symptom relief should be expected in 6–9 visits, allowing a decision to be made to progress the patient to a general upper-extremity strengthening and conditioning exercise program at home.

If surgical management is elected to release the first extensor compartment, early active wrist and thumb motion is advocated to minimize the risk of scar adherence. The patient performs tendon gliding exercises, isolating the APL and EPB with the wrist in ulnar deviation (see figure *B, next page*) and performing composite thumb flexion with the wrist in radial deviation (see figure *C*). A custom, volar, forearm-based, thumb-hole splint that sup-

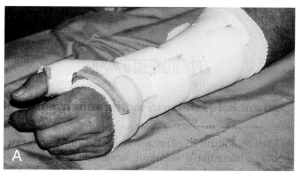

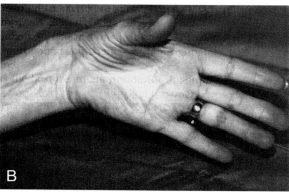

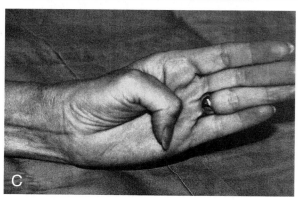

ports the wrist in 15° extension may be worn between exercise sessions for up to 2 weeks to protect the APL and EPB tendons. Scar massage can also be performed, once sutures are removed. Exercise progression should include a general upper extremity strengthening and conditioning program.

Hand Therapy Pearl

When fabricating a thumb spica splint for managing de Quervain's tenosynovitis, the patient should be capable of composite flexion of the medial four fingers to the palm, and of tip-to-tip opposition of the thumb to the medial four fingers.

REFERENCES
1. Cannon NM: de Quervain's tenosynovitis. In Diagnosis and Treatment Manual for Physicians and Therapists, 3rd ed. Indianapolis, Hand Rehabilitation Center of Indianapolis, 1991, pp 168–169.
2. Eaton RG. Entrapment syndromes in musicians. J Hand Ther 5:91–96, 1992.
3. Kirkpatrick WH, Lisser S. Soft tissue conditions: Trigger fingers and de Quervain's disease In Hunter JM, Mackin EJ, Callahan AD (eds): Rehabilitation of the Hand: Surgery and Therapy, 4th ed. St. Louis, Mosby, 1995, pp 1007–1016.

PATIENT 24

A 46-year-old woman with an asymptomatic lesion on hand x-ray

A 46-year-old woman is referred to you for evaluation. Her original complaint was of persistent thumb pain after a fall. She presented to her family physician, who ordered a hand x-ray to rule out a fracture. Although no thumb fracture or dislocation was identified, a lytic lesion was noted at the distal phalanx of her fifth finger. She denies any knowledge of injury or problems with this digit, and she is not experiencing any current symptoms related to the fifth finger.

Physical Examination: Her fifth finger has full active and passive range of motion without pain or limitation. There is no edema, nor any erythema. There is no tenderness, nor any laxity with radial or ulnar deviation of the distal phalanx. Sensation is intact and normal. She is afebrile. No epitrochlear or axillary lymphadenopathy. In summary, the physical examination is completely normal.

Laboratory Findings: WBC 6200/μl, hemoglobin 11 g/dl, hct 33%, ESR 6 mm/hr. Radiograph: see figure.

Questions: What is the diagnosis? What treatment would you recommend?

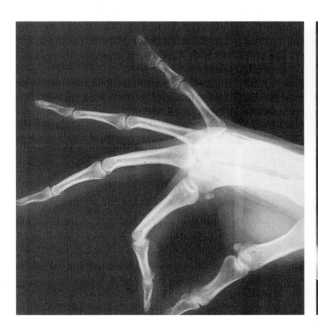
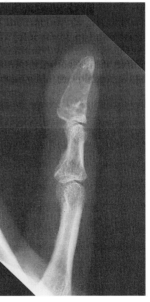

Answers: Enchondroma. Recommend elective curettage and cancellous bone grafting.

Discussion: Enchondromas are benign tumors of cartilaginous origin that originate within the medullary cavity, most often at the tubular bones of the hands and feet: the metacarpals, metatarsals, and phalanges. They are the most common benign bone tumor of the hand. These lesions are better characterized as dysplasias of the central growth plate, resulting from a failure of normal endochondral ossification. They most frequently present with a pathologic fracture: a fracture diagnosed radiographically in a patient who had minimal or no trauma to the bony area. Enchondromas are usually completely asymptomatic unless associated with a pathologic fracture (see figure).

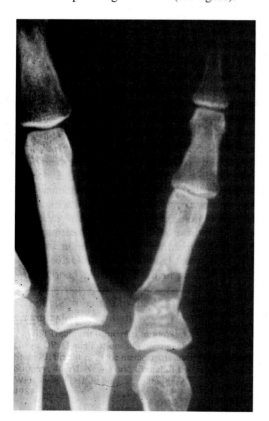

Less than 2% of isolated enchondromas undergo malignant transformation to chondrosarcoma. In patients who have multiple lesions (such as in Ollier's disease), there is a much higher risk of malignant transformation, approaching 25% by the time the patient reaches 40 years of age.

Diagnosis of an enchondroma is usually straightforward using plain radiographs. They typically present as a lytic (radiolucent) lesion with a mildly thickened bony margin. If a bone scan is obtained, it may show increased uptake in this bony margin (depending on how active the lesion currently is).

Treatment entails immobilization to allow the fracture to heal, after which time curettage of the enchondroma can be elected. The cortical shell is left intact. This space is then packed with cancellous bone graft from either the distal radius or iliac crest (see figure next page, *left*). Long-term results are typically quite good, and complete bony healing without recurrence is common (see figure next page, *right*). If a patient with a single lesion is reluctant to undergo surgical resection, treatment can be expectant, monitoring with yearly x-rays. If the lesion becomes symptomatic, or begins to enlarge, biopsy is indicated to rule out malignant degeneration. If a patient presents with a pathologic fracture, the best method is immobilization/casting to first allow it to heal. After bony healing, curettage and bone grafting is indicated on an elective basis.

Multiple enchondromatosis (Ollier's disease) is a condition characterized by multiple enchondromas throughout the body, involving the long bones of the extremities as well as the more typical location at the tubular bones of the hands and feet. These lesions are much more likely than solitary lesions to produce palpable masses, angular deformities of the bone, or alterations in growth of the bone. Lesions that cross the growth plate are much more likely to produce growth disturbances, which can be severe enough to require surgery to correct limb length inequality.

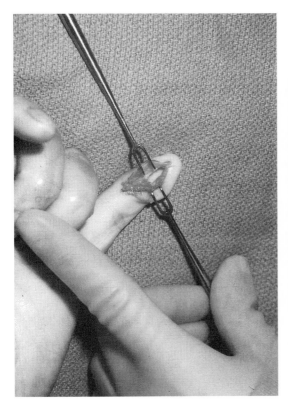
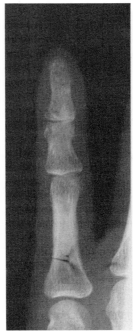
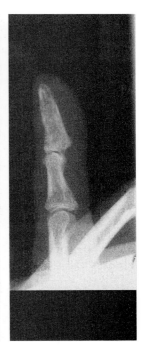

Clinical Pearls

1. Individual enchondromas are benign processes, which are largely asymptomatic unless the bone is weakened to such a degree that it fractures. In the situation of a pathologic fracture, immobilization to allow fracture healing should be done prior to definitive treatment of the enchondroma (curettage and bone grafting).

2. There are two syndromes involving multiple enchondromatosis: Ollier's disease (multiple enchondromas only) and Maffucci's syndrome (multiple enchondromas with overlying vascular malformations). In both of these syndromes, the growth disturbances and impact on function are much more significant than in individuals with isolated enchondroma lesions. The risk of malignant transformation is approximately 25% in patients with Ollier's; the risk for patients with Mafucci's approaches 100%.

3. Malignant degeneration should be considered (particularly in a patient with multiple lesions) if the tumors become painful, begin to enlarge, or are associated with progressive deformity. In this scenario, biopsy is required to rule out malignancy.

REFERENCES

1. Bauer H, Brosjo O, Kreicsbergs A, Lindholm J: Low risk of recurrence of enchondroma and low-grade chondrosarcoma in extremities: 80 patients followed for 2–25 years. Acta Orthop Scand 66:283, 1995.
2. Schwartz HS, Zimmerman NB, Simon MA, et al: The malignant potential of enchondromatosis. J Bone Joint Surg 69:269–274, 1987.
3. Shapiro F: Ollier's disease. An assessment of angular deformity, shortening, and pathological fracture in 21 patients. J Bone Joint Surg 64:95–103, 1982.

Hand Therapy Pearls

1. Initiate gentle active motion of the involved finger following discontinuation of closed reduction.

2. Splint use between exercise sessions is advisable to protect the patient's involved finger, particularly during anticipated vigorous activities.

3. Passive motion and dynamic splinting are contraindicated in these patients secondary to concerns about decreased bone stock. There is a risk of refracture and formation of a pseudoarthrosis or fibrous joint.

4. Should the patient receive bone grafting, he or she may report significant complaints of pain at the donor site. Uneventful wound healing at both the donor and recipient sites is a prerequisite of case management.

5. Providing there are no contraindications, active motion, as opposed to passive, is preferred for patients having undergone bone grafting.

REFERENCE

Meyer FN, Wilson RL. Management of nonarticular fractures of the hand. In Hunter JM, Mackin EJ, Callahan AD (eds): Rehabilitation of the Hand: Surgery and Therapy, 4th ed. St. Louis, Mosby, 1995, pp 353–375.

PATIENT 25

A 46-year-old woman with an injured index finger

A 46-year-old woman was leading her horse by its bridle when the horse startled and attempted to flee, frightened by a snake. The patient notes pain throughout her whole hand, but is most symptomatic at the index finger. She complains of tenderness on the volar aspect of the finger, some swelling, and pain with attempted flexion.

Physical Examination: Neurologic: adequate perfusion and sensation of all digits. Musculoskeletal: no limitation to full passive ROM; pain with full extension of index finger; active flexion of index finger PIP joint possible with long and ring fingers held in full extension; active flexion of distal phalanx not possible while holding index finger middle phalanx (see figure, *left*). Palpation: tender mass at distal mid-palm (see figure, *right*).

Laboratory Findings: Radiographs: no fractures or dislocations.

Questions: What is the diagnosis? What is the recommended treatment?

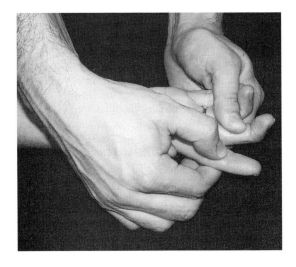

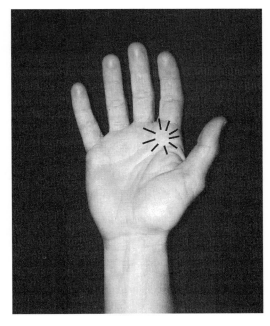

Answers: Rupture of the flexor digitorum profundus tendon, index finger. Surgical repair should be attempted if diagnosed early enough; if diagnosed after 2 weeks consider DIP joint fusion.

Discussion: Flexor digitorum profundus (FDP) rupture occurs when there is forceful hyperextension of the distal interphalangeal (DIP) joint while the FDP is maximally contracted (in this example, the fingers curled around the horse bridle). A classic example of this injury is a football player who catches his finger on an opponent's jersey during a tackle, avulsing his ring finger FDP. The tendon may rupture directly from the bone, or may remain attached to a bony chip. This bony fragment may be visible on x-ray as a small chip fracture, or a displaced fragment proximal to the distal phalanx. Seventy-five percent of FDP ruptures involve the ring finger, due to a weaker insertion point on that digit than the adjacent fingers.

The degree of proximal retraction may be limited by the bony chip (preventing migration proximal to Camper's chiasm, the split insertion of the flexor digitorum superficialis [FDS]), or by an intact vinculum. If the tendon is caught at this level, the patient typically presents with a flexion contracture of the PIP joint. The farthest proximal extent that the tendon can retract is the midpalm: further proximal retraction is limited by the lumbrical muscle attachment to the profundus tendon. If the proximal tendon is at the midpalm, it is often palpable as a tender mass.

These type of injuries have been classified based on the degree of retraction noted at surgery:

Type I: retracted into the palm

Type II: retracted to the PIP joint

Type III: the bony fragment remains distal to the A4 pulley.

Note that the radiographic position of the bony fragment *does not* reliably locate the retracted position of the tendon.

The FDP is difficult to repair if it is retracted into the palm longer than 7 days. It becomes edematous, and it is difficult to replace the tendon within the fibro-osseous tunnel without compromising PIP movement. Typically, efforts to repair the tendon after 2 weeks are not successful. It is usually a good idea (if the tendon has retracted into the palm) to discuss possible tendon excision and DIP fusion with the patient preoperatively, in case a direct tendon repair can't be performed.

Another option for the treatment of late injuries is tendon reconstruction, which may require the use of Hunter rod placement prior to tendon reconstruction with a graft.

Reinsertion of the tendon into the distal phalanx can be performed using either a pullout nylon suture or wire (tied over a button on the fingernail) until healing is completed. Another option is to reinsert the tendon directly with a bone anchor.

Another potential cause of the inability to flex the distal phalanx of the index or long fingers is proximal nerve palsy (anterior interosseous nerve injury). While not likely (particularly in the setting of acute onset of symptoms after trauma), it can be easily ruled out by checking the **tenodesis effect** of the intact tendons. With the patient's fingers completely relaxed, wrist extension by the examiner causes the fingers to gently curl (due to the tenodesis effect of the flexor tendons). If the tendon is intact, the affected finger will curl in a standard cascade with the adjacent digits; if the tendon is ruptured, the cascade will be altered, and the finger will not curl to the regular degree (see figure, *below*).

Of course, the tenodesis effect may be observed in multiple fingers (see figure, *next page:* here, transection of the flexor tendons to the ring and 5th fingers caused loss of the normal resting flexion cascade in the index and long fingers. Further wrist extension would result in slightly increased flexion of the index and long, but no movement of the ring and 5th fingers).

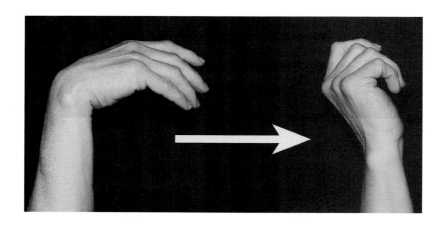

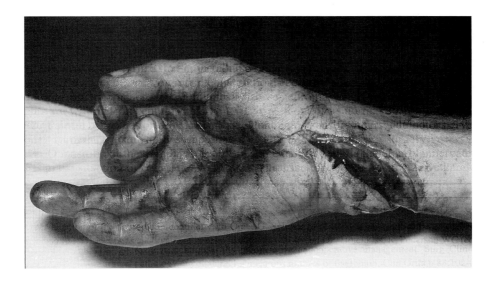

Clinical Pearls

1. Flexor digitorum profundus tendon ruptures are most common in the ring finger, due to a weaker insertion on that digit than the other fingers.

2. If these injuries are not addressed relatively quickly (within 2 weeks of the injury) with surgical intervention, direct repair of the tendon becomes significantly more difficult to perform. If direct repair is not possible, consider fusion of the DIP joint.

REFERENCES

1. Leddy JP, Packer JW: Avulsion of the profundus tendon insertion in athletes. J Hand Surg 2A:66–69, 1977.
2. Lunn PG, Lamb DW: "Rugby finger": Avulsion of the profundus of the ring finger. J Hand Surg Br 9:69–71, 1984.
3. Trumble TE, Vedder NB, Benirschke SK: Misleading fractures after profundus tendon avulsions: A report of six cases. J Hand Surg 17:902–906, 1992.

Perspectives For Therapy

Flexor tendon repairs in Zone 1 require hand therapy treatment distinct from that used for Zone 2 repairs. Zone 1 extends from the broad insertions of FDS on P2 to the insertion of FDP on the volar surface of the base of P3. Accordingly, Zone 1 includes the A5, C3, and A4 pulleys. The volar surface of P2 bounded by the A4 pulley represents a *transitional area* where FDS and FDP are in contact with one another.

Ideally, referral to hand therapy should be made on the third day following surgery, and this provides an opportunity for postoperative edema to subside. Because these treatment guidelines introduce a component of active exercise within the initial 3 weeks postoperatively, a further prerequisite is that a Kessler or modified Kessler core suture, with an epitendinous peripheral suture, be used for tendon repair. These guidelines are also appropriate for patients whose FDP tendon is reattached onto the distal phalanx.

Early intervention requires protection of the repair using a custom-fabricated, forearm-based, dorsal block splint. The patient's wrist is immobilized in 30–40° flexion, MCP joints in 30° flexion, and IP joints, with the exception of the injured finger, at 0° within the confines of the splint. A distal strap is used to support the medial four fingers between exercise sessions.

In contrast to hand therapy treatment for Zone 2 flexor tendon repairs, a second splint is created for the injured finger. This is a dorsally-based finger splint that positions the DIP joint in 40–45° flexion. The splint extends over the nailplate and ends just distal to the PIP joint such that it does not interfere with PIP extension. The finger-based splint is secured to the middle phalanx with porous paper tape. The rationale for splinting the DIP in 40–45° flexion is to immobilize the repaired FDP tendon *proximal* to its lengthened position, thereby minimizing the risk of gap formation where end-to-end tendon or tendon-to-bone repairs are performed.

Patient education regarding the need to protect the repaired tendon and to comply exactly with the exercise regimen are mandatory for a positive outcome—Zone 1 flexor tendon repairs demonstrate a significant complication rate. Tendon rupture, scar adherence, gap formation, and interference with the A4 pulley are cited as reasons for poor outcomes. Strict upper extremity elevation, uneventful wound healing, and use of cohesive dressings are the focus of the initial treatment session.

The patient is instructed in a written home-exercise program with the following components. Each waking hour, within the confines of both dorsal block splints, the patient performs 20 repetitions of passive DIP flexion through his or her full range of motion, followed by active extension to the limit of the finger-based dorsal block splint. This is sufficient to create 3–4 mm of proximal glide required to promote intrinsic tendon healing and minimize adherence of the FDP to the FDS. However, the repair may be positioned beneath the A4 pulley, which is a potential site of interference with tendon gliding. The hand therapist should review with the hand surgeon whether the A4 pulley was released or "vented" to achieve free gliding of the repair.

The patient also performs 20 repetitions each of passive composite finger flexion to the mid-palm and isolated PIP flexion. Exercises are done within the confines of both dorsal block splints, and each passive maneuver is followed by active extension to the limit of the forearm-based dorsal block splint. Mobilization of the PIP of the injured finger performed by the hand therapist is also desirable to minimize the risk of flexion contracture.

The IP joints of the uninjured fingers are positioned in extension using the distal strap of the forearm-based dorsal block splint. The patient then performs a place-hold maneuver of the PIP of the injured finger, recruiting the FDS. Differential recruitment of the FDS helps minimize tendon adherence between FDS and FDP and between FDS

and the flexor tendon sheath. Differential recruitment of FDS may also help to minimize PIP flexion contracture.

Under therapist supervision, the forearm-based dorsal block splint is removed and the patient is led through wrist tenodesis exercises. The therapist then positions the patient's wrist in 20° extension. The MCP joint of the injured finger is positioned in 75–80° flexion and PIP in 70–75° flexion. The DIP remains in 40–45° flexion within the finger-based dorsal block splint. It may be advisable for the hand therapist to fabricate a thermoplastic exercise template to help guide the patient's hand and wrist into the desired position.

The patient is then asked to generate the minimal amount of muscle tension required to hold this posture; from 15–20 gmf is generated at the fingertip, and this can be confirmed by using a Haldex strain gauge. It has been shown experimentally that this controlled active exercise creates approximately 41 gmf and 605 gmf internal tension within the FDP and FDS, respectively. These internal forces appear to be well within the tensile strength of the two-strand Kessler (or modified Kessler) suture technique.

The finger-based dorsal block splint is discontinued at 21–25 days postoperatively, and the forearm-based splint is revised to place the wrist at neutral. Passive DIP extension is not initiated until after 28 days. Tendon gliding exercises are added between 3–4 weeks postoperatively, and these are introduced to the patient by the hand therapist as place-hold maneuvers. The patient continues to perform isolated active composite flexion exercises for the injured finger, gradually increasing the amount of end-range flexion. Isolating the finger of interest prevents trapping by the uninvolved fingers.

The forearm-based splint may be discontinued at 6 weeks postoperatively. Joint-blocking exercises are initiated at this time, also. At 8 weeks, the patient is progressed to light, resistive exercises using theraputty with gradual resumption of preinjury activities at 12 weeks postoperatively.

Hand Therapy Pearls

1. Zone 1 extends from the broad insertions of FDS on P2 to the insertion of FDP on the volar surface of the base of P3, and includes the A5, C3, and A4 pulleys. The volar surface of P2, bounded by the A4 pulley, represents a *transitional area* where FDS and FDP are in contact with one another.

2. In contrast to hand therapy treatment for Zone 2 flexor tendon repairs, Zone 1 treatment requires fabrication of a dorsally based finger splint that positions the DIP of the injured finger in 40–45° flexion.

3. The sanctity of the A4 pulley has been questioned because of the potential for FDP tendon impingement and/or adherence. The hand therapist should not necessarily expect free excursion of the repair if the A4 pulley is intact.

4. Early active mobilization of the FDS should not exceed adherence to the FDP and to the flexor sheath, and reduces risk of PIP flexion contracture.

5. Controlled active exercise for the repaired FDP should not exceed the strength of two-strand FDP repairs; however, precise positioning of the patient's hand is required. A thermoplastic template molded to the patient's hand is recommended.

REFERENCES

1. Evans R: A study of the zone I flexor tendon injury and implications for treatment. J Hand Ther 3:133–148, 1990.
2. Evans R: Rehabilitation techniques for applying immediate active tension to zone I and II flexor tendon repairs. Tech Hand Upper Extremity Surg 1:286–296, 1997.
3. Moieman NS, Elliot D: Primary flexor tendon repair in zone 1. J Hand Surg 25B:78–84, 2000.

PATIENT 26

A 71-year-old woman with rheumatoid arthritis and a weak grip

A 71-year-old woman with rheumatoid arthritis presents with a new left thumb problem. Approximately 5 years ago she underwent synovectomy of a significant amount of dorsally located hypertrophic synovium around her extensor retinaculum, as well as trigger-finger releases of her thumb and ring fingers on the left hand. She has done well since that operation, with reasonably good hand function. Her rheumatologist is currently managing her rheumatoid arthritis, and she has been relatively happy with her ability to perform her normal activities of daily living.

While weeding her garden last week, she noticed difficulty making a fist, because her left thumb felt "weak." She denied any cuts or other injury to that hand. She has not noticed any increase in pain, or change in subjective sensation.

Physical Examination: Skin: well-healed dorsal incision from prior surgical procedure. Neurologic: adequate perfusion of hand; intact arch with inflow from both ulnar and radial arteries; moving two-point sensory 5–6 mm on volar fingertips of all five digits. Musculoskeletal: fingers actively adduct and abduct; volar and dorsal interossei intact; flexion of distal phalanx strong at index, long, ring, and small fingers; thumb actively opposes to touch 5th fingertip, but actively flexing distal phalanx of thumb is difficult (see figure); all other fingers actively flex into a full fist.

Questions: What is the diagnosis? What are her treatment options?

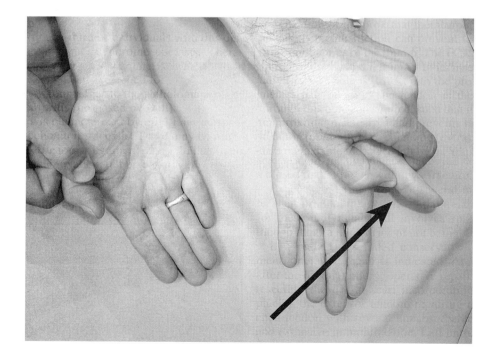

Answers: Rupture of the flexor pollicis longus. Best treatment option is tendon transfer to restore active thumb flexion.

Discussion: The flexor pollicis longus (FPL) is the most common *flexor* tendon to be ruptured in patients with rheumatoid arthritis. The pathogenesis of this injury involves the abrasion and ultimate attrition rupture of the tendon over the rough volar surface of the scaphoid (typically on a volar osteophyte): this is also known as the "Mannerfelt lesion." The loss of this tendon produces an acute inability to actively flex the IP joint of the thumb.

When examining these patients, it is important to carefully test the anterior interosseous branch of the median nerve, because an entrapment of this nerve can also cause loss of thumb IP flexion. This nerve also innervates the flexor digitorum profundus (FDP) to the index and long fingers, and the pronator quadratus. Therefore, patients with *palsy of the anterior interosseous nerve* will also be unable to actively flex the DIP joint of the index and long fingers, and will have difficulty pronating their forearm with the elbow flexed.

Treatment options for tendon reconstruction include either tendon grafting or transfer. Because of the etiology of the tendon injury (chronic abrasion and wearing down of the tendon), direct tendon repair is usually not possible. Tendon transfer (for example, transferring the motor from one of the flexor digitorum superficialis [FDS] tendons)

is a very nice option that affords a reliably good result.

However, in this patient population, due to disease involvement of the wrist and other digits, tendon transfer may not be advisable, or would result in too much donor morbidity. An alternative option is to reconstruct the loss of tendon length with a section of tendon graft. This is attractive because tendon from relatively noninvolved areas (i.e., plantaris tendon from the leg) can be harvested without worry of adversely affecting hand function. If tendon grafting is performed, it is important to completely resect the frayed and damaged tendon ends both proximally and distally. Active range of motion is started at about 3 weeks to prevent recalcitrant stiffness and the formation of tendon adhesions.

If there are no good options in regards to tendon reconstruction, then fusion of the thumb IP joint should be done to provide stabilization. If reasonable range of motion remains at the thumb MCP and CMC joints, this can afford a functional result. During surgical reconstruction (regardless of the technique used) the volar wrist should be explored, and any osteophytes debrided to prevent recurrence, as well as to prevent injury to the flexor tendons to the index finger.

Clinical Pearls

1. The flexor pollicis longus tendon is the most commonly ruptured *flexor* tendon in patients with rheumatoid arthritis. In this patient population, extensor tendons (especially the extensor pollicis longus) rupture much more frequently than flexor tendons.

2. The best treatment option for these patients is tendon transfer, if a suitable donor is available. Direct tendon repair is rarely (if ever) possible or advisable.

3. During surgical reconstruction, exploration and removal of the offending anatomic structure (usually an osteophyte that has eroded through the volar wrist capsule) is also warranted to prevent recurrence or injury to other tendons.

REFERENCES
1. Ertel AN: Flexor tendon ruptures in rheumatoid arthritis. Hand Clin 5:177–190, 1989.
2. Mannerfelt L, Norman O: Attrition ruptures of flexor tendons in rheumatoid arthritis caused by bony spurs in the carpal tunnel. A clinical and radiographic study. J Bone Joint Surg 51:270–277, 1969.
3. Schneider LH, Wiltshire D: Restoration of flexor pollicis longus function by flexor digitorum superficialis transfer. J Hand Surg 8:98–101, 1983.
4. Stark HH, Anderson DR, Zemel NP, et al: Bridge flexor tendon grafts. Clin Orthop 242:51–59, 1989.

Perspectives for Therapy

Fusion of the thumb IP joint may require that the patient be fitted with a custom hand- or forearm-based spica splint that protects the distal joint

during interval bone healing. The splint is worn for 4–8 weeks during waking hours.

The patient should be instructed in a home program of exercises for the uninvolved joints of the operated extremity. He or she may benefit from the use of a volar, finger-based gutter splint to support the thumb IP during active MCP and CMC motion, that is, during opposition exercises. Attention to wound care of both the operated thumb and wrist, patient instruction in pin care, and edema management are important components of patient treatment.

Assuming this patient has also been followed by a hand therapist preoperatively, she may continue use of her resting hand splint at bedtime, providing the splint offers a thumb component. Otherwise, the thumb spica splint may also be worn at bedtime.

The manner in which a tendon graft is secured to the distal and proximal ends of the salvaged FPL may qualify this patient for early, protected active motion. For example, the four-strand and Pulvertaft tenorraphies are especially strong constructs permitting tenodesis exercises—active wrist extension coupled with place-hold thumb flexion, and passive wrist flexion coupled with passive thumb extension. An ideal progression for tenodesis exercise is to have the patient use the compositely flexed fingers as a natural motion stop for the thumb. The exercise is progressed by allowing the thumb to make palmar contact.

A dorsal block splint that immobilizes the wrist in 20–30° flexion, thumb CMC in 20–25° abduction, and thumb MCP and IP in 15° flexion is fabricated to protect the grafted FPL between exercise sessions for 6 weeks. The fingers may be omitted from the splint design and permitted unrestricted active motion.

The dorsal block splint is revised to neutral at the wrist at 3 weeks postoperatively. Differential gliding of the FPL, that is, CMC and MCP extension combined with IP flexion, may be added at 4–5 weeks postoperatively, and this exercise, as well the wrist-thumb tenodesis exercises, can be performed outside of the dorsal splint. The patient then returns to the splint for continued protection between exercise sessions.

Blocking exercises for the FPL can be added at 6 weeks postoperatively. To facilitate a mechanical advantage for the FPL, the patient's wrist should be positioned in about 30° extension during gliding and blocking exercises. Light resistive exercises are initiated at 8 weeks, and the patient may gradually resume their preinjury level of activity at 12 weeks postoperatively.

Tendon transfer of the ring finger FDS, to substitute for the FPL, requires fabrication at 3 weeks postoperatively of a dorsal block splint that immobilizes the wrist and thumb as previously described. The patient attempts active flexion of the ring finger simultaneously with thumb flexion, within the confines of the dorsal splint. This is accomplished simply during tip-to-tip opposition of the thumb and ring finger. This exercise is progressed by having the patient actively flex the thumb in a palmar-ward direction, along the volar surface of the flexed ring finger.

Thumb IP blocking exercises, muscle stimulation with instrument settings appropriate for transfer education, and scar management to minimize tendon adherence, are relevant components of hand therapy following muscle transfer. At 4–5 weeks postoperatively, the wrist component of the dorsal block splint is revised to neutral. The splint is discontinued at 6 weeks, and active composite thumb, finger, and wrist extension may be initiated at this time. It may be necessary for the hand therapist to provide adjunctive, static-progressive extension splinting to counteract shortness of the extrinsic flexors, secondary to a relatively prolonged interval of immobilization in flexion.

At 8 weeks, progression to gentle strengthening may commence, with gradual return to the patient's preinjury level of activity at 12 weeks postoperatively.

Hand Therapy Pearls

1. The most important point is that the hand therapist and hand surgeon be in communication regarding the nature and status of surgical management of FPL rupture.

2. The hand therapist should be poised to provide adjunctive splinting, wound care, and patient education.

3. Uninvolved upper extremity joints should be permitted unrestricted, active motion while protecting operated structures.

4. Augmented techniques of tenorraphy should permit consideration of early active thumb motion, performed under therapist supervision.

REFERENCES

1. Cannon N: Tendon transfers. Diagnosis and Treatment Manual for Physicians and Therapists, 3rd ed. Indianapolis, The Hand Rehabilitation Center of Indiana, 1991, p 185.
2. Strickland JW: The Indiana method of tendon repair. Atlas of the Hand Clin 1:77–103, 1996.
3. Strickland JW, Cannon N: Flexor tendon repair-Indiana method. Indiana Hand Center Newsletter 1:1–17, 1993.

PATIENT 27

A 26-year-old woman with a mass on her right wrist

A 26-year-old woman presents to your office complaining of a mass on her volar wrist. She has been aware of it for the past 2 years, but she is now becoming concerned because it is getting larger. Her mother and a maternal aunt both had breast carcinoma. The patient is concerned that the mass may be a malignancy, particularly since it has increased in size.

Physical Examination: General: small, 2-centimeter mass on volar radial wrist (see figure); moderately soft and compressible. Palpation: slightly tender with direct compression over mass. Neurologic: no epitrochlear or axillary lymphadenopathy. Musculoskeletal: Allen's testing demonstrates vascular arch not intact (no perfusion of thumb and index fingers on manual compression of radial artery).

Questions: What is the diagnosis? What is your treatment recommendation?

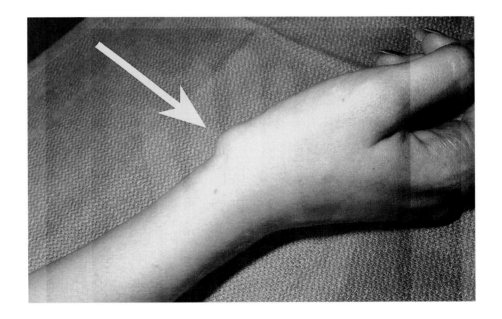

Answers: Ganglion cyst. Recommend surgical excision.

Discussion: Ganglion cysts are perhaps the most common benign, soft tissue tumor found in the hand. They occur most commonly in women (at a ratio of 3 to 1) and typically present between the ages of 20 and 40. The cyst walls are formed microscopically by compressed collagen fibers and fibroblasts, as opposed to the synovial or epithelial lining found in the true cysts. Ganglion cysts are actually **pseudocysts,** formed by leakage of joint synovial fluid into the surrounding soft tissue. The content of the ganglion cyst is a sticky, thick, mucous fluid that is high in hyaluronic acid.

The pathogenesis of the formation of these cysts remains controversial. It is thought that they occur at areas of degeneration at the wrist capsule, forming a physiologic "one-way valve" at the capsule. For example, if dye is injected into the wrist joint, it will freely flow into the ganglion cyst. In contrast, dye injected into the cyst will not flow into the wrist joint. This has implications for the surgeon: simple excision of the ganglion cyst (without resection of its origin from the wrist capsule) is *destined to fail.* Obliteration or destruction of the ganglion's origin and degenerative capsule is required to prevent recurrence.

Dorsal wrist ganglia typically arise from the scapholunate ligament (see left figure, *top*); volar wrist ganglia typically arise from either the trapeziometacarpal or the scaphotrapezial ligaments. The typical lesion is a thin-walled cyst containing clear, viscous material (see left figure, *bottom*).

Aspiration of the cyst has little long-term effect. Fluid will almost certainly reaccumulate, since this treatment does not address the underlying problem at the wrist capsule. Multiply aspirated cysts may make ultimate surgical resection more difficult secondary to scarring. Volar wrist ganglions may be intimately associated with the radial artery (see *top* figure on next page, *arrow*). For this reason, they may appear to be pulsatile on examination, due to a *transmitted* pulse (rather than because they are true vascular lesions). More importantly, this close association needs to be kept in mind during surgical resection, to prevent inadvertent injury to the artery. Allen's testing should be performed prior to volar ganglion excision, to assess vascular perfusion of the thumb and index finger via the ulnar artery in case the radial artery is damaged during dissection.

If the radial artery is injured during the dissection of the ganglion cyst, vascular repair may be necessary. Patients should be warned of this preoperatively, and the surgeon needs to be prepared for this possibility as well. Dorsal wrist ganglia are often adjacent to one or two terminal branches of the radial nerve (see *bottom* figure: radial nerve after ganglion resection—*white arrow;* ganglion location—*black arrows*). Care needs to be taken to avoid injury to these nerve branches, as they are prone to troublesome, painful, and treatment-resistant neuroma formation.

Nonoperative treatment, including aspiration, steroid injection, or manual rupture, is doomed to recurrence for the same reasons that incomplete surgical resection is—these methods do not address the underlying pathology and etiology of the cyst and its communication with the wrist capsule. In particular, injection or aspiration of volar ganglions should be performed with a great deal of caution (if at all) because of the intimate association with the radial artery.

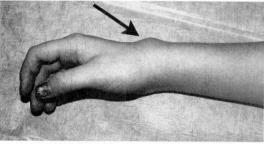

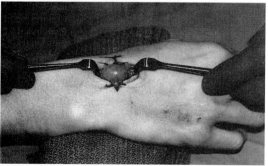

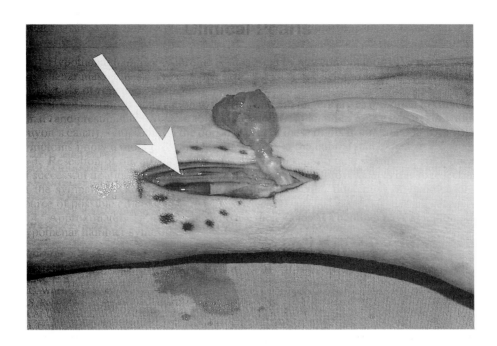

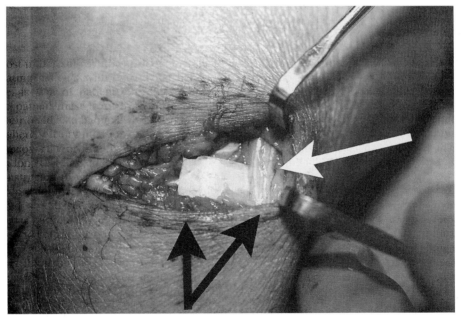

Clinical Pearls

1. Ganglion cysts represent the most common benign "tumor" of the hand; about 75% arise at the dorsal wrist, and 25% arise volarly.

2. Volar ganglion cysts are frequently closely associated with the radial artery. Transmission of the radial pulse through the cyst may give the examiner the incorrect impression that this is a vascular lesion.

3. Surgical resection remains the mainstay of treatment, but care needs to be taken to protect the radial artery from injury.

4. The rate of recurrence of these cysts after surgical resection is 5–10%. This number is higher when the originating stalk from the underlying wrist ligament is not respected at the time of surgery.

Hand Therapy Pearls

1. Emphasize early, active wrist motion for patients who have undergone excision of either a dorsal or volar ganglion cyst.

2. After sutures are removed, scar management is appropriate. Pay particular attention to skin territories supplied by terminal branches of sensory nerves. Desensitization in these areas may be indicated.

3. Passive range-of-motion exercises are relatively contraindicated in these patients, particularly if capsulodesis, or capsular shortening, has been performed. Discussion with the referring hand surgeon can clarify the extent of surgery required to excise the cyst and manage the resulting capsular defect.

REFERENCES

1. Angelides AC: Ganglions of the hand and wrist. In Green DP, Hotchkiss R, Pederson WC (ed): Green's Operative Hand Surgery, 4th ed. New York, Churchill Livingstone, 1999, pp 2157–2171.
2. Angelides AC, Wallace PF: The dorsal ganglion of the wrist: Its pathogenesis, gross and microscopic anatomy, and surgical treatment. J Hand Surg 1:228–235, 1976.
3. Lister GD, Smith RR: Protection of the radial artery in resection of adherent ganglions of the wrist. Plast Reconstr Surg 61:127–129, 1978.

PATIENT 28

A 65-year-old man with a painful and swollen index finger

You are called to the emergency department to evaluate a 65-year-old with a 2-day history of pain and swelling of the left index finger. He denies any lacerations or other injury to the digit. He does have a history of heart disease: on a recent physical examination by his primary care physician, he was noted to be hypertensive, and was started on hydrochlorothiazide. Other medications include allopurinol and sublingual nitroglycerin (prn chest pain).

Physical Examination: Temperature 98.6° F. Skin: finger moderately edematous and erythematous; no obvious fluid collection or evidence of abscess formation; no new or healing lacerations or open wounds. Musculoskeletal: tender; decreased range of motion, largely limited by pain.

Laboratory Findings: Radiographs: normal. CBC, WBC normal; ESR elevated.

Questions: What is the likely diagnosis? What is your treatment recommendation?

Answers: The most likely diagnosis is an acute exacerbation of gout. Recommend administration of colchicine for the acute attack.

Discussion: While the patient did not volunteer a history of gout, he was already being treated for it (allopurinol). Acute gout attacks are often misdiagnosed as an infection because the symptoms are so similar. In this patient an infectious etiology was less likely in the absence of a laceration or other trauma. You may consider discussing alternative antihypertensive medications with his primary care physician: thiazide diuretics can precipitate acute attacks of gout.

Gout is caused by increased production of uric acid; insufficient elimination by the body; or increased intake of foods that are high in purines (purines are broken down into uric acid). Foods high in purines include certain meats, seafood, dried peas, and beans. Alcohol can precipitate an acute attack by inhibiting excretion of uric acid via the kidneys. The symptoms of gout arise from the precipitation of uric acid crystals at the joints and soft tissues. The typical patient is a man aged 30–50 years. Gout is uncommon in premenopausal women.

The differential diagnosis of patients presenting with erythema, edema, and pain includes hand infection, rheumatoid arthritis, pseudogout (the deposition of calcium pyrophosphate crystals, rather than urate), and bony tumor. The diagnosis of gout can be definitively made by examination of synovial fluid. Under compensated, polarized light microscopy, needle-like intracellular and extracellular monosodium urate crystals can be observed. They are birefringent and have negative elongation. Observation of these crystals engulfed by neutrophils makes the diagnosis.

Treatment of the acute attack involves medical management only, usually with colchicine. Two milligrams of colchicine should be administered via slow IV push. If the patient remains symptomatic, additional colchicine can be given (0.5 mg every 6 hours). Due to potential serious toxicity, it is not recommended to administer more than 4 mg in a 24-hour period, and after a full course of IV therapy (4 mg maximum) no further colchicine is recommended for at least 7 days.

After the acute attack has resolved, chronic medical management (using allopurinol, probenecid, and/or colchicine) can be started or resumed. Allopurinol (a xanthine oxidase inhibitor) prevents the breakdown of xanthine and hypoxanthine into uric acid, therefore keeping uric acid levels low. Note that allopurinol and probenicid may actually worsen symptoms if given during an acute attack.

Most patients can be managed medically with this condition, but occasionally patients present with painful and destructive masses (see figure below, *arrows*) of this precipitate. In severe cases, these tophi can erode through cartilage, tendon, and even bone, causing significant deformity and loss of function (see figure, *next page;* consistency of precipitated uric acid in gouty tophus within a flexor tendon). Surgical resection of these can often significantly decrease local pain, and limit further damage and loss of function.

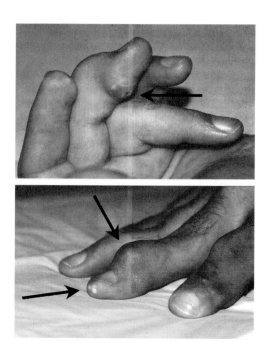

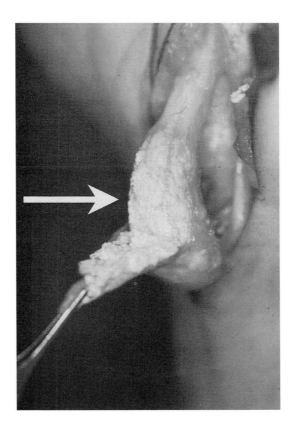

Clinical Pearls

1. The mainstay of treatment for gout is medical management: allopurinol and probenicid for long-term management; colchicine for acute attacks.

2. Patients with medically resistant gout may experience tophi—painful masses formed by the precipitation of urate crystals. Relief of significant pain (and, ideally, prevention of additional local tissue damage can be obtained via surgical resection.

3. The differential diagnosis for a painful and erythematous digit includes infection, rheumatoid arthritis, pseudogout, gout, and bony tumor. Infection is by far the most common of these diagnoses.

REFERENCES
1. Louis DS, Jebson PJ: Mimickers of hand infections. Hand Clin 14:519–529, 1998.
2. Pal B, Foxall M, Dysart T, et al: How is gout managed in primary care? A review of current practice and proposed guidelines. Clin Rheumatol 19:21–25, 2000.
3. Pascual E: Gout update: From lab to the clinic and back. Curr Opin Rheumatol 12:213–218, 2000.

PATIENT 29

A 19-year-old maintenance worker with acute onset of severe bilateral forearm pain

A 19-year-old man at a local glass etching factory presents to the emergency department with acute onset of severe pain at his bilateral hands and forearms. He was brought in via ambulance from his work: the pains started rapidly, without warning. When asked about his activities while at work, he replies that his duties are routine (e.g., emptying trash, mopping floors) except for a liquid spill that he had to clean several hours ago. As the current time is 2 AM, there is only a skeleton crew working at his plant. No supervisory personnel are available to assist you in identifying the caustic substance that he may have come into contact with.

Physical Examination: General: extreme pain at hands and forearms. Skin: some splotchy whitish areas; erythematous; a few blisters diffusely. Otherwise, skin is largely intact. Musculoskeletal (cursory): excellent range of motion and motor strength.

Laboratory Findings: Hemoglobin 12 g/dl, hematocrit 36%, platelets 342,000/μl, WBC 8400/μl. Drug screen: trace cannaboids, trace ethanol, otherwise negative. Also see table below.

Element	Patient	Normal
Sodium	140 mEq/L	(136–148)
Potassium	6.7 mEq/L	(3.7–5.4)
Chloride	106 mEq/L	(96–111)
CO2	28 mEq/L	(23–33)
Creatinine	0.6 mg/dl	(0.4–1.5)
BUN	12 mg/dl	(10–20)
Glucose	96 mg/dl	(70–110)
Calcium	6.5 mg/dl	(8.9–10.6)
Total bilirubin	0.5 mg/dl	(0.1–1.5)
Magnesium	1.4 mg/dl	(1.8–2.4)

Questions: What is the probable agent that this young man has encountered? What is your recommended treatment?

Answers: Hydrofluoric acid burn. Administer calcium.

Discussion: Hydrofluoric acid is one of the strongest acids, and is used primarily in industry (glass etching, electronics manufacturing, and metal cleaning). It can also be found in widely available rust removers. Symptoms may not present for several hours after exposure. The time of onset is related somewhat to the concentration of the acid: symptoms are delayed with exposure to more dilute solutions, allowing the acid to penetrate more deeply into the soft tissues (with more widespread damage).

The fluoride ions bind to intracellular calcium and magnesium, resulting in cell death. That is why these patients present with hypocalcemia, hypomagnesemia, and hyperkalemia. Potassium, the major intracellular cation, is released into the serum after the cell dies. At the same time, fluoride ion is released into the surrounding tissue, causing further cellular destruction.

When examining the patient, the skin involvement may seem minor; this is deceptive, and is particularly true with exposure to more dilute concentrations (less than 7%). The patient may present with signs and symptoms related to hypocalcemia, including tetany, Chovstek's sign (hypersensitivity of the facial nerve to gentle tapping), or Trousseau's sign. The patient should be placed on telemetry, because until the hypocalcemia is corrected he or she is at risk for cardiac arrhythmias (the primary cause of death in these injuries).

Treatment involves initial copious lavage with water, followed by direct application of 2.5% calcium gluconate gel to bind the fluoride ion. If a prepackaged gel is not available, it can be "manufactured" by combining one part 10% calcium gluconate solution with three parts water-soluble gel (such as K-Y gel). Calcium chloride is not used because it can irritate the tissue. If the topical gel application is not effective at relieving pain, subeschar infiltration of 10% calcium gluconate is the next step, with pain relief being the indicator to titrate the end-point of therapy. Other delivery options include intravenous or intra-arterial injection. Anesthesia and analgesia are contraindicated, because pain is followed to determine the amount of calcium injected.

Note that these injuries can be quite serious and even lethal. Patients should be admitted to intensive care (ICU) for close observation and correction of any electrolyte imbalances.

In the present patient, the diagnosis was suggested by the fact that he worked at a glass-etching factory: hydrofluoric acid is widely used in that industry. Additionally, his serum calcium and magnesium levels had already begun to drop, and potassium had begun to rise, which is characteristic of hydrofluoric acid burns. Calcium was administered both intravenously and injected directly into the damaged tissue. He was admitted to the ICU, and eventually made a full recovery.

Clinical Pearls

1. Treatment of hydrofluoric acid burns centers around calcium gluconate administration to bind the damaging fluoride ion.

2. Treatment is titrated to relief of pain: analgesia and anesthesia are not indicated in these patients.

3. Laboratory abnormalities include hypocalcemia, hypomagnesemia, and hyperkalemia. Cardiac arrhythmias are a significant concern, and the major cause of mortality in these injuries.

REFERENCES

1. Bertolini JC: Hydroluoric acid: A review of toxicity. J Emerg Med 10:163–168, 1992.
2. Concannon MJ: Common Hand Problems in Primary Care. Philadelphia, PA, Hanley & Belfus, Inc, 1999, pp 159–163.
3. Greco RJ, Hartford CE, Haith Jr LR, et al: Hydrofluoric acid-induced hypocalcemia. J Trauma 28:1593–1596, 1988.
4. Ryan JM, McCarthy GM, Plunkett PK: Regional intravenous calcium—an effective method of treating hydrofluoric acid burns to limb peripheries. Emerg Med J 14:401–404, 1997.

Perspectives For Therapy

The hand is the most common site of thermal injury, and thermal injuries rank second among upper extremity injuries requiring hospitalization.

Although the burn agent in this case is a chemical, rather than thermal energy per se, the soft tissue injuries resulting from chemical exposure herald a similar process of wound healing that culminates in scar formation. Hand therapy management is therefore guided by: (1) the depth of the burn, (2) an inventory of involved tissues and affected skin surfaces, and (3) knowledge of when the burn occurred.

Burn depth has been classified as follows. A **superficial partial-thickness (SPT) burn,** or first-degree burn, involves the epidermis to the depth of the dermal papillae. SPT burns are glistening pink or bright red because the dermal vascular plexus is intact and markedly vasodilated. Blisters may be present, and the patient is exquisitely sensitive to pain because the dermal sensory receptors are also intact. SPT burns heal spontaneously, due to the presence of germinative tissues, and they have a good functional and cosmetic prognosis.

Deep partial-thickness (DPT) burns, or second-degree burns, involve the epidermis and variable thicknesses of the dermis. While the neurovascular plexuses are extensively damaged, the epidermal appendages (hair follicles and glands) are spared. The soft tissues are edematous, soft, and elastic. DPT burns have the potential to heal spontaneously; however, their functional and cosmetic prognosis tends to be less favorable than that of SPT burns.

Full-thickness (FT) burns, or third-degree burns, result in injury to epidermal, dermal, and subcutaneous tissues. Though the skin need not be lost, it is devitalized and forms a dry, leathery eschar that can be white to dark brown. Massive edema is evident. Because there is loss of the neural plexus, cutaneous sensory perception is absent. FT burns do not heal spontaneously due to the absence of germinative tissues, and require soft-tissue grafting for wound closure. Accordingly, FT burns have the greatest potential to result in functional loss and poor-quality cosmesis.

It is important for the hand therapist to understand that the integument is of variable thickness throughout the hands and upper extremities. This is largely due to variation in the thicknesses of the stratum corneum and subcutaneous tissue layer. Thus, identical amounts of thermal energy or, as in this case, identical durations of contact with a chemical agent can cause quite different presentations of a patient's burns, depending upon the precise location of skin contact. A complete inventory of involved tissues and skin surfaces is therefore mandatory.

Burn care is synonymous with uneventful wound healing. The hand therapist must be capable of matching treatment modalities with each phase of wound repair—inflammation, fibroplasia, and remodeling. Minimizing the duration of the inflammatory stage, controlling edema, and maintaining optimal health of the wound environment during granulation and epithelialization are paramount for modifying scar tissue. Treatment design varies as a function of when the burn occurred and when the patient is referred to hand therapy.

Always clear mechanical debridement of burns with the referring hand surgeon. Debridement is desirable when hematoma, eschar, or blisters interfere with or block motion. However, debridement should *never* interfere with neovascularization or epithelialization. Choice of wound dressings and medications is also made by the referring hand surgeon. The purpose of their use, frequency of change, and appearance of the wounds should be clearly understood by the hand therapist, patient, and family. In general, dressings and medicines are used to protect the wound environment and apply gentle pressure. They also help to position the joints, and they may serve to limit or promote motion, depending upon the stage of wound healing.

Splinting the burned hand or upper extremity is done for a specific purpose. For example, a splint may be indicated to: (1) rest healing tissues and optimize hand position, (2) minimize mechanical faults, and (3) promote sensorimotor function of uninvolved tissues. The hand therapist is required to make ongoing evaluations of hand anatomy and function as wounds heal, and modify splints accordingly.

Exercise for the burn patient improves joint motion, mobilizes edema, and ensures tendon gliding. However, exercises should be done slowly through the patient's full, active range. In some situations, passive motion is contraindicated due to the increased risk of soft tissue damage—for example, when tendons are attenuated or when joint injury is possible due to impaired afference.

Pressure therapy is a mainstay for all phases of rehabilitation of the burned hand and upper extremity. Pressure therapy controls edema, protects fragile healing skin, and minimizes hypertrophy of healing soft tissues and scar. A variety of materials are available. Cohesive materials can be applied to healing wounds with appropriate nonadherent interfaces such as Xeroform or Adaptic. Elastomer; silicone gel sheeting, tubes, caps, and pads; and compression garments, such as Tubigrip and gloves, can be applied to healed wounds for scar compression. Each material has relative advantages that must be matched to the specific needs of each patient. For example, elastomer can be combined with custom splints to provide conforming pressure in conjunction with hand positioning. Gloves can be used to provide even, generalized scar compression over large areas while allowing hand mobility.

Hand Therapy Pearls

1. Burns are classified according to the depth of integumentary injury. This classification scheme has prognosticatory value and guides hand therapy treatment.

2. Uneventful wound healing is synonymous with burn care. Treatment modalities are matched with the stage of wound healing to optimize neovascularization and epithelialization.

3. Splinting the burned hand is indicated to rest healing tissues, optimize hand position, mimimize mechanical faults, and promote sensorimotor function.

4. Active exercise helps mobilize edema, improve joint motion, and ensure tendon gliding.

5. Pressure therapy is one of the mainstays of burn rehabilitation. A variety of materials are available and these can help influence healing wounds and scar tissue.

REFERENCES

1. Grigsby deLinde L, Miles WK: Remodeling of scar tissue in the burned hand. In Hunter JM, Mackin EJ, Callahan AD (eds): Rehabilitation of the Hand: Surgery and Therapy, 4th ed. St. Louis, Mosby, 1995, pp 1267–1294.
2. Howell JW: Management of the acutely burned hand for the nonspecialized clinician. Phys Ther 69:1077–1090, 1989.
3. Howell, JW: Management of the burned hand. In Richard RL, Staley MJ (eds). Burn Care and Rehabilitation: Priniciples and Practice. Philadelphia, FA Davis, 1994, pp 531–575.

PATIENT 30

A 16-year-old girl with metacarpophalangeal joint pain

A 16-year-old girl presents with pain at her right, long-finger MCP joint after falling 3 days ago. She was riding a combination skate board-scooter and fell forward on her outstretched hand. She does not have any other complaints except for her chief symptom of pain and an abrasion over the distal forearm.

Physical Examination: Skin: intact; swelling and tenderness over MCP joint. Musculoskeletal: decreased range of motion at that joint, largely because movement makes patient uncomfortable. Neurologic: normal.

Laboratory Findings: Radiograph: see figure.

Questions: What is the diagnosis? What is your recommended treatment?

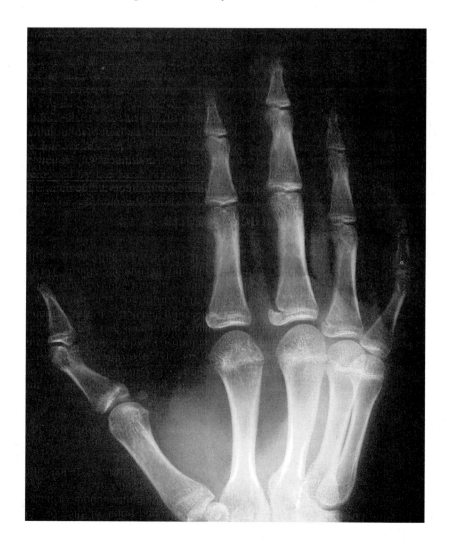

Answers: Intra-articular fracture of the proximal phalanx of the index finger. Recommend open reduction and internal fixation.

Discussion: In this patient, a relatively large percentage of the articular surface is involved in the fracture. In situations of significant comminution with multiple small bony fractures within the joint (see x-ray), internal fixation is neither possible nor practical, and prolonged immobilization is almost doomed to result in a difficult, stiff joint. Application of dynamic traction is more appropriate. In contrast, when a single (relatively large) fragment exists, it may be possible to reduce and fix the fracture using very small screws currently available, such as the 0.8-mm screw (see figures below). In this patient, failure to reduce this fragment into anatomic position would almost certainly lead to late arthritic changes of the joint.

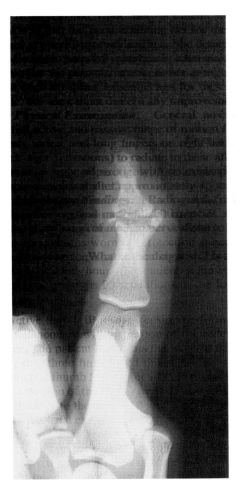

During the surgical reduction, care must be taken to obtain a precise restoration of the articular surface, without impinging on the joint space with hardware. The fracture segment is identified and maneuvered into position with the forceps (see figure below, *A*). Care is taken to preserve as much of the soft tissue attachment to the fragment as possible, to preserve vascularity and viability of the segment. The fracture is reduced and held in reduction with the forceps (*B*). Correct reduction is confirmed by evaluating the joint surface, to ensure that there are no contour irregularities. A single screw is placed across the fracture (*C*) to fix it in anatomic position.

When the joints of the hand are exposed surgically, special attention needs to be paid to postoperative therapy. These patients are at risk for recalcitrant stiffness if after open reduction and placement of internal hardware they are kept immobilized for an extended period. Therefore, every attempt needs to be made during the surgical procedure to obtain a fixation that is secure enough to allow *early supervised* ROM exercises within 7 to 10 days, if at all possible. That is easier said than done, due to several factors: the delicate screw size and small thread; the small bony fragments with which you must work; and limited options for screw placement (cannot be intra-articular). Thus, reduction is precarious.

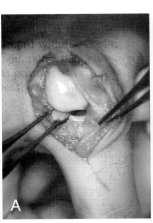
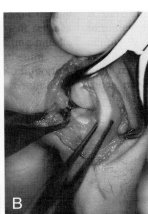
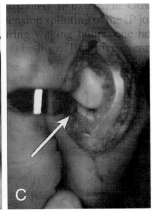

A

B

C

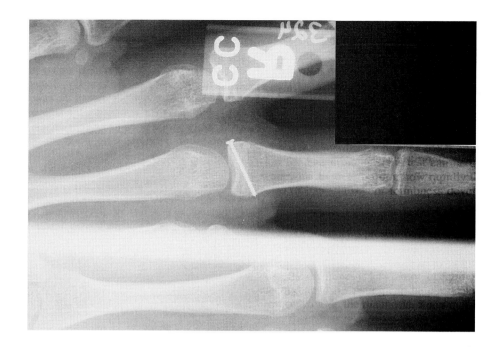

Clinical Pearls

1. A significant risk of intra-articular fractures is ultimate stiffness or decrease in mobility, and treatment needs to be aimed at avoiding this outcome as much as possible.

2. Removing the soft-tissue attachments from the fracture fragment risks devascularizing it. Instead of removing the tissue, consider placing the screw or K-wire directly through it.

3. Directly visualize and reduce the articular surface. Do not attempt to align the external surface of the bone to facilitate accurate fracture reduction.

4. If the fracture involves multiple, small fragments, or if the fracture cannot be secured with internal fixation, consider dynamic skeletal traction to preserve maximal ultimate joint motion.

REFERENCES
1. Hastings II H, Carroll IV C: Treatment of closed articular fractures of the metacarpophalangeal and proximal interphalangeal joints. Hand Clin 4:503–527, 1988.
2. Margles SW: Intra-articular fractures of the metacarpophalangeal and proximal interphalangeal joints. Hand Clin 4:67–74, 1988.
3. McElfresh EC, Dobyns JH: Intra-articular metacarpal head fractures. J Hand Surg 8:383–393, 1983.

Perspectives For Therapy

Intra-articular fractures of the MCP joints are relatively uncommon. Yet, when they occur, they can cause severe hand impairment. The patient loses the enhanced mobility originally enjoyed by the MCP joints. He or she cannot adapt the hand to the variety of sizes and shapes of objects encountered during normal grasping and prehension, and is instead constrained by limited MCP motion. Hand function is especially impaired when the MCP joints of the highly mobile border

digits (thumb, ring, and small fingers) are injured. Early referral to hand therapy for this patient should include supervised active motion, static splinting to protect the repaired fracture, wound care, and edema management.

The dorsum of the hand is the bellwether for edema. Relatively thin, stretchable, and loosely connected to deeper tissues, distension of dorsal skin caused by edema will significantly reduce distal gliding required for finger flexion. The

MCP joints therefore tend to be postured in extension in the edematous hand. The sequela of prolonged MCP joint extension is adaptive shortening of the MCP collateral ligaments, and this limits full MCP flexion. Clinically, this is described as an *extension contracture.*

It is imperative that the hand therapist measure and document edema when present, and initiate prompt, progressive measures to control it through elevation, use of cohesive dressings, and retrograde massage while sutures are placed. In the geriatric patient, retrograde massage must be performed gently. Exuberant compression over fragile dorsal skin can cause extensive ecchymosis, soft tissue trauma, and increased inflammation. Following suture removal, contrast baths are a useful adjunct to improve hand circulation and decrease edema.

The extensor tendons are prone to restraint from dorsal scar formation, with resulting limitations in extension and flexion of the MCP and IP joints. After sutures are removed, gentle scar massage may be initiated, and this is effective for mobilizing superficial and deep soft tissues. As healing skin becomes thicker and stronger, scar massage can become more vigorous.

The anatomy of the MCP joints ensures that the collateral ligaments are brought into tension as these joints are flexed. Thus, flexion is the optimal position for splinting this patient's hand because it maintains ligament length while protecting the repaired fracture. A hand-based, ulnar gutter or volar resting hand splint, incorporating the small and ring fingers, is most desirable. The MCP joints should be flexed 60–70° and the IP joints immobilized at absolute 0°, which is the intrinsic-plus hand position. In this manner, the patient may continue to use the radial three digits for activities of daily living without jeopardizing the repaired fracture.

During fabrication of the splint, it may be difficult for the patient to maintain the MCP joints in the required amount of flexion, due to dorsal edema and passive restraint of the extrinsic extensors. Supinating the patient's forearm allows the wrist to passively extend, and a tenodesis effect is produced, resulting in passive MCP joint flexion. This position will be an aid during splint fabrication.

Early referral to hand therapy and initiation of supervised active hand motion is most desirable for reasons alluded to previously. Intrinsic-plus hand positioning lends itself well to both composite finger extension and to straight fisting. Intrinsic-minus exercise recruits the ED, FDP, and FDS, and stretches the hand intrinsics. Active motion also helps decrease edema through the pumping action of skeletal muscle on venous and lymphatic flow. Passive motion exercises are contraindicated due to the risk of damaging delicate hardware, with loss of fracture reduction.

In the older pediatric patient sustaining an MCP injury, there may be a very slight risk of impaired hand growth, as a function of injury to the epiphyseal plates at the base of P1 and the metacarpal head. Review of x-rays permits an appraisal of the presence of epiphyseal lines, and discussion of objective findings can ensue with the patient and family.

Hand Therapy Pearls

1. The dorsum of the hand is the bellwether for edema. Failure to appreciate and rigorously control edema will lead to induration, fibrosis, and impaired hand function.

2. Scar massage may be initiated once sutures are removed. The vigor of application can be increased as soft tissues become thicker and stronger.

3. The patient's hand is splinted in the intrinsic-plus position to protect the repaired fracture and optimize MCP joint collateral ligament length. As an aid to hand splinting, the patient's forearm should be supinated, allowing the wrist to extend and MCP joints to flex by tenodesis.

4. Active hand exercises, such as composite extension, straight fist, and intrinsic-minus, are prioritized. Passive exercises are contraindicated due to the risk of hardware failure and loss of fracture reduction.

REFERENCES

1. Dubousett JF: The digital joints. In Tubiana R (ed): The Hand. Vol 1. Philadelphia, WB Saunders, 1981, pp 191–201.
2. Flowers KR: Edema: Differential management based on the stages of wound healing. In Hunter JM, Mackin EJ, Callahan AD (eds): Rehabilitation of the Hand: Surgery and Therapy, 4th ed. St. Louis, Mosby, 1995, pp 87–91.
3. Hunter JM, Mackin EJ: Edema: Techniques of evaluation and management. In Hunter JM, Mackin EJ, Callahan AD (eds): Rehabilitation of the Hand: Surgery and Therapy, 4th ed. St. Louis, Mosby, 1995, pp 77–85.
4. Light TR, Bednar MS: Management of intra-articular fractures of the metacarpophalangeal joint. Hand Clin 10:303–314, 1994.
5. Moran CA: Anatomy of the hand. Phys Ther 69:1007–1013, 1989.
6. Thomine J-M: The skin of the hand. In Tubiana R (ed): The Hand, Vol. 1. Philadelphia, WB Saunders, 1981, pp 107–115.

PATIENT 31

A 35-year-old quadriplegic man with poor hand function

A 35-year-old man is referred to you for assistance improving his hand function. Approximately 9 months earlier, he was involved in a motor vehicle accident in which he was an unrestrained passenger. He suffered a fracture of his cervical spine at the C7–8 level, with spinal cord injury and tetraplegia. He has completed an extensive course of rehabilitation. The patient denies any prior hand injuries or surgery. His main complaint is that he cannot grasp or hold onto objects. He realizes that fine manipulation of objects will not be possible, but he is hopeful that if he can obtain even a rudimentary grip he will be much more independent in his activities of daily living (ADLs).

Physical Examination: Upper extremity function (see figure): strong elbow flexion and extension; strong extension of wrist; fingers cannot actively extend or flex; wrist flexes weakly. Neurologic: some sensation over dorsal and volar radial hand; very little effective sensation on ulnar aspect.

Question: What procedure can you offer this patient that would provide him with more function?

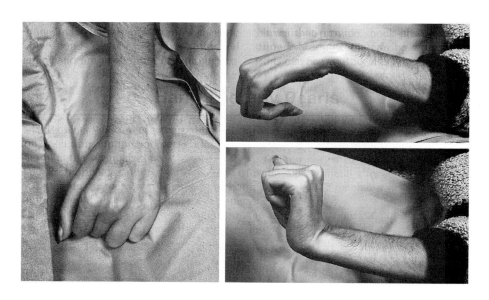

Answer: Moberg key-pinch procedure

Discussion: This procedure is an elegant surgical option for tetraplegics to improve their hand function. A prerequisite is that the candidate must have strong wrist extension; this is what powers the "key pinch."

There are several components involved in this procedure: fusion of the thumb IP joint, division of the annular pulley of the thumb (to allow bowstringing of the flexor pollicis longus [FPL] tendon), and tenodesis of the FPL to the distal radius. The overall effect of this procedure is to secure the proximal FPL to the distal radius, such that when the patient actively extends the wrist, the thumb will be forcefully adducted to the index finger, providing strong key pinch. This ability to grasp can dramatically improve the functional capacity of the hand, and does not require the sacrifice of an additional (and often scarce) active motor unit.

Dividing the proximal FPL tendon and securing it to the distal radius causes a "tenodesis effect" of wrist extension, which in turn causes the thumb to be drawn to the radial index finger. The tenodesis effect is commonly observed in normal individuals, and can be exploited to ascertain whether a tendon is intact in an unconscious patient in a trauma evaluation. For example, at rest with wrist flexion, the fingers assume a characteristic posture of slight flexion. With wrist extension, the tenodesis effect of the flexor tendons causes the fingers to be gently drawn into the palm (see figure). If the flexor tendons have been transected, the fingers will remain extended, and will not flex with wrist extension.

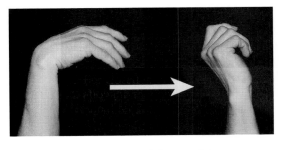

Fusion of the thumb IP joint provides more stability for grasp (see *top* figure, next page). As orig-inally described, a formal fusion was not performed; the thumb IP joint was merely fixed in position with a buried percutaneous K-wire. However, after having seen several patients present with broken K-wires as a late (several years postop) complication, this author (MC) has changed his approach and now fuses this joint at the original surgery.

Division of the annular pulley (A1) of the thumb (allowing bowstringing) gives more power to thumb flexion, at the cost of decreased excursion—which is always the effect of dividing a pulley (see *middle* figure). The decreased excursion is not an issue in regards to functional loss in these patients, partially because the IP joint is fused. Sufficient excursion remains to provide full adduction of the thumb with wrist extension, and the additional power helps maintain meaningful grasp for these patients.

An additional component to this procedure that has been proposed is a dorsal tenodesis of the extensor mechanism at the level of the thumb MCP joint. The purpose of this is to prevent hyperflexion at the MCP joint. This is relatively simple to perform: using a dorsal approach, the periostium at the MCP joint is abraded, and the extensor hood sutured to the periosteum using two to four sutures. If the tenodesis does not maintain this support (and the patient does exhibit hyperflexion at the MCP joint), an arthrodesis can be used to maintain the joint position.

Tenodesis of the FPL is requires division of the tendon at the musculotendinous junction (see *bottom* figure). The tendon is then passed through two holes placed in the distal radius, and then preliminarily sutured to itself. Prior to completing the procedure, the tenodesis is tested by flexing and extending the wrist to judge the adequacy of the tendon tension. After adjusting the FPL tenodesis to the proper position, the procedure is completed and the patient is splinted in a position to reduce tension on the tendon repair: wrist flexed and thumb adducted. This position is maintained for at least 4 weeks, at which time the patient may begin an active exercise program as a component of postoperative therapy.

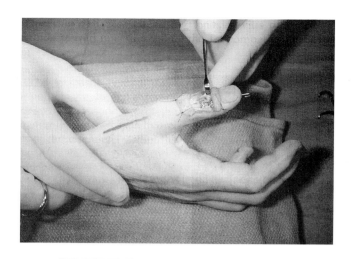

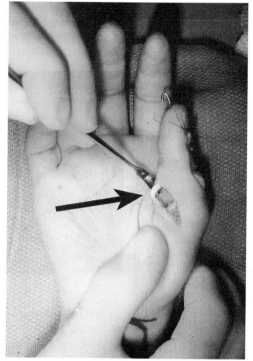

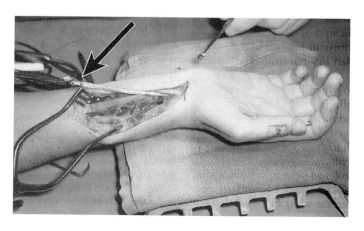

Clinical Pearls

1. The most important criterion for the Moberg key-pinch procedure is the preoperative ability to strongly extend the wrist: this surgery capitalizes on FPL tenodesis to provide strong key-pinch grasp without sacrifice of another functioning motor donor.

2. Although not described in the original procedure, fusion of the thumb IP joint (rather than simply holding it in position with a buried K-wire) provides a stronger and more lasting result.

3. Loss of any pulley results in greater power at the expense of excursion. This principle is used in this procedure to improve the power of the key pinch.

REFERENCES

1. Hentz VR, Brown M, Keoshian LA: Upper limb reconstruction in quadriplegia: Functional assessment and proposed treatment modifications. J Hand Surg 8:119–131, 1983.
2. McDowell CL: Tetraplegia. In Green DP, Hotchkiss R, Pederson WC (eds): Green's Operative Hand Surgery, 4th ed. New York, Churchill Livingstone, 1999.
3. Moberg EA: The present state of surgical rehabilitation of the upper limb in tetraplegia. Paraplegia 25:351–356, 1987.
4. Moberg EA: The Upper Limb in Tetraplegia: A New Approach to Surgical Rehabiliation. Stuttgart, Thieme, 1978.

Perspectives For Therapy

Postoperative hand therapy consists of teaching the patient a new hand motor pattern—namely, *active* wrist extension to achieve *passive* key pinch. This novel hand motor pattern should be broken down into separate steps to facilitate patient learning.

The **first step** is preparatory: the patient performs wrist flexion with gravity to position the thumb in relative abduction. In the **second step,** the patient positions the hand in space using proximal upper extremity muscles (in this case, as far distally as the elbow flexors and extensors). For most tasks, the patient's forearm will either be in neutral rotation or pronated, providing the pronator teres has been spared, in part. The **third step** consists of active wrist extension to accomplish passive key pinch. In this manner, the patient learns to use his or her operated hand to grasp and hold objects.

While the optimal duration and timing of practice required to learn new hand motor skills in quadriplegia has not been documented, an empirical 10 minutes per waking hour is suggested. A volar, forearm-based, thumbhole splint may be used by the patient between exercise sessions and at bedtime for 3–4 weeks to support the operated wrist in extension. This will help maintain the adequacy of the FPL tenodesis.

The above-described hand motor pattern may, with practice, become automatic fairly quickly as the patient learns the relationships among cutaneous sensation, proprioception, and the amounts of thumb abduction and muscle power available. These variables are important because they determine the weight and size of the object to be grasped and held. It may be efficient for the patient to store routinely used objects such as eating utensils and writing implements in a manner that minimizes energy expenditure.

In a retrospective survey of 18 quadriplegic patients (21 hands) examining postoperative hand function as it relates to ADLs, 1–10 years following a Moberg procedure, all patients reported a significant increase in independence and in ADLs. All patients would have the procedure done again, and would strongly recommend it to other patients.

Hand Therapy Pearls

1. New hand motor skills, made possible by muscle transfers, must be learned by the patient. The optimal duration and timing of practice required to learn these skills in quadriplegia is not known; however, 10 minutes of practice each waking hour is suggested to start.

2. Motor skills should be broken down into steps to facilitate learning of new hand functions. The individual steps must be matched to the available cutaneous sensation, proprioception, joint motion, and muscle power.

3. Postoperative splint use supports the operated wrist and maintains the adequacy of tenodesis.

REFERENCES

1. Dahl AL, House JH, Comadoll C. Functional outcome following one-stage key pinch and release with thumb carpal metacarpal fusion in tetraplegia. J Hand Ther 4:25, 1991.
2. Ejeskar A, Dahllof A-G, Moberg E. Upper limb surgery in tetraplegia. In Hunter JM, Mackin EJ, Callahan AD (eds): Rehabilitation of the Hand: Surgery and Therapy, 4th ed. St. Louis, Mosby, 1995, pp 1413–1421.

PATIENT 32

A 68-year-old man with a nail deformity and mass on his index finger

A 68-year-old gentleman presents to your office complaining of a mass on the dorsal aspect of his dominant index finger. He claims that it has slowly gotten larger over the past 8–12 months, but denies any pain associated with it. He cannot recall any trauma to that finger, or any significant trauma to the hand. He smokes about one pack per day, and had coronary bypass surgery a year and a half ago, but denies any other medical problems.

Physical Examination: Skin: small, cystic mass on radial aspect of dominant index finger (see figure); skin somewhat thinner over mass; groove (or depression) on fingernail, also on radial aspect. Fingers and nails otherwise appear completely normal.

Questions: What is your diagnosis? How can the nail deformity be fixed?

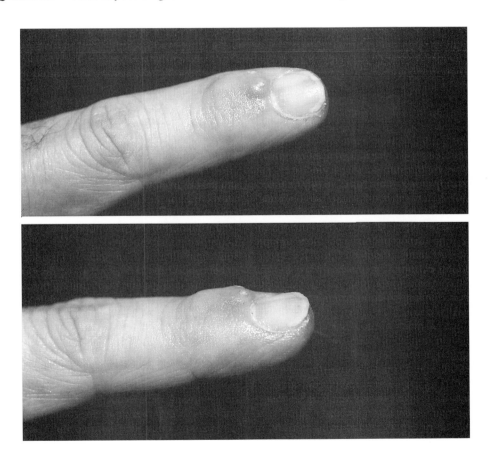

Answers: Mucous cyst. Recommend surgical treatment.

Discussion: Mucous cysts are actually ganglion cysts, but the former always arise at the DIP joint and are almost universally associated with an osteophyte at that joint. The cyst may or may not have an identifiable stalk, or connection to the underlying joint. A significant percentage cause the secondary nail deformity (fingernail depression) by placing pressure on the germinal matrix of the nail bed. The skin overlying the cyst is often thinned out considerably, and more often than not needs to be resected at the time of mucous cyst excision.

It is important to document the patient's preoperative range of motion at the DIP joint, because these lesions are associated with osteophytes and arthritic changes. If the cyst ruptures spontaneously and becomes secondarily infected, there is a risk of a septic joint developing.

Excision requires the creation of a relatively large dorsal rotation flap (over the middle phalanx; see figures) to allow closure of the defect. Resection of the underlying osteophyte is recommended during surgical resection of the cyst, to prevent recurrence. Some surgeons have demonstrated that, in some cases, resection of the osteophyte is *all* that is required in the treatment of these lesions: after debriding the offending pathology, the cyst and nail deformity may resolve without further treatment.

Prior to seeking medical attention, the individual pictured below had drained his cyst on multiple occasions, which led to a more scarred appearance over the recurrent cyst itself. Note the characteristic nail deformity distally. In the figure below, the *left* image shows the planned resection of skin overlying the mucous cyst and the dorsal rotation flap for coverage. The *right* image shows the defect after skin, cyst, and osteophyte resection. The complete removal of the cyst and its associated osteophyte is easier to accomplish after elevation of the dorsal flap, which gives the surgeon a much wider exposure to the underlying structures.

The level of flap dissection is just above the paratenon of the extensor mechanism—the same plane used when elevating a crossfinger flap (next page, *left image*). The *right* image shows the thumb after flap advancement and final closure.

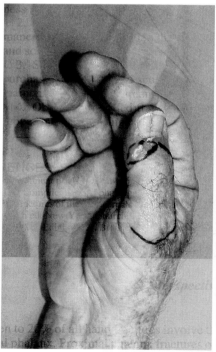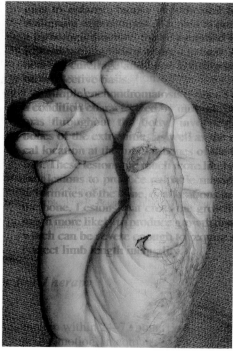

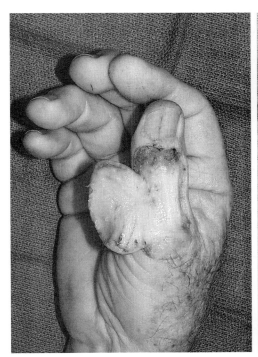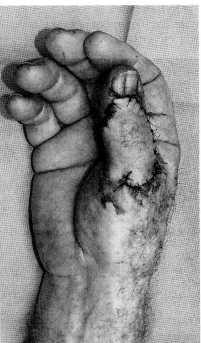

Clinical Pearls

1. Resection of the cyst typically allows resolution of the nail deformity, which exists as a secondary lesion.

2. Resection of the underlying osteophyte is mandatory in the surgical treatment of these lesions, or the recurrence rate will be much higher.

3. The attenuated skin typically found over these cysts requires planning for a dorsal rotation flap (or other arrangement for skin coverage), to be placed during resection.

4. Take care to avoid injury to the insertion of the distal extensor tendon, or a mallet finger deformity may result.

REFERENCES

1. Brown RE, Zook EG, Russell RC, et al: Fingernail deformities secondary to ganglions of the distal interphalangeal joint (mucous cysts). Plast Reconstr Surg 87:718–725, 1991.
2. Fritz GR, Stern PJ, Dickey M: Complications following mucous cyst excision. J Hand Surg [Br] 22:222–225, 1997.
3. Gingrass MK, Brown RE, Zook EG: Treatment of fingernail deformities secondary to ganglions of the distal interphalangeal joint. J Hand Surg 20:502–505, 1995.
4. Kasdan ML, Stallings SP, Leis VM, Wolens D: Outcome of surgically treated mucous cysts of the hand. J Hand Surg 19:504–507, 1994.

Perspectives For Therapy

Postoperative management of a patient having undergone excision of a mucous cyst, with placement of skin coverage (in this case, a dorsal rotation flap), requires that minimal tension be placed on healing tissues. Mechanical stress fosters prolonged inflammation, which, in turn, heralds fibroblast recruitment and collagen synthesis. The end result is hypertrophic scar formation. Whereas hypertrophic scar formation in the region of the proximal nailfold may not be functionally debilitating, it may be cosmetically unfavorable to the patient.

The patient should be encouraged to maintain mobility of the uninvolved hand joints immediately after surgery. Active motion of the index finger DIP joint can usually be initiated at 3 weeks postoperatively. When resuming active motion for the involved joint, it is important to ensure that the patient achieves full, active DIP extension secondary to the proximity of the surgical site to the terminal extensor tendon.

This patient will benefit from scar massage, to help mobilize the proximal nail fold and adjacent skin, and from scar compression supplied by a silicone digital gel pad or finger cap. These appliances offer a number of advantages: they are flexible, reasonably unobtrusive, simple to use, and easy to keep clean. The pad or cap is recommended for use at bedtime, or when the patient is not actively using his or her operated hand; it is placed in contact with the proximal nailfold clearing the DIP joint flexion crease.

Educate the patient that after surgery, which is a planned injury, the rate of nail growth slows. It may take up to 1 year, or even longer, for the nailplate to regain its normal appearance.

Hand Therapy Pearls

1. The risk of hypertrophic scar formation can be minimized by limiting tension on healing wounds.

2. Pay attention to achieving full DIP joint extension of the operated finger.

3. Circumferential silicone gel pads or caps provide an effective means of scar compression.

4. Educate the patient regarding the physiology of nail growth—it can take up to 1 year, or more, to regain a normal-appearing nailplate following surgery.

REFERENCES

1. Repair of skin wounds. In Peacock EE, Van Winkle W: Wound Repair. Philadelphia, WB Saunders, 1976, pp 237–240.
2. Zook EG. Understanding the perionychium. J Hand Ther 13:269–275, 2000.

PATIENT 33

A 45-year-old man with wrist and finger limitations after a humerus fracture

A 45-year-old man fell while working at a construction site 3 months ago and fractured his left humerus. The injury was treated with cast immobilization after reduction by his orthopedic surgeon. Following removal of the cast, the patient was unable to perform certain activities with that hand. He also complains of numbness in areas of his hand and forearm. He is referred to you for diagnosis and treatment. There were no other injuries other than the arm fracture.

Physical Examination: Musculoskeletal: not tender over upper arm (site of humerus fracture); strong finger and wrist flexion, as well as elbow flexion and extension; strong pronation, but weak supination of forearm. Patient is unable to actively extend fingers without assistance, but if he holds his MCP joints in flexion, he can actively extend his middle and distal phalanges. He cannot actively extend his thumb. He cannot extend his wrist. Neurologic: anesthetic at dorsal-radial aspect of hand.

Laboratory Findings: Radiograph (obtained at time of injury): see figure.

Questions: What is your diagnosis? What is the suggested treatment?

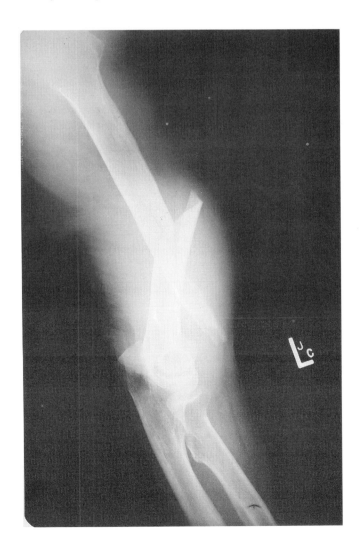

Answers: Proximal radial nerve injury. Recommend radial nerve exploration and possible repair.

Discussion: As many as 18% of patients with humerus fractures have an associated radial nerve palsy—most commonly when the fracture occurs on the middle third of the bone. The nerve can be lacerated (usually in association with a distal spiral humerus fracture), or entrapped at the fracture site. Typically, the nerve injury is incomplete (neuropraxia) and will spontaneously recover.

The radial nerve innervates the musculature that extends the wrist and fingers, and also provides sensation to the dorsal-radial aspect of the hand (see figure, *arrow*). In this patient, extension of the PIP and DIP joints of the fingers (when the MCP joints were held in flexion) was accomplished via the ulnar nerve–innervated hand intrinsic musculature.

If the original injury was a closed humerus fracture, radial nerve function returns within 3–4 months in nearly 90% of patients. If there has not been a return of function by 3 months, surgical exploration is warranted. Return of function is manifest earliest by return of function of the extensor carpi radialis longus (ECRL; the most proximally innervated of the muscles supplied by this nerve). When this muscle regains activity, the patient is able to extend the wrist with radial deviation. This radial deviation will be observed because of the

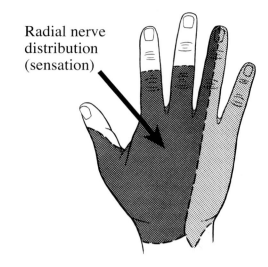

Radial nerve distribution (sensation)

persistent weakness of the extensor carpi ulnaris, which is innervated more distally.

If a patient presents with symptoms of radial nerve injury in the setting of an open humerus fracture, immediate exploration is warranted. Similarly, if the symptoms begin after fracture reduction (perhaps due to impingement within the fracture) immediate exploration is required.

Clinical Pearls

1. Most radial nerve lacerations occur with spiral fractures of the distal third of the humerus.

2. Radial nerve neuropraxia usually occurs with injuries at the junction of the middle and distal third of the humerus: here the nerve is emerging from the spiral groove, and it is tethered as it pierces the intramuscular septum.

3. If no function has returned within 3 months, operative exploration is warranted. If the nerve has been transected, strongly consider tendon transfers to reconstruct wrist, finger, and thumb extensor function.

REFERENCES

1. Amillo S, Barrios H, Martinez-Peric R, Losada JI: Surgical treatment of the radial nerve lesions associated with fractures of the humerus. J Orthop Trauma 7:211–215, 1993.
2. Bostman O, Bakalim G, Vainionpaa S, et al: Immediate radial nerve palsy complicating fracture of the shaft of the humerus: When is early exploration justified? Injury 16:499–502, 1985.
3. Colditz JC: Splinting for radial nerve palsy. J Hand Ther 1:18, 1987.
4. Samardzic M, Grujicic D, Milinkovic ZB: Radial nerve lesions associated with fractures of the humeral shaft. Injury 21:220–222, 1990.

If the clinician suspects a radial nerve lesion, he or she should perform a detailed assessment of the strength of the posterior compartment muscles, including the triceps. This examination, which should proceed distally, will determine the approximate location of the nerve lesion.

Splinting for proximal radial nerve injury should incorporate the wrist in up to 30° extension and in neutral with respect to radial and ulnar deviation. Discontinuation of splinting is usually indicated when the patient is able to achieve motion against gravity, usually in the 3/5 range.

Hand Therapy Pearls

1. In the preferred muscle testing position for pinpointing the ECRL, the patient extends and radially deviates the wrist of interest *with the elbow extended.* The examiner applies resistance to the dorsum of the patient's hand as if to flex and ulnarly deviate the patient's wrist.

2. In the testing position that distinguishes the ECRB from the ECRL, the patient extends and radially deviates the wrist of interest *with the elbow flexed.* The examiner applies resistance to the dorsum of the patient's hand as if to flex and ulnarly deviate the patient's wrist.

REFERENCE
Kendall FP, McCreary EK, Provance PG: Muscles, Testing and Function, 4th ed. Baltimore, Williams and Wilkins, 1993.

PATIENT 34

A 56-year-old woman with ulcerations at her distal fingertips

A 56-year-old woman complains of painful ulcerations at the volar distal aspects of her left ring and right long fingers. There is no history of any drainage or other purulence from the digits. She denies any history of trauma or other injury to her hands. Three weeks ago she had a complete workup and evaluation by her internist and a rheumatologist: both gave her a clean bill of health.

Physical Examination: General: digits somewhat cool to touch; moderately tender, but not exquisitely so. Skin: dried eschars over ulcerations (see figure); erythema around each eschar, but no other evidence of infection; fingernails evidently uninvolved—no pathology at dorsal nails; ulcerations approximately 1–1.5 cm. Upon cold water immersion of hand, skin is initially pale white and then a mottled purplish color; after several minutes, fingers are bright red and flushed.

Questions: What is the diagnosis? What treatment would you recommend?

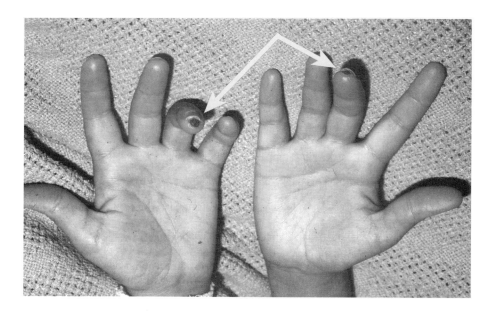

Answers: Raynaud's disease. Treatment options include biofeedback therapy, pharmacologic therapy, and distal digital sympathectomy.

Discussion: This patient exhibits and describes symptoms of chronic ischemia of her fingers. Particularly classic in this disorder is the ulcer formation at the distal fingertips. The patient also demonstrates the classic "Raynaud's phenomenon": blanching of the skin upon exposure to cold, followed by venous congestion, cyanosis, and finally erythema. The color changes of the skin (white, blue, and finally red) mirror the underlying vasoconstriction and reperfusion. Initial attacks are succeeded by an intense hyperemia, and then a gradual return to "normal."

Raynaud's phenomenon is very common in association with connective tissue disorders, such as the collagen diseases, including scleroderma, polyarteritis, rheumatoid arthritis, systemic lupus erythematosus, dermatomyositis, and polymyositis. It is one of the primary symptoms in CREST syndrome, a form of scleroderma. When these symptoms of vasoconstriction and cyanosis are associated with a disease (such as a connective tissue disorder), the term used is Raynaud's *syndrome*. In the absence of an associated autoimmune disease, this process is termed Raynaud's phenomenon or Raynaud's disease. As an idiopathic entity, Raynaud's disease typically causes more morbidity than Raynaud's syndrome.

Whenever the symptoms of Raynaud's phenomenon are encountered, a thorough work-up and search for an underlying cause must be undertaken. The initial work-up should be in collaboration with an internist or rheumatologist to confirm or rule out any associated autoimmune process. Assessment of the arterial anatomy of both hands also is indicated: the gold standard remains angiography. Typically, angiography of the hands demonstrates diffuse narrowing of the digital vessels. Depending on the duration of the disease, collateral vessel formation may be visualized as well. Note that the vascular anatomy should be analyzed over the entire upper extremity to insure that no proximal vascular obstruction contributes to the patient's symptoms.

Severe Raynaud's disease (see figure) results in loss of hand and finger vacularity. Here, the radial artery is completely absent, and the common and proper digital arteries demonstrate diffuse narrowing and even distal loss. This patient experienced necrosis of the thumb secondary to ischemia from this process. The thumb was amputated after demonstrating dry gangrene.

Once the disease process has been confirmed using angiography, the mainstay of treatment is distal digital sympathectomy (as originally advocated by Flatt) to all of the affected digits. If more proximal regions exist at the ulnar or radial arter-

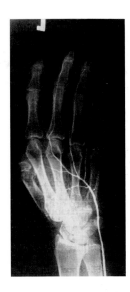

ial levels, vascular reconstruction at that level may be indicated as well. Revision amputation of the digits (if required due to substantial soft tissue loss) should be deferred until healing has occurred after sympathectomy, as the augmentation of blood flow may ameliorate the symptoms making further treatment unnecessary.

Biofeedback training has been shown to be effective in some of these patients, and there have been successful reports of amelioration of symptoms using pharmacologic agents. The most commonly used class of drug for this disorder is the calcium channel blockers, which diminish sympathetically driven vasoconstriction. Other classes of drugs that have been employed include tricyclic antidepressants, serotonin reuptake inhibitors, and sympatholytics.

Pharmacologic Agents Successfully Used To Treat Raynaud's Disease

Calcium channel blockers
  Nifedipine, 10–30 ml tid
  Amlodipine besylate (Norvasc), 5–10 mg qd
Tricyclic antidepressants
  Amitriptyline, 25–75 mg QHS
Serotonin reuptake inhibitors
  Fluoxetine hydrochloride (Prozac), 20 mg qd
  Sertraline (Zoloft), 25–50 mg qd
  Paroxetine (Paxil), 20–50 mg qd
Sympatholytic drugs
  Prazosin hydrochloride, 1–2 mg bid
  Terazosin hydrochloride, 1–2 mg qd
  Clonidine, 0.1 mg bid*

*Also available in transdermal patch

Clinical Pearls

1. The most effective treatment for fingertip ischemia secondary to Raynaud's disease is distal digital sympathectomy.

2. Biofeedback significantly reduces symptoms in patients with adequate circulation (i.e., those who are more symptomatic secondary to vasospasm, rather than fixed thrombosis).

REFERENCES

1. Coffman JD, Davies WT: Vasospastic diseases: A review. Prog Cardiovasc Dis 18:123–146, 1975.
2. Flatt AE: Digital artery sympathectomy. J Hand Surg 5:550–556, 1980.
3. Jones NF: Ischemia of the hand in systemic disease: The potential role of microsurgical revascularization and digital sympathectomy. Clin Plast Surg 16:547–556, 1989.
4. Machleder H: Vaso-occlusive disorders of the upper extremity. Curr Probl Surg 25:1–67, 1988.

Perspectives For Therapy

In the present patient, meticulous care of the volar ulcerations on the patient's ring and long fingers and any postoperative wounds should be prioritized. For example, open wounds can be treated with a minute amount of triple antibiotic ointment, nonadherent interface dressing, dry dressing, and a protective splint made from 1/16-inch thermoplastic.

From the standpoint of hand therapy, conservative and postoperative treatment for Raynaud symptoms primarily involves behavioral modification to reduce symptoms. For example, vibratory occupational trauma should be avoided because vibration induces vasocontriction. This occurs for two reasons; the first is anatomical and the second is physiological. First, vibration causes endothelial cells to proliferate within the digital arteries, which results in luminal narrowing. These structural changes can diminish blood flow. Second, vibration appears to lower the threshold of smooth muscle response to norepinephrine, resulting in vasoconstriction. These mechanisms, occuring alone or in combination, result in arterial obstruction and ischemia.

Abstinence from vasocontrictive compounds such as caffeine and nicotine is mandatory, although compliance may be difficult. Patients should dress for warmth and minimize contact with all forms of cold to retain hand warmth.

Adaptive padding through the use of properly fitted anti-vibration gloves and essential equipment and handles will help protect soft tissues and provide hand warmth.

Hand Therapy Pearls

1. The hand therapist's first line of treatment for the patient with Raynaud's symptoms is behavioral modification.

2. Vibratory stresses, exposure to cold, and vasoconstrictive compounds should be avoided.

3. Wound care consists of antibiotic ointment, nonadherent interfaces, and a dry dressing. Light-weight splints may be used to support the dressings.

REFERENCES

1. Brown AP. The effects of anti-vibration gloves on vibration-induced disorders: A case study. J Hand Ther 3:94–100, 1990.
2. Levin LS, Moore RS. Vascular disorders of the hand: Surgeons' perspective. J Hand Ther 12:152–159, 1999.
3. Melvin JL. Scleroderma (systemic sclerosis): Treatment of the hand. In Hunter JM, Mackin EJ, Callahan AD (eds): Rehabilitation of the Hand: Surgery and Therapy, 4th ed. St. Louis, Mosby, 1995, pp 1385–1397.
4. Talley M. Vascular disorders of the hand: Therapist's commentary. J Hand Ther 12:160–163, 1999.
5. Taras JS, Lemel MS, Nathan R. Vascular disorders of the upper extremity. In Hunter JM, Mackin EJ, Callahan AD (eds): Rehabilitation of the Hand: Surgery and Therapy, 4th ed. St. Louis, Mosby, 1995, pp 959–978.

PATIENT 35

A 70-year-old man with chronic wrist pain

A 70-year-old man complains of right wrist pain of 10-year duration. While the pain is not excruciating, this stoic individual is wondering if there is anything that can be done to relieve it. Upon questioning, he notes that he suffered a significant wrist injury nearly 10 years ago, during a fall while at work. Unfortunately, he never sought medical attention, so there are neither old records nor earlier radiographs to examine. The patient is very active and works as a farmer. He desires to maintain his current level of activity if at all possible.

Physical Examination: Musculoskeletal: wrist flexion and extension limited (25° flexion, 20° extension); wrist diffusely tender with direct pressure—most tender area is at anatomic snuffbox; palpation of scapholunate joint just proximal to 3rd metacarpal is painful. While holding wrist in flexion, active finger extension is painful at dorsal wrist.

Laboratory Findings: Radiograph: see figure.

Question: What is the diagnosis?

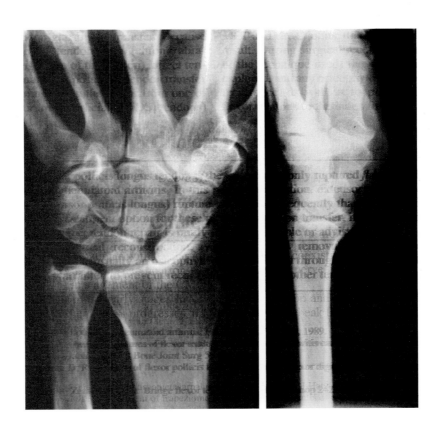

Diagnosis: Scapholunate advanced collapse (SLAC wrist)

Discussion: SLAC wrist refers to a specific pattern of osteoarthritis and subluxation that results from untreated, chronic scapholunate dissociation, or from chronic scaphoid nonunion. The degenerative changes appear most notably in areas of abnormal loading: the radioscaphoid joint is involved earliest, but if left untreated can be followed by degeneration of the capitatolunate joint, as the capitate subluxes dorsally on the lunate. As this process progresses, the midcarpal joint collapses under this compression, and the lunate assumes an extended (dorsiflexed) position. This end-stage SLAC is termed dorsal intercalated segment instability (DISI).

On a lateral radiographic view (see figure below), if the lunate (*outline*) has slipped into an extended (dorsiflexed) position ($> 10°$), it is diagnostic for DISI. Compare this image to the figure at right, in which the lunate is in a normal configuration. The DISI deformity is also present when the scapholunate angle is $> 70°$. When evaluating these x-rays, it is important to ensure that the wrist was not dorsiflexed during the x-ray.

The surgical options depend on the quality of the remaining cartilage of the wrist: if the triangular fibrocartilage complex (TFCC) and proximal capitate have maintained good articular surfaces, a proximal row carpectomy may preserve reasonable (although certainly decreased) wrist motion while relieving pain. Another option for SLAC salvage is four-corner fusion. The most reliable method for pain relief is total wrist fusion, although the decreased function that comes with *no wrist motion* is generally unattractive to patients.

A **proximal row carpectomy** involves resection of the scaphoid, lunate, and triquetrum. The proximal capitate then is seated within the lunate fossa at the TFCC and becomes the major hinge point for motion at the wrist. Significant cartilage loss of either the proximal articular surface of the capitate or of the TFCC (where the capitate will seat) is a contraindication to proceeding with this surgical procedure. One advantage of the proximal row carpectomy is that it is relatively easy to perform, and often allows better preservation of strength and motion as compared to limited carpal arthrodesis. Patients can expect 33–75% of their normal range of motion (ROM) compared to their opposite wrist (total arc) and 50–90% of their normal grip strength.

If there is significant capitolunate arthrosis, a limited carpal fusion (**four-corner fusion**) may be an option. This involves preservation of the radiolunate joint and stabilization of the midcarpal row; it is usually combined with scaphoid excision to address the radioscaphoid arthrosis. With this option, patients may expect up to 75% of retained grip strength, but $< 50\%$ of wrist ROM will be retained. In addition, approximately 30% of patients will experience persistent pain after this procedure. Regarding ROM and strength after these limited-fusion options, it is worthwhile to keep the following in mind: all other things being equal (patient motivation, surgeon's skills, hand therapist's skills, etc.), ROM and grip strength outcomes will depend upon the type/severity of the original injury, time interval to surgery, and reinjury prior to definitive management.

A final option for the relief of pain is **total wrist fusion**. While this can be very satisfactory in regards to pain relief, the loss of wrist mobility often is very troubling, and its effect on the patient's lifestyle should be strongly considered prior to proceeding.

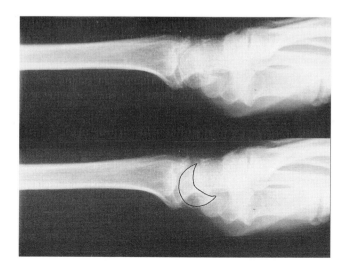

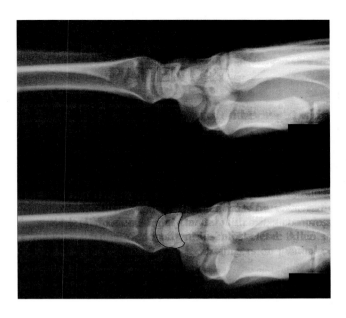

Clinical Pearls

1. The radioscaphoid is usually the first location to develop degenerative changes visible on x-ray. With advanced disease, the capitate will migrate proximally, and the lunate will begin to assume a characteristic dorsiflexed position on lateral x-ray views.

2. When evaluating for dorsal angulation of the lunate, ensure that the x-ray is a true lateral (i.e., not rotated) and that the wrist is not extended, to get accurate visualization of the lunate position.

3. The DISI deformity is the result of end-stage scapholunate advanced collapse. It most often arises from previous scaphoid fracture, scapholunate dissociation, or trans-scaphoid perilunate dislocation.

REFERENCES

1. Culp RW, McGuigan FX, Turner MA, et al: Proximal row carpectomy: A multicenter study. J Hand Surg 18:19–25, 1993.
2. Imbriglia JE, Broudy AS, Hagberg WC, McKernan D: Proximal row carpectomy: Clinical evaluation. J Hand Surg 15:426–430, 1990.
3. Tomaino MM, Delsignore J, Burton RI: Long-term results following proximal row carpectomy. J Hand Surg 19:694–703, 1994.
4. Wyrick JD, Stern PJ, Kiefhaber TR: Motion-preserving procedures in the treatment of scapholunate advanced collapse wrist: Proximal row carpectomy versus four-corner arthrodesis. J Hand Surg 20:965–970, 1995.

Perspectives For Therapy

Active motion of the digits and thumb can begin immediately, with strict elevation of the operated extremity above the level of the patient's heart. Patients are typically taken out of their postoperative dressing at 10–14 days for a wound check, and then returned to a short arm cast. The hand therapist may follow-up with the patient once per week or more regularly, depending upon the patient's ability to perform composite digital flexion and extension within the confines of the cast.

At 4–6 weeks postoperatively, the cast is discontinued and the patient is returned to a custom-fabricated, volar, forearm-based wrist support splint. Scar management should now be initiated, in addition to active wrist and forearm ROM exercise, and the patient continues to rely on the splint between exercise sessions. Depending on the hand surgeons's confidence regarding the strength of the dorsal capsular repair and wound condition, the patient may be returned to a custom splint and started on active wrist and forearm exercises as early as 2–4 weeks postoperatively.

The patient should be weaned from the wrist support splint at 6–8 weeks postoperatively, and progressive, resisted strengthening exercises may be initiated. It is anticipated that the patient will return to work on a light duty basis at this time, also. Most patients will return to full-time work with modified duty 12–24 weeks postoperatively.

Proximal row carpectomy (PRC) is a surgical procedure that places maximal adaptive demands, both structural and functional, on the patient's musculotendinous system, because it results in significantly altered wrist structure and mechanics. From the standpoint of outcomes following surgery and therapy, patients should be educated that they may not achieve maximum strength or motion for up to 1 year postoperatively. It is also important for the hand therapist to appreciate the significant mismatch that results between the lengths of the extrinsic wrist and hand musculature and carpal height, secondary to PRC. This mismatch contributes to decreased wrist and finger excursion, and reduction in grip strength, for several reasons.

Effect of PRC on wrist and finger excursion:
- There is decreased total motion available at the carpus because there are fewer articulating elements available to participate.
- The multiarticular muscles ECRL/B, ECU, FCR/U, FDP/S, and FPL are relatively length-ened by PRC. The active elements of skeletal muscle—sarcomeres—have some capacity to adjust to the "slack" position of their respective whole muscles. However, the potential mismatch between muscle length and carpal height represents a form of active insufficiency in skeletal muscle, and it results in decreased motion.
- The distal edge of the redundant dorsal capsule of the wrist is advanced during PRC to effect a secure repair, and this may contribute to decreased wrist flexion.
- Scar adherence may limit gliding of the wrist extensor tendons, and this may result in decreased wrist excursion.

Effect of PRC on grip strength:
- Extrinsic wrist and hand muscles will contribute a fraction of the tension they normally develop simply to "reel in" or reset the lengths of their respective whole muscles, leaving reduced tension fraction available for functional grip.
- The normal synergistic relationship among the extrinsic wrist extensors (ECRL/B and ECU) permits the extrinsic finger/thumb flexors (FDP/S and FPL) to produce peak tension near, or at, the resting lengths of the whole muscles, and this results in a strong, functional grasp. There is less wrist extension available following PRC; thus, the FDP/S and FPL are constrained to develop force along the *ascending* limbs of their length-tension curves, resulting in diminished peak tension and translating directly into decreased grip strength.

Hand Therapy Pearl

The hand therapist must fully appreciate the anatomical and biomechanical consequences of PRC, and educate the patient with regard to ROM and grip strength outcomes.

REFERENCES
1. Degnan GC, Lichtman DM. Soft tissue arthroplasty about the wrist. In Lichtman DM (ed): The Wrist and its Disorders. Philadelphia, WB Saunders, 1997, pp 609–615.
2. Jebson PJL, Engber WD. Proximal row carpectomy. Tech Hand Upper Extremity Surg 3:32–36, 1999.
3. Proximal row carpectomy. In Cannon NM (ed): Diagnosis and Treatment Manual for Physicians and Therapists 3rd ed. Indianapolis, Hand Rehabilitation Center of Indianapolis, 1991, pp 221–222.
4. Van Heest AE, House JH. Proximal row carpectomy. In Gelberman RH (ed): Master Techniques in Orthopaedic Surgery, The Wrist. New York, Raven, 1994, pp 331–344.

PATIENT 36

A 20-year-old man with a snakebite

While hiking on a vacation in Colorado, you notice a young man surrounded by several very anxious people. Evidently he had bent over to tie his shoes while on a scenic wooded trail, and suddenly felt a sharp pain at his left distal forearm: a snake had bitten him. He cannot recall any specific details about the snake itself. He thinks it was brown, and does recall hearing a rattling sound that he originally did not think was a snake. He does not know how big it was. He has no other medical problems. You observe fresh fang marks on his distal forearm approximately 3 cm apart. He reports a metallic taste in his mouth, and he feels nauseated. His brother has placed his belt as a tourniquet on the proximal arm at the level of the biceps. You contact the emergency medical service via your cell phone and volunteer to ride back with him to the clinic.

Physical Examination: Skin: no active bleeding; erythema surrounds fang marks; mild swelling. Neurologic: distal sensation intact. Musculoskeletal: good range of motion; active, full extension and flexion of fingers and wrist.

Questions: What treatment options did you initiate in the field? What treatment do you recommend at the medical clinic?

Answers: Early treatment—removal of the tourniquet, facilitation of transport to a medical facility, and support of airway, breathing, and circulation, if required. Later management—continued support, hydration, and possible administration of antivenom.

Discussion: Pit viper snakebites are the most common poisonous snakebites in the United States. Approximately 65% of all venomous snakebites are caused by rattlesnakes, 25% by copperheads, and 10% by cottonmouths. In many bites (up to 50%) there may be no envenomation.

Patients will complain of pain and swelling at the bite site. They may experience nausea, vomiting, and dizziness, and there is often a complaint of taste changes ("metallic taste"). Fang marks are typically evident on physical examination. The distance between the puncture sites can be used to estimate the size of the snake: a larger snake is more likely to have envenomated the victim. Other signs on physical exam are erythema and edema (very common). Bruising, blister formation, and bleeding from the puncture sites may also be observed. Systemically, the patient may demonstrate muscular fasciculations as well as circulatory changes (either hypotension or hypertension).

Rattlesnake venom produces a coagulopathy, although it is rarely associated with clinically significant hemorrhage or bleeding. It is characterized by a benign defibrination (low serum fibrinogen, elevated fibrin split products) and a venom-induced thrombocytopenia. The prothrombin time may be elevated; laboratory derangements are usually not evident for 2–3 days.

Laboratory tests should include CBC with platelet count, prothrombin time and partial thromboplastin time, fibrinogen and fibrin split products, type and cross, urinalysis, electrolytes, and CPK. Rhabdomyolysis may occur, and can lead to renal failure secondary to myoglobinuria. CPK and urinalysis may be helpful to identify patients at risk for rhabdomyolysis and guide further treatment (such as alkalinization of the urine to prevent myoglobin precipitation).

In the pre-hospital setting, it may be helpful to mark the level of erythema directly on the arm, to gauge progression. Studies have shown that venom extraction devices are of no benefit to the patient, and actually could result in additional injury. Creating an incision across the fang marks and/or providing mouth suction are contraindicated. Tourniquets are not recommended: while they definitely can restrict lymphatic spread, no clear improvement in outcome has been shown. In addition, the restriction of spread of the venom may increase the local tissue damage. Other early (field) maneuvers or treatments to avoid include topical alcohol, placing ice packs on the wound, or administration of antivenom.

Hospital care initially involves aggressive hydration for circulatory support; vasopressor support may be required in severe cases. Patients with evidence of bleeding/hemorrhage, significant necrosis, compartment syndrome, rhabdomyolysis (possible renal failure), or evidence of other system failure (such as respiratory failure) require administration of antivenom.

Quite commonly, the hand surgeon only meets the snakebite victim after all supportive measures have been taken, in order to assess for possible fasciotomy. In reality, compartment syndrome is rare in these injuries, because most bites remain at the subcutaneous level. Nevertheless, the edema of the soft tissue can be quite severe and dramatic in appearance, and compartment pressures in these patients should be closely monitored to prevent late Volkman's contracture.

Clinical Pearls

1. Tourniquets or venom extraction devices are not indicated in the acute treatment of snakebites. The most important first-aid maneuver is facilitating the patient's transfer to a healthcare facility.

2. The application of ice or ice packs to a snakebite will actually increase the local necrotic effect of the venom, and should be avoided.

3. If there is enough soft tissue swelling (on occasion, the edema is massive), the patient may benefit from skin release (dermotomy)—even in the absence of compartment syndrome. Local tissue necrosis (typically the entrance points of the fangs) can be debrided during this procedure.

REFERENCES

1. Bush SP, Hegewald KG, Green SM, et al: Effects of a negative pressure venom extraction device (Extractor) on local tissue injury after artificial rattlesnake envenomation in a porcine model. Wilderness Environ Med 11:180–188, 2000.
2. Hurlbut KM, Dart RC, Spaite D, McNally J: Reliability of clinical presentation for predicting significant pit viper envenomation. Ann Emerg Med 17:438–439, 1988.
3. Sullivan Jr JB, Wingert WA, Norris Jr RL: North American venomous reptile bites. In Aurbach PS (ed): Wilderness Medicine: Management of Wilderness and Environmental Emergencies, 3rd ed. St. Louis, Mosby, 1995, pp 680–709.
4. Wingert WA, Chan L: Rattlesnakebites in southern California and rationale for recommended treatment. West J Med 148:37–44, 1988.

PATIENT 37

An infant boy with conjoined fingers

A 9-month-old boy is brought into your office by his parents. They are concerned about his congenital hand deformity and are quite anxious, particularly in regards to treatment options and possible surgical risks. They are also curious as to the risk of this deformity occurring in subsequent children (they are currently pregnant with their second child). The mother wants to know if she should obtain amniocentesis for her current pregnancy. There is no family history of any other congenital hand problems, or other congenital defects. The patient's medical records, forwarded by his pediatrician, indicate that he is otherwise completely healthy, with no cardiac, pulmonary, or central nervous system congenital defects.

Physical Examination: General: happy, healthy. Musculoskeletal: can grasp and manipulate objects with both hands without problems; left ring and long fingers are attached to each other by soft tissue along entire length (see figure, *left*); excellent (full) range of motion of the MCP, PIP, and DIP joints of these fingers. Other than the cutaneous connection, they appear normally formed.

Laboratory Findings: Radiograph: see figure, *right*.

Questions: What is the diagnosis? What is your recommended treatment?

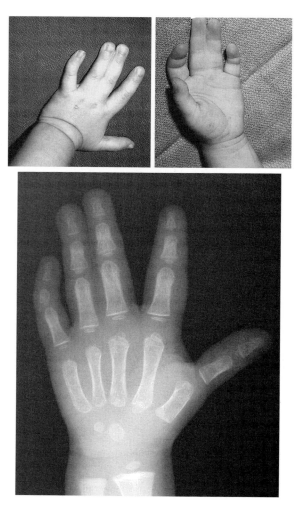

Answers: Complete simple syndactyly. Surgical separation of the affected digits is the accepted treatment.

Discussion: Syndactyly is one of the most common congenital hand deformities. It can be classified and characterized based on the degree of soft tissue and bony involvement between the affected digits. When the digits are connected by skin and soft tissue along their entire length, it is termed a **complete syndactyly**. If there is only a partial connection along the length, it is termed an **incomplete syndactyly** (see figure; *top* is incomplete toe syndactyly, *bottom* is complete).

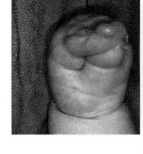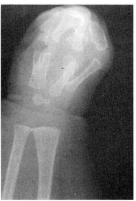

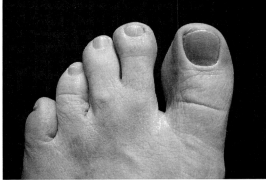

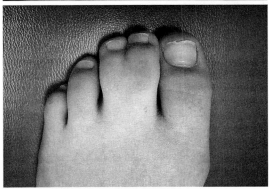

If the adjacent bony phalanges are connected, it is termed a **complex syndactyly**. Children with Apert's syndrome typically present with severe complex syndactyly of *all* of their digits; this is known as "mitten hand" deformity (see figure, *upper right*). If there is no bony involvement, the disorder is termed **simple syndactyly**. The surgeon is much more likely to encounter altered anatomy of the neurovascular bundles, as well as rudimentary or vestigial structures, in cases of complex syndactyly.

Syndactyly occurs in the general population with a frequency of approximately 1/2000 births. Nearly 80% of all isolated cases (i.e., not associated with another congenital syndrome) occur sporadically, with approximately one-fifth passed as a familial trait. In the latter situation, it is usually passed as an autosomal dominant gene. Syndactyly is also a component of the following congenital syndromes: Apert's syndrome (as mentioned above), Poland syndrome, Jarcho-Levin syndrome, oral-facial-digital syndrome, Pfeiffer syndrome, and Edwards syndrome. Less frequently, it may be associated with Gordon syndrome, Fraser syndrome, Greig cephalopolysyndactyly, phenylketonuria, Saethre-Chotzen syndrome, Russell-Silver syndrome, and triploidy.

Surgical separation of the digits can be performed when the child is 12–24 months old. Timing of the surgical release is related to several factors, one of which is that correction is easier when when the child is older and the fingers are larger. Typically there is no advantage to releasing the syndactyly in an early infant. However, if it begins to impact on the growth of one of the conjoined digits, surgical separation should not be further delayed. The most common example of this is in syndactyly of the ring and 5th fingers: since the 5th is significantly shorter than the ring, the ring finger may be pulled ulnarly by the tethering effect of the soft tissue of the 5th finger. Overall, the optimal timing of surgical correction remains controversial, with no clear advantage except perhaps surgeon preference.

There are a myriad surgical techniques for the syndactyly release, but most of these methods share two common elements: careful creation of skin flaps to maximize efficient use of the available skin, and full-thickness skin grafts to provide additional coverage. As in most cases of pediatric hand surgery, the child needs to be immobilized in an above-elbow cast postoperatively to protect the repair and prevent escape. The elbow should be flexed slightly more than 90°. Note that during cast manufacture, it is imperative that the elbow *already* be in the flexed position. If a dressing and cast padding is placed circumferentially on the child's arm in extension, and *then* the arm is flexed for plaster placement, significant pressure and compression may be placed at the antecubital fossa, potentially compromising tissue viability and perhaps even distal circulation.

The present patient appeared to be affected by sporadic syndactyly (as opposed to familial transmission). The parents were informed that the risk to subsequent siblings would be the same as to the general population: approximately 1/2000. Amniocentesis would not be of assistance in prenatal diagnosis, and was not recommended. Surgical release was performed at 16 months of age, and the boy was doing fine 1 year postoperatively (see figure).

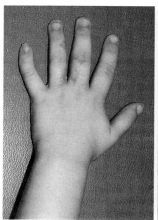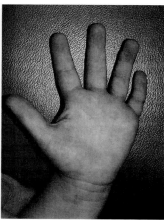

Clinical Pearls

1. The incidence of syndactyly in the general population is 1 per 2000 births; the majority of these cases occur sporadically.

2. Syndactyly is the most common congenital hand anomaly; the second most common is polydactyly.

3. The timing of surgical release is controversial. The majority of hand surgeons would agree that release at 12–24 months of age is appropriate (assuming there are no other indications for surgery, such as development of a rotational or lateral deviation deformity).

REFERENCES

1. Dobyns JH, Wood VE, Bayne LG: Congenital Hand Deformities. In Green DP, Hotchkiss R, Pederson WC (eds): Green's Operative Hand Surgery, 4th ed. New York, Churchill Livingstone, 1999.
2. Eaton CJ, Lister GD: Syndactyly. Hand Clin 6:555–575, 1990.
3. Flatt AE: The Care of Congenital Hand Anomalies. St. Louis, CV Mosby, 1977.

Perspectives For Therapy

Normally, the fingers are individuated during the seventh week of gestation as two companion processes occur. First, the developing limb bud, including the hand, grows in length in a proximal-to-distal direction. Second, at discrete regions in the developing hand, mesenchymal and ectodermal cells undergo programmed death in a distal-to-proximal direction. As a result of these companion processes, the fingers and thumb grow in length, and they normally become separated by four distinct incisions.

Syndactyly results from the failure of ectodermal and mesenchymal tissues to undergo programmed breakdown. The degree of tissue connection, both in terms of its completeness and complexity, provides an indication of which tissues had abnormal development.

Surgical release involves the creation of individuated fingers and thumb, if involved, by separating the joined structures. Surgical treatment improves hand function and appearance, and contributes to normal digit growth.

Some degree of skin grafting is performed by the hand surgeon; thus, postoperative hand rehabilitation emphasizes wound care and scar management. Static splinting, to maintain surgically created webspaces, can be accomplished by using elastomer inserts galvanized to the splint-base. These inserts passively abduct the released digits and also offer scar compression. Overly vigorous soft-tissue compression, with concommitant vas-

cular compromise, is to be avoided. Splints must be large enough to offer support, yet they should never block motion of uninvolved joints. Splint fit must be revised as hand growth dictates.

Cohesive dressings or well-placed straps are advisable for maintaining splint position, and the splint is worn at all times, except during exercise and hygiene activities, for up to 9 weeks. "Exercise" includes feeding, developmentally appropriate play, and motor tasks that challenge the use of the individuated digits. By increasing exercise duration, the child is gradually weaned from the splint while at the same time encouraged to use the operated hand. Bedtime splint use for up to 1 year is advisable and will contribute to scar management. Again, splint revisions to accommodate changes in hand size and shape are mandatory.

Hand Therapy Pearls

1. As in any pediatric hand condition, active parental involvement is the key to the child's functional use and acceptance of the operated hand.

2. Uneventful wound care is paramount following surgical release of connected digits; there will often be extensive soft-tissue revision as the surgical team takes advantage of available skin and uses skin grafts to provide additional coverage.

3. Hand splinting to maintain webspaces, scar management, and therapeutic exercise—all matched to the developmental status of the child—play an important role in postoperative rehabilitation.

REFERENCES

1. Development of mesodermal organs in vertebrates. In Balinsky BI: An Introduction to Embryology, 3rd ed. Philadelphia, WB Saunders, 1970, pp 438–439.
2. Fuller M: Treatment of congenital differences of the upper extremity: Therapist's commentary. J Hand Ther 12:174–177, 1999.
3. Lourie GM: Treatment of congenital differences of the upper extremity: Surgeon's perspective. J Hand Ther 12:164–173, 1999.

PATIENT 38

A 9-month-old child who doesn't extend his left thumb

Your neighborhood pediatrician has sent over a 9-month-old patient of hers for evaluation. The parents are concerned because the child does not use his left thumb. The thumb stays within the palm, and it is even difficult to extend the finger passively. This is their first child, and they report that the pregnancy and postpartum course have been uneventful. The family history is unremarkable except that the father did have a syndactyly repair of his ring and long fingers as a child: he has had no other problems with his hands since that time.

Physical Examination: General: patient developmentally appropriate, sitting up without assistance and using hands to pick up and manipulate both large and small objects. Musculoskeletal: evenly developed on both arms, with no evidence of atrophy or nonuse; full active extension and flexion of right thumb; left thumb remains within palm during these activities; passive extension of left thumb only partial; pea-sized, nontender mass palpated over volar MCP joint of thumb (see figure, *arrow*).

Laboratory Findings: Radiograph: normal, and demonstrate normal ossification for patient's age.

Questions: What is your diagnosis? What treatment options do you recommend?

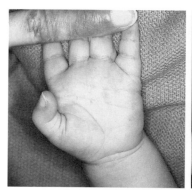 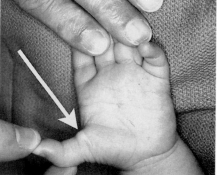

Answers: Congenital trigger thumb. Recommend surgery if not resolved by 12 months of age.

Discussion: In contrast to trigger fingers in adults, congenital triggering is most common at the thumb. The underlying pathologic process remains the same: a nodular swelling of the flexor tendon blocks gliding under the A1 pulley of the involved digit. In children, this stenosing tenosynovitis is present at birth, although the diagnosis is typically not made until the child is around 6 months old. It is not uncommon for this disorder to present bilaterally. Nearly one-third of those cases that are present at birth spontaneously resolve by the time the child is 1 year old. If it does not resolve spontaneously, surgical division of the A1 pulley is indicated, because the condition could develop into a persistent flexion contracture.

The swelling of the tendon that causes the obstruction at the pulley (often palpable, as in this child) is termed "Notta's node." This can be palpated, and its movement appreciated with thumb flexion and extension.

Surgical release is relatively straightforward, with the proximal constriction of the A1 pulley divided under direct vision (with the child under a general anesthetic). The incision is made transversely at the level of the volar MCP joint (a longitudinal incision is not indicated across a flexor surface). The largest risk is injury to the digital nerves, which lay relatively superficially and close to the tendon sheath. Some authors have proposed performing a reduction tenotomy of the tendon nodule, but this is not necessary and merely adds further risk to the procedure. The tendon swelling will resolve spontaneously after division of the pulley.

The differential diagnosis for patients presenting with a thumb deformity such as this should include clasped thumb. The underlying cause of the clasped thumb deformity typically involves hypoplasia or absence of the extensor pollicis brevis, and occasionally the extensor pollicis longus.

Clinical Pearls

1. The palpable swelling of the involved tendon is termed "Notta's node." On physical examination this can be appreciated to move with gentle extension and flexion of the distal phalanx of the thumb.

2. The diagnosis of clasped thumb (hypoplasia or absence of the thumb extensors) needs to be considered when evaluating infants with this thumb position: the presence of Notta's node can confirm the diagnosis of trigger thumb.

3. In infants, one-third of cases of trigger thumb resolve spontaneously by the time they are 1 year old. If it has not resolved by then, surgical release should be strongly considered to prevent permanent flexion contracture.

REFERENCES
1. Flatt AE: The Care of Congenital Hand Anomolies, 2nd ed. St. Louis, Quality Medical Publishing, Inc, 1994, pp 89–95.
2. Ger E, Kupcha P, Ger D: The management of trigger thumb in children. J Hand Surg 16:944–947, 1991.
3. Steenwerckx A, De Smet L, Fabry G: Congenital trigger digit. J Hand Surg 21:909–911, 1996.

Perspectives For Therapy

Postoperative treatment of the pediatric patient with release of a congenital trigger thumb may include fabrication of a custom splint, worn at bedtime, to maintain composite MCP and IP extension. A well-padded, volar, forearm-based splint with a volar gutter that conforms to the thumb is fabricated from 1/16-inch or 3/32-inch material. The splint is secured to the patient's extremity with Coban, and the parents are instructed in splint application/removal and skin precautions. Depending upon the age of the patient, the splint can be molded in an Isolet.

At home, hand exploration/play, locomotion, and self-feeding are encouraged during waking hours. Functional activities that encourage the manipulation of a variety of different-sized objects will provide the infant ample opportunities to explore the environment while emphasizing composite MCP and IP extension and radial digital grasp using the operated thumb in opposition.

Depending upon the age of the patient when the FPL tendon is released, structured hand therapy may be indicated in a clinic setting. This is true particularly if the patient was older at surgery, between the ages of 9 months and 3 years; was required to make prolonged compensatory use of more proximal hand joints during interval observation; and experienced an extended period of thumb IP joint flexion posturing. Accordingly, static splinting may also be indicated for a longer duration of time, with the goal to discontinue splint use once the child can achieve and sustain active MCP and IP extension and thumb opposition in a consistent manner that is task-appropriate.

The use of absorbable sutures will make wound care largely a matter of observation. Scar massage may be indicated to manage the surgical site and also to help mobilize first webspace soft tissues.

REFERENCES

1. Case-Smith J. Grasp, release, and bimanual skills in the first two years of life. In Henderson A, Pehoski C (eds): Hand Function in the Child: Foundations for Remediation. St. Louis, Mosby 1995, pp 113–135.
2. Dobyns JH. Management of congenital hand anomalies. In Hunter JM, Mackin EJ, Callahan AD (eds): Rehabilitation of the Hand: Surgery and Therapy, 4th ed. St. Louis, Mosby, 1995, pp 1425–1442.
3. Ger E, Kupcha P, Ger D. The management of trigger thumb in children. J Hand Surg 16A:944–947, 1991.

PATIENT 39

A 27-year-old man with an amputated finger

A 27-year-old carpenter suffered an acute amputation of his right index finger while working with a circular saw. He is right-handed, and is a nonsmoker. He has no other hand injuries, and no other medical problems.

Physical Examination: Index finger completely amputated at mid-proximal phalanx level. No active bleeding. Digital vessels visible at base of wound, in vasospasm (see figure).

Laboratory Findings: Radiographs: No other bony injury revealed.

Question: What is the best treatment option?

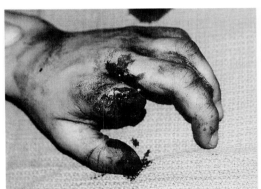 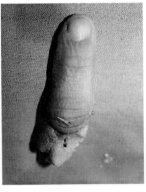

Answer: Ray amputation.

Discussion: There are no absolute "right or wrong" answers when dealing with issues such as when to perform replantation. There are several *relative* indications and contraindications for and against finger replantation. Therefore, prior to embarking on a lengthy operative procedure and even lengthier rehabilitation process, it is important to carefully evaluate each patient, discuss the treatment options and goals with him or her, and decide on an appropriate treatment course. The individual situation and details of injury must be carefully considered.

When microsurgery and finger replantation were in their infancy, early evaluation of success centered on **biologic survival:** as long as the finger was *alive,* the operation was considered a success. Replanted fingers with poor mobility and/or poor sensation (often negatively impacting adjacent, uninjured fingers) prompted a closer look at the goals and indications for replantation. Several general situations have been identified in which it is *usually* beneficial to the patient to proceed with replantation; situations in which it is not beneficial have also been determined. Note that these are only general criteria—each case must be carefully considered in the context of the patient in total.

The relative indications for replantation are:

1. Injury in a child. Children often have very good recovery of function after replantation, much more so than would be expected in an adult with an amputation at the same level. Recovery of even very proximal injuries (such as arm amputation), in which meaningful motor reinnervation is much less likely in an adult, can be remarkable in a child (see figure *A;* this child regained forearm, wrist, and even some independent finger flexion and extension after arm replantation at the mid-humerus level).

2. Injuries within zone 1 (*distal* to the insertion of the FDS tendon). Since these injuries lie distal to the fibro-osseous tunnel, replantations are not as prone to troubling adhesions between the FDS and FDP tendons, and postoperative stiffness of the finger is not as much of a problem as in replantations within "no-man's land" (zone 2).

3. Amputation at the level of the midpalm (metacarpal level). Similar to those injuries at zone 1 (distal to the insertion of the FDS tendon), amputations at this level are not troubled with tendon adhesions nearly as much as those in zone 2.

4. Multiple finger amputations. Hand function is greatly impacted by the loss of multiple digits. Therefore, attempted replantation may be advisable (see figure *B;* this individual has both a relative indication for replantation [multiple digits] as well as a contraindication [level at zone 2]).

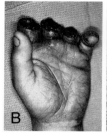
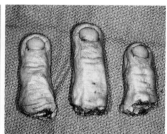

5. Amputations of the thumb (see figure C). The thumb contributes so much to the overall function of the hand, and its loss is therefore so devastating, that every effort should be made to salvage it if at all possible. In addition, even if there is some amount of stiffness of the replanted thumb, it will not impact the other fingers negatively (in contrast to a stiff index finger, which may impede motion of the adjacent long finger).

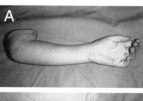
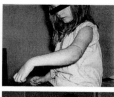
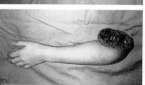
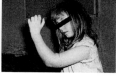
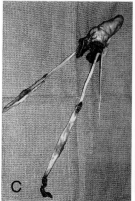
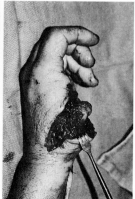

The relative contraindications for replantation are:

1. Single digit amputation within zone 2 (at the level of the fibro-osseous tunnel, see figure previous page). These digits are very prone to developing scarring between the tendons and the bone within the fibro-osseous tunnel ("no-man's land"). The resultant stiff finger will actually limit mobility of the adjacent digits (through interconnections such as the junctura tendinae, or common muscle origins such as the FDP). The end result is a hand that is *less functional* than one with a simple revision amputation.

2. Multiple levels of injury on the same digit. Fingers that have been cut at several levels are destined to have poor recovery of sensation and much stiffness.

3. Avulsion/crush injuries (refer back to figure C). An avulsive mechanism of injury severely damages the arterial structure, in particular its intimal layer. If the damaged section of the artery is not resected and replaced with a vein graft (even with successful microvascular anastomosis), the artery is destined to thrombose. The area of arterial damage often extends significantly beyond the level of the amputation itself, and defining injury-free vessels distal to the level of the amputation is often the most difficult part of this procedure (and often not possible).

4. Amputations in patients with other serious injuries or diseases. Medical issues such as heart or pulmonary disease may make a lengthy operative procedure too risky to undertake. Smokers have an increased risk of replantation failure due to their propensity for profound postoperative vasospasm at the replanted digital artery level.

5. Prolonged warm ischemia. This depends on the level of the amputation. Digits are composed of tissue that is relatively resistant to ischemia (bone, tendon, skin) and therefore are more tolerant of longer periods of ischemia than amputated parts with significant skeletal muscle (such as hand or proximal forearm amputation). The ischemia is better tolerated if the part is properly stored (see discussion below).

6. Mentally unstable patients. The postoperative course for replantation patients requires extensive therapy; patients need to be able to commit to a lengthy and often painful process of rehabilitation or very poor results are nearly guaranteed. Mentally unstable patients are unlikely to be able to protect the digit in the early postoperative period, nor commit to the extensive rehabilitation required.

7. Arteriosclerotic vessels. Although not nearly as common in the upper extremity as the lower extremity, if the vessels have significant atherosclerotic disease, prospects of successful replantation are significantly diminished.

Very rarely will an individual present with a clear indication or contraindication in regards to replantation: usually there are one or two indications and/or contraindications. The patient needs to be informed of the risks and benefits of either replantation or revision amputation. He or she looks to the surgeon for guidance as to the best course to take. A desire to surgically correct traumatic injury needs to be tempered with a realistic eye toward projected outcome for the patient.

Storage of the amputated part is an important component of the care of these patients until the decision for surgery has been made. The amputated part should be wrapped in saline-soaked gauze, and then placed in a watertight container (a urine specimen cup will do for a digit; a zip-lock bag for larger parts). This container should then be floated in a bath of ice and water. This method ensures that only an isotonic solution comes into contact with the part (if floated directly in ice water, a hypotonic injury can occur). It also protects the part from direct freezing injury, which can occur if placed in direct contact with ice.

When performing ray amputation of the long or ring fingers, attention should be paid to securing the remaining metacarpals at the level of the distal metacarpal head. This is accomplished by suturing the deep intervolar plate ligaments securely with several sturdy, nonabsorbable, braided sutures. Additionally, a K-wire is placed across the metacarpals during the healing phase (3–4 weeks) to provide further support. Although there are many different techniques described for accomplishing ray amputation (including metacarpal repositioning of the remaining digits) this author (MC) been quite satisfied with the results afforded by simply removing the affected metacarpal at the proximal metaphyseal flare. This maintains the carpometacarpal relationships, limiting further difficulties and instability.

Ray amputations typically provide the patient with a very functional hand. Patients can expect to resume nearly all of their preinjury activities, even typing. Aesthetically, hands with ray amputations appear more normal in appearance than those with a deleted digit at the proximal phalangeal or MCP joint level. In the present patient (see figure D), the long finger easily assumes the "trigger finger" function of the index finger. The volar skin of the index finger remained viable, and so it was used to provide coverage of the dorsal hand as a filet flap. The ray amputation preserved a wide 1st web space, allowing the hand to maintain normal grasp.

Figure E shows a failed revascularization attempt prior to ray amputation of the long finger. Note the postoperative appearance of this same patient (figure F). She remains fond of rings, despite the ring avulsion injury that cost her her long finger.

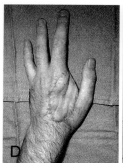
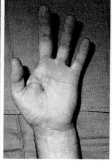
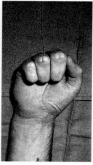

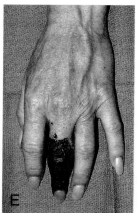
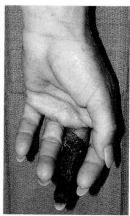

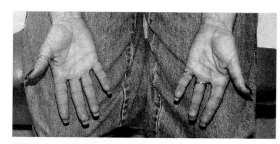
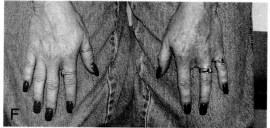

Clinical Pearls

1. The decision to replant is based on relative indications and contraindications; the patient's occupation and hobbies; and general medical health. In some cases, successful replantation may actually *decrease* hand function.

2. Ray amputation results are most gratifying in the index finger. The large 1st web space facilitates grasp, and the long finger easily and with little therapy naturally assumes the function of "trigger finger."

3. When performing ray amputation of the long or ring fingers, attention should be paid to securing the remaining metacarpals at the level of the distal metacarpal head.

REFERENCES

1. Concannon MJ: Finger replantation. In Kenter K, Anglen JO (eds): Hospital Physician—Orthopaedic Surgery Board Review Manual. Wayne, PA, Turner White Communications, Inc., 5(2):12–20, 1999.
2. Concannon MJ: Amputations and soft tissue loss. In: Common Hand Problems in Primary Care. Philadelphia, PA, Hanley & Belfus, 1999.
3. Saies AD, Urbaniak JR, Nunley JA, et al: Results after replantation and revascularization in the upper extremity in children. J Bone Joint Surg 76:1766–1776, 1994.
4. Tamai S: Twenty years' experience of limb replantation: Review of 293 upper extremity replants. J Hand Surg 7:549–556, 1982.
5. Urbaniak JR, Roth JH, Nunley JA, et al: The results of replantation after amputation of a single finger. J Bone Joint Surg 67:611–619, 1985.

Of all upper extremity amputations, one-third involve the fingers and of those, 97% are caused by trauma. When an amputated finger is deemed irretrievable, ray amputation is a viable alternative procedure. The hand therapist's goal is exactly that of the hand surgeon's—to preserve the patient's hand function.

Strict upper extremity elevation and attention to wound care are vital in the early stages of postoperative rehabilitation. Desensitization exercises including scar massage, texture, and percussion techniques are instituted following suture removal. These modalities are particularly important after index finger resection because of the prevalence of neuroma formation in the sensory branches of the median and superficial radial nerves.

The patient is instructed in early active motion for the uninvolved fingers of the operated hand. Unless contraindicated, due to skin grafting or neurovascular repairs, active motion may be initiated within 3–5 days after surgery. The patient and family must understand that full motion in the remaining digits is to be expected. Passive range-of-motion and progressive resisted exercises may be initiated as soon as wounds are well healed, usually at 3–6 weeks postoperatively.

Splinting between exercise sessions, for up to 6–8 weeks, may be indicated to provide support for the patient's transverse and longitudinal palmar arches. If the first dorsal interosseous muscle has been transfered to the extensor mechanism of the long finger, a P1 block is added to the palmar splint and used for approximately 1–2 weeks. This prevents MPC flexion, which could stretch the transferred muscle.

Ray resection results in decreased hand area and strength, and the hand therapist should educate patients, family members, and employers accordingly. Following single ray amputation, patients experience 17–57% loss of grip strength, 4–48% loss of pinch strength, and require 8–31% more time to complete timed function tests. Patients undergoing primary ray resection fare better quantitatively in the above three measures than do their counterparts undergoing secondary procedures. Patients in whom central, long, and ring fingers are resected experience less deficits in both pinch strength and in timed function tests than do their counterparts undergoing resection of the border, index, and small fingers.

There may be a role for the use of an aesthetic prosthesis to restore a more normal appearance to the hand in patients with loss of a finger. Despite the fact that these structures offer no moving parts and may actually hinder the patient's sensory appreciation of the residual hand, it cannot be overemphasized that, for some patients, the appearance of the hand plays a significant role in determining the ease with which activities of daily living are resumed.

Hand Therapy Pearls

1. Hand therapy is directed at preserving the function of the remaining hand and upper extremity parts. While dynamic, serial-static, and static-progressive splints can be used, patients treated with ray resection must be encouraged to regain full, active motion of their remaining digits.

2. Strict upper extremity elevation at the level of the heart and uneventful wound healing are mandatory following amputation of an upper extremity part.

3. Desensitization takes on a central role following amputation because of the tendency to form neuromas.

4. Patients, their family members, and employers must be educated to expect decreased hand area and strength following ray resection.

5. For some patients, there may be great psychological benefit gained through the use of an aesthetic prosthesis. However, educate patients that these structures have no moving parts and may actually *limit* sensory appreciation of the residual hand.

REFERENCES

1. Peimer CA, Wheeler DR, Barrett A, et al. Hand function following a single ray amputation. J Hand Surg 24A:1245–1248, 1999.
2. Pillet J, Mackin EJ. Aesthetic hand prosthesis: Its psychologic and functional potential. In Hunter JM, Mackin EJ, Callahan AD (eds): Rehabilitation of the Hand: Surgery and Therapy, 4th ed. St. Louis, Mosby, 1995, pp 1253–1263.
3. Ray resections. In Cannon NM (ed): Diagnosis and Treatment Manual for Physicians and Therapists, 3rd ed. Indianapolis, Hand Rehabilitation Center of Indianapolis, 1991, pp 158–159.

PATIENT 40

A 17-year-old boy with an injury to his fifth proximal interphalangeal joint

This 17-year-old, varsity football player suffered an acute injury to his dominant fifth finger while attempting to catch a pass during a scrimmage. Although he cannot remember the exact details, he was tackled, and suffered the fifth when his hand hit the ground. Immediately after the tackle he complained of pain at the fifth PIP joint, and was unable to either actively extend or flex it (it had assumed the posture of flexion). Multiple attempts by the trainers and coaches to "pull out" and therefore reduce his "jammed finger" were unsuccessful.

Physical Examination: General: right fifth finger flexed at PIP joint (see figure, *left*). Musculoskeletal: finger swollen and very tender; little active motion of PIP, largely due to pain. Neurologic: sensation intact; adequate perfusion distally. Proximal hand and other fingers are atraumatic and asymptomatic.

Laboratory Findings: Radiograph: see figure, *right*.

Questions: What is the diagnosis? What treatment (if any) is indicated?

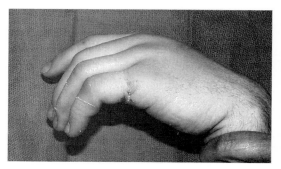

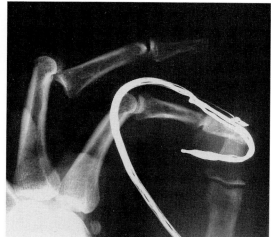

Answers: Volar PIP dislocation. Open (operative) reduction and possible extensor tendon repair is indicated.

Discussion: Dislocations are classified as either dorsal or volar, describing the relationship of the middle phalanx to the proximal phalanx. Volar PIP dislocations are very rare; the vast majority of dislocations at this level are dorsal, meaning that the middle phalanx is dislocated *dorsal* to the proximal phalanx (see figure).

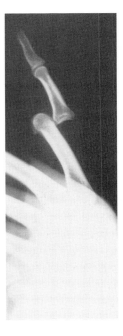

In a volar dislocation, the distal aspect of the proximal phalanx often tears through the extensor mechanism (see figure below, *arrow;* the extensor mechanism prevented closed reduction of this dislocation). The central slip may be avulsed, or the condyle may tear between the central slip and the lateral band. It is this configuration of the torn extensor tendon holding the proximal phalanx out of position that makes closed reduction difficult (compare the intraoperative finding to the preoperative x-ray, which shows the relationship of the proximal phalanx to the middle phalanx and the extensor mechanism).

Management of these injuries is controversial: many authors advocate operative reduction so that the extensor tear can be repaired (see figure, *next page;* after reduction and prior to tendon repair). The extensor tendon can trap the proximal phalanx, such that with simple distraction of the middle phalanx, the extensor tendon holds the proximal phalanx even more tightly, blocking reduction.

The method of closed reduction for volar dislocations differs from that for dorsal dislocations because of the entrapped proximal phalanx through the extensor mechanism. Flexion of the MCP and PIP joints has been advocated t o relax the lateral band that holds the proximal phalanx out of anatomic position. Simultaneous wrist extension can further relax the extensor tendon. In this position, gentle traction with a rotary motion can disengage the condyle and allow reduction. As with all reductions, confirmation of adequate reduction is accomplished by observing gentle range of motion as well as post-reduction x-rays.

If closed reduction is not successful after *one or at most two* attempts, operative exploration and manipulation or removal of the anatomic structure blocking reduction is indicated. In the present patient, multiple attempts at reduction had already been performed, and therefore surgical repair is warranted. Exploration revealed the sling effect of the torn extensor mechanism: the condylar head had pushed through and become entrapped within the extensor tendon, preventing closed reduction. Open reduction also allowed direct repair of the torn extensor mechanism.

Post-reduction management should address possible central slip injury and boutonnière deformity. After 7 days of immobilization in extension, an extension splint (maintaining PIP extension but allowing MCP and DIP mobility) will prevent volar migration of the lateral bands and a secondary boutonnière deformity from occurring.

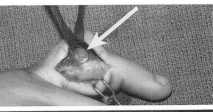

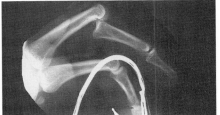

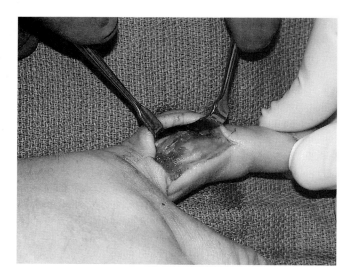

Clinical Pearls

1. Volar PIP dislocations are very rare, but are important to recognize because they are treated differently than dorsal dislocations.

2. The extensor mechanism is torn by the distal aspect of the proximal phalanx. The lateral band often acts as a "sling" that makes closed reduction difficult, if not impossible.

3. After reduction, these injuries should be treated to avoid the progression to a boutonnière deformity (assuming the central slip has been disrupted). This is done by maintaining the PIP in extension (either in a dynamic or static splint) to prevent volar migration of the lateral bands.

REFERENCES

1. De Smet L, Vercauteren M: Palmar dislocation of the proximal interphalangeal joint requiring open reduction: A case report. J Hand Surg 9:717–718, 1984.
2. Dray GJ, Eaton RG: Dislocations and ligament injuries in the digits. In Green DP, Hotchkiss R, Pederson WC (eds): Green's Operative Hand Surgery, 4th ed. New York, Churchill Livingstone, 1999.
3. Peimer CA, Sullivan DJ, Wild DR: Palmar dislocation of the proximal interphalangeal joint. J Hand Surg 9:39–48, 1984.
4. Thompson JS, Eaton RG: Volar dislocation of the proximal interphalangeal joint. J Hand Surg 2:232, 1977.

Perspectives For Therapy

With referral to hand therapy, the patient is provided a custom-fabricated, volar, finger-based gutter splint to maintain the PIP joint in extension. This is worn continuously for up to 5 weeks. It is good practice to provide the patient with two splints: one is worn during hygiene and can be replaced with a dry splint. Perforated thermoplastic is optimal for skin health, and soft tissues should be inspected regularly for maceration and erythema. Baby powder or corn starch absorbs excess moisture. Edema management is accomplished with cohesive dressings.

After 5 weeks of extension splinting, the patient is instructed in active PIP flexion. However, extension splinting is continued between exercise sessions and at bedtime. Providing that the patient has no PIP extension lag $\geq 30°$, he or she may begin passive PIP flexion at 8 weeks postoperatively. Dynamic flexion splinting may also be initiated at this time in addition to light resistive exercises.

Open reduction to restore PIP congruity may require some form of skeletal fixation to maintain the reduction. It is therefore important for the hand therapist to understand that the patient will be immobilized for up to 5 weeks. Should the extensor tendon central slip *also* have been repaired, this case evolves into a complex hand injury. Accordingly, the prognosis may not be as favorable as that expected for a patient referred to hand therapy for early mobilization following repair of an isolated central slip injury.

In a volar PIP joint dislocation, the mechanism of injury involves disruption of one collateral ligament, volar plate damage, and disruption of the central slip. When these tissues are immobilized for a prolonged interval following surgical release, scar adherence of the extensor mechanism central slip and lateral bands, and the volar plate and collateral ligaments is practically assured, and leads to predictable decreases in IP joint flexion and in IP extension lags. Moreover, it has been documented clinically that a patient with a chronic, volar PIP dislocation—defined as 4 weeks between injury and treatment—has the least favorable prognosis.

Hand Therapy Pearls

1. Volar PIP dislocation represents a complex hand injury involving the extensor mechanism central slip and lateral bands, collateral ligaments, and volar plate. There may also be an associated intra-articular P2 fracture.

2. Medical management involves prolonged immobilization of the injured finger. From the standpoint of hand therapy, the patient can be expected to have decreased IP joint motion.

3. Hand impairments become more pronounced as the amount of time increases between injury and treatment.

REFERENCES

1. Volar PIP fractures/dislocations. In Cannon NM (ed): Diagnosis and Treatment Manual for Physicians and Therapists. Indianapolis, Hand Rehabilitation Center of Indianapolis, 1991, p 108.
2. Rosenstadt BE, Glickel SZ, Lane LB, Kaplan SJ: Palmar fracture dislocation of the proximal interphalangeal joint. J Hand Surg 23:811–820, 1998.
3. Glickel SZ, Barron OA: Proximal interphalangeal joint fracture dislocations. Hand Clin 16:333–344, 2000.

PATIENT 41

A 60-year-old gardener with a stiff finger

A 60-year-old woman who is an avid gardener presents complaining that her right index finger has been "locking up" for the past 5–6 months. She is a retired librarian, and is right-hand dominant. She denies any injury to the hand, and does not recall any sticks or punctures of the skin while gardening. She relates that the finger is usually worst in the morning: when she awakes, it is stuck in a flexed position, and she cannot actively extend it. She can only extend the digit by pulling it out with her other hand, and she can feel a "snap" when she does this. After regaining mobility in the early morning, she can resume active extension and flexion of the finger, but it "catches" upon flexion; with a lot of movement (e.g., weeding her garden) her distal palm and finger become sore and tender.

Physical Examination: Neurologic: normal. Musculoskeletal: active full flexion of right index finger possible, but difficult; visible "catch" as finger is flexed and extended. Palpation: pea-sized mass on palm (see figure); moderately tender; mass moves with index finger flexion and extension.

Questions: What is your diagnosis? What treatment options do you offer her?

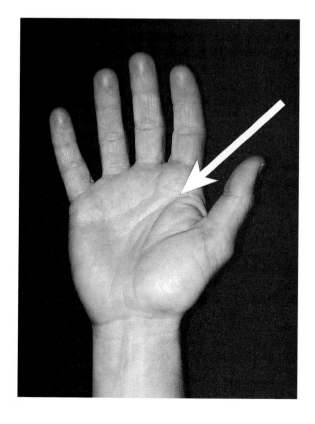

Answers: Stenosing tenosynovitis of the index finger (trigger finger). Treatment can consist of either steroid injection or open release of the A1 flexor pulley.

Discussion: Trigger finger (stenosing tenosynovitis) can be a troubling cause of pain and motion limitation. However, it is easily treated successfully on an outpatient basis or in the clinic. The inflammation occurs between the flexor tendons and A1 pulley at the distal palm and can be brought on by repetitive motion or trauma. This condition involves a vicious cycle, which begins with tenosynovitis and inflammation of the tendons and their surrounding sheath at the palmar pulley. The tendons become secondarily thickened in response to the inflammation, further limiting gliding and causing additional irritation when motion is attempted. This tendonous thickening can progress to a nodular enlargement. This nodule ("Notta's node") blocks movement of the tendon within the pulley system, and the patient ultimately is unable to actively extend or flex the tendon past the obstruction.

Although stenosing tenosynovitis is not the only cause of finger "catching" with motion, it certainly is the most common. PIP osteophytes (including "joint mice") can also restrict normal joint motion of the digit.

Trigger finger most commonly presents in women 60–70 years old, and is associated with de Quervain's tenosynovitis and carpal tunnel syndrome. Patients who have diabetes, rheumatoid arthritis, or Dupuytren's disease are more likely than the general population to develop stenosing tenosynovitis.

There are several different treatment options: steroid injection, percutaneous release of the A1 pulley, and open release of the A1 pulley. Steroid injection within the palm at the level of the A-1 pulley can be an effective means of addressing this problem in adults, sparing the patient a surgical procedure. It is not recommended for use in the pediatric population. Typical application is 0.25 cc of depomethylprednisolone acetate (80 mg/cc) or triamcinolone acetonide (40 mg/cc) diluted with 0.5 cc of 1% lidocaine.

Extreme care must be taken not to inject directly into the tendon, because the steroid can irrevocably weaken it and potentially lead to an attritional rupture. One way to avoid this complication is to ask the patient to *gently* flex and extend the fingers after you've placed the needle in the desired position. If (after advancing the needle) the needle tip moves with flexion, it is stuck within the tendon.

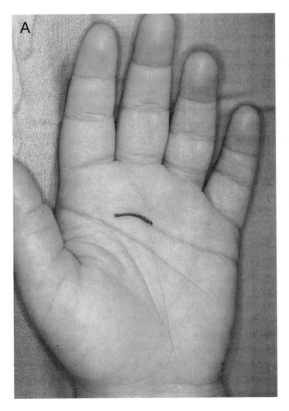

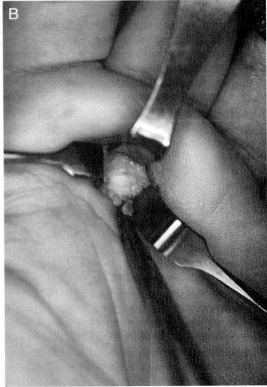

Simply withdraw the needle slightly and ask the patient to repeat the maneuver to confirm the tip position outside of the tendon.

Percutaneous release of the A1 pulley has little advantage over simple open release, but does carry additional risk of tendon or digital nerve injury. For that reason, we do not advocate this method of treatment.

Simple open release involves creation of a small (1.0–1.5 cm) incision, transversely oriented over the proximal palmar crease (at the level of the A1 pulley). The proposed incision for release of the A1 pulley is directly over the pulley at the proximal palmar crease (see figure A). The pulley is exposed at the base of the incision and divided longitudinally under direct vision, eliminating obstruction to tendon gliding (see figure B). The procedure is conducted under wrist tourniquet control, using local anesthesia. Full active flexion and extension (without triggering) is confirmed prior to skin closure. Injury to the digital nerves or tendon is possible, but not as likely as with percutaneous release, since direct visualization and protection of these important structures is possible.

Clinical Pearls

1. When performing steroid injection for stenosing tenosynovitis, it is important to not inject into the substance of the tendon, to prevent possible late tendon rupture.

2. Nearly two-thirds of patients with trigger finger present with (or have a history of) some other kind of tenosynovitis. The more common forms include de Quervain's tenosynovitis and carpal tunnel syndrome. Approximately 25% of patients present with bilateral symptoms.

3. *Congenital* trigger finger most commonly affects the thumb. The thumb is the least commonly involved digit in *adult* stenosing tenosynovitis.

4. The population at risk for developing Dupuytren's (Norwegian, British Isles–Celtic ancestry) is also at risk for developing secondary thickening of the palmar fascia after A1 pulley release. Excise a section of the visible palmar fascia at the time of open pulley division to prevent this occurrence.

REFERENCES
1. Bain GI, Turnbull J, Charles MN, et al: Percutaneous A1 pulley release: A cadaveric study. J Hand Surg 20:781–784, 1995.
2. Chammas M, Bousquet P, Renard E, et al: Dupuytren's disease, carpal tunnel syndrome, trigger finger, and diabetes mellitus. J Hand Surg 20:109–114, 1995.
3. Murphy D, Failla JM, Koniuch MP: Steroid versus placebo injection for trigger finger. J Hand Surg 20:628–631, 1995.
4. Sampson SP, Badalamente MA, Hurst LC, Seidman J: Pathology of the human A1 pulley in the trigger finger. J Hand Surg 16:714–721, 1991.

Perspectives For Therapy

When conservative measures for treatment of trigger finger, such as splinting and exercise, have been exhausted, surgical management becomes a viable option. Patients may then be referred to hand therapy for instruction in active motion exercises. The "hook fist" or "intrinsic-minus" position creates maximum differential gliding between the FDS and FDP tendons, and between the extrinsic flexors and the synovial sheath. It is also essential that the patient achieve full IP joint extension to maximize distal gliding of the FDS and FDP, and to prevent PIP joint flexion contracture. Up to 10 repetitions of exercise may be performed every other waking hour.

If the FPL is released, differential gliding consists of isolated IP flexion and extension while maintaining the MCP in extension. In all surgical releases, scar management is indicated to mobilize soft tissues and to desensitize the surgical site(s).

While it may be impractical for the patient to avoid repetitive activities following surgery, it generally is feasible for them to build up or otherwise modify the handles of frequently used work implements and tools to lessen the magnitude of contact forces required for sustained gripping. A variety of materials, such as cylindrical foam and foam tape, are readily available, relatively inexpensive, and easily applied.

If strengthening and conditioning are desired, a program should be developed for the patient that emphasizes the major upper extremity muscle groups. Programs using graded rubber-bands with the following components are well-tolerated: shoulder abduction, extension, external/internal rotation, flexion, horizontal abduction/adduction, and diagonal patterns; elbow extension and flexion; and forearm rotation. Isolated wrist- and finger- strengthening exercises are contraindicated precisely because they encourage repetitive grasping, power grip, and high contact forces.

Hand Therapy Pearls

1. Following surgical release of a trigger finger or thumb, tendon gliding exercises that maximize differential gliding are prioritized. It is important for the patient to achieve full active flexion *and* extension.

2. Scar management is useful for mobilizing soft tissues and desensitization.

3. Building up the handles of commonly used tools is a practical and cost-effective solution for lessening contact forces.

4. Consider developing a strengthening and conditioning home exercise program that targets the large muscle groups of the patient's upper extremity.

REFERENCES

1. Evans RB, Hunter JM, Burkhalter WE: Conservative management of the trigger finger: A new approach. J Hand Ther 1:59–68, 1988.
2. Kirkpatrick WH, Lisser S: Soft-tissue conditions: Trigger fingers and de Quervain's disease. In Hunter JM, Mackin EJ, Callahan AD (eds): Rehabilitation of the Hand: Surgery and Therapy, 4th ed. St. Louis, Mosby, 1995, pp 1007–1016.

PATIENT 42

A 20-year-old man with a mass on his volar forearm

A 20-year-old prisoner at the local penitentiary is brought into your office for evaluation of a new mass on his right volar forearm. He has noticed it for the past month or so, and he thinks it is getting larger. Two months ago he had been taken to the infirmary after a fight in which he had suffered multiple lacerations to his face, hands, and bilateral forearms. The guards have brought the medical records from that visit; according to these records the arm lacerations were very superficial (no deep structure involvement). The patient's past medical history is significant for tuberculosis and hepatitis C.

Physical Examination: Skin: 3-cm mass on mid-forearm (see figure); well-healed incision (from recent altercation) overlying mass. Palpation: mass pulsatile, with bruit. Vascular: good hand perfusion from both radial and ulnar arteries on Allen's test. Musculoskeletal: all muscular and tendonous units intact; intact FDS, FDP, and FPL; full active and passive range of motion of wrist and fingers. Neurologic: sensation intact throughout median, ulnar, and radial nerve distributions. No epitrochlear or axillary lymphadenopathy.

Questions: What other tests would you recommend? What is your differential diagnosis?

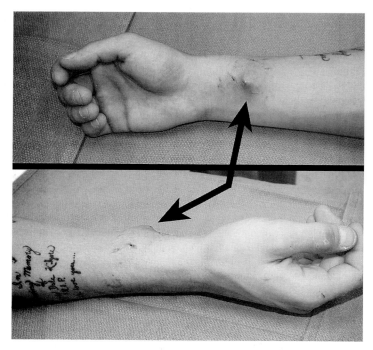

See color panels.

Answers: Since this appears to be a vascular lesion, vascular studies such as duplex or (preferably) angiography are indicated. Suspect relation between mass and laceration (i.e., pseudoaneurysm or arterial venous malformation of the radial artery). Other (less likely) possibilities include inclusion cyst and any of the other soft tissue tumors (e.g., lipoma, sebaceous cyst).

Discussion: The angiogram of the patient's arm revealed that the previous laceration had extended down into the radial artery: a pseudoaneurysm had formed (see figure A). A *true* aneurysm (in contrast to what this individual had) is composed of all three layers of the arterial wall (intima, media, adventitia), whereas a pseudoaneurysm is contained by a fibrous encapsulation and usually arises as a result of rupture or laceration of the artery. At surgical exploration, after removal of the pseudoaneurysm, the original arterial defect is visible (see figure B, *arrow*).

Partial arteriotomies are, at least theoretically, one of the few potentially lethal injuries to the upper extremity. Unable to control bleeding via vasospasm (the physiologic response to a complete arterial transection), the hemorrhage may continue unless stopped by the tamponade effect of the resultant hematoma. If the skin envelope does not contain the blood, a massive amount of blood could be lost if not stopped medically.

The lacerated artery leaks blood through the arteriotomy, which forms a hematoma that is ultimately contained by perivascular tissues. With time, the hematoma lyses, forming a hollow chamber through which the blood may enter (see figure, *next page*). Ultimately, the walls of the pseudoaneurysm become organized by deposition of collagen by perivascular fibroblasts. The formation of a pseudoaneurysm is most common after penetrating arterial injury, such as with a needle or knife, while true aneurysm formation (rare in the upper extremity) is a common result of longstanding arteriosclerosis (e.g., aortic).

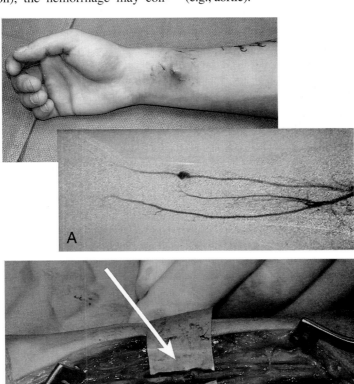

A

B

Treatment involves resection of the pseudoaneurysm, and either direct repair of the vessel (if the vessel ends can be mobilized sufficiently to repair without tension) or repair with vein graft. Theoretically, if the arterial supply to the hand was sufficiently supplied by the ulnar artery, arterial repair or reconstruction would not be mandatory, as ligation of the radial artery does not result in critical ischemia of the hand. The determination of whether to reconstruct or repair the artery is made on an individual basis, and in a young individual most surgeons would opt to repair the vessel to maintain as robust a circulation in the hand as possible.

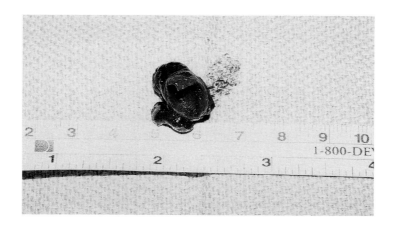

Clinical Pearls

1. The presence of a pulsatile mass can indicate a vascular mass (such as an aneurysm or pseudoaneurysm), or may simply represent a mass *overlying* an artery. The latter is very common with volar wrist ganglions, which often arise in close association with the radial artery.

2. Pseudoaneurysms are much more common than true aneurysms in the upper extremity, and are typically the result of penetrating trauma. True aneurysms typically form as an end result of atherosclerosis, a disease process that to a large degree spares the upper extremity.

3. The most common sequelae of pseudoaneurysm formation are rupture and hemorrhage; both are best treated with direct pressure and operative repair.

REFERENCES
1. Ho PK, Weiland AJ, McClinton MA, Wilgis EF: Aneurysms of the upper extremity. J Hand Surg 12:39–46, 1987.
2. Louis DS, Simon MA: Traumatic false aneurysms of the upper extremity: A diagnostic problem. J Bone Joint Surg 56:176–179, 1974.
3. Mays ET: Traumatic aneurysm of the hand. Am Surg 36:552–557, 1970.
4. Milling MA, Kinmonth MH: False aneurysm of the ulnar artery. Hand 9:57–59, 1977.

PATIENT 43

A 15-year-old boy with progressive finger flexion contracture

A 15-year-old boy is brought to your office by his parents for evaluation of a progressive finger flexion deformity. The parents have noticed that he is unable to completely extend his small fingers. The deformity originated approximately 2 years ago, and they think it is worsening. The boy is adamant that he has no functional problem: he was reluctant to come and is anxious to leave your office. Both patient and parents deny any recent history of trauma to his hands. No other siblings or relatives have noticed similar problems.

Physical Examination: Musculoskeletal: fifth finger PIP joints cannot be actively or passively extended beyond 20° of flexion (see figure); positioning MCP joint in flexion or extension does not change range of motion at PIP joint; full and strong flexion of all fingers. Neurologic: both FDP and FDS of fifth digits intact bilaterally.

Laboratory Findings: Radiographs: normal.

Questions: What is your diagnosis? What treatment options do you recommend?

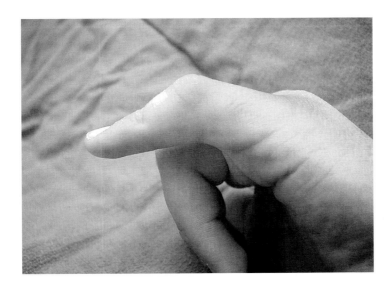

Answers: Camptodactyly. At this stage, no treatment is recommended, as none is particularly helpful.

Discussion: Camptodactyly is an idiopathic flexion contracture of the PIP joints. Usually it affects the fifth fingers and is bilateral. It has two peaks of presentation: one in early childhood and secondarily in the adolescent years (corresponding to growth spurts).

In most cases, the defect has very little functional impact and is largely an aesthetic concern. Attempts to surgically release the contracture may give some early improvement, but late recurrence is typical. If the PIP flexion contracture does limit normal hand function (similar to the situation for patients with PIP involvement in Dupuytren's contracture, who are unable to wear gloves or place their hands in their pockets), another option may be to fuse the PIP in a position of function.

Myriad causes for camptodactyly have been documented, including fibrous bands limiting full extension, anomalous insertions of the lumbrical muscles, anomalous flexor tendons, and underdeveloped extensor tendons. Perhaps the only configuration that lends itself to surgical repair is the situation in which there is an anomalous insertion of the lumbrical. In these patients, the PIP can be fully extended when the MCP is flexed, but with MCP extension full PIP extension is blocked. In these cases, the lumbrical muscle either arises from or inserts into the FDS tendon, and acts to block motion at the A1 pulley (the lumbrical is too bulky to pass under the pulley). Resection of the lumbrical (and reinsertion into the lateral band if possible) can restore the digit to normal mobility.

Prior to any surgical treatment, prolonged splinting is advisable. This may overcome some flexion contracture, and in particular may prevent further progression of the contracture, which is particularly important during active growth phases in adolescence. Care must be taken not to apply pressure at the distal phalanx; such pressure could create a concurrent hyperextension deformity at the DIP joint.

In the present patient, a conservative wait-and-see approach was adopted. For more severe cases, surgical release can be attempted, but results are typically disappointing. If severe contracture limits a patient's function, PIP fusion may ultimately be the best option.

Clinical Pearls

1. Camptodactyly affects both sexes equally at birth; in cases presenting in the teens, females predominate. Only 13% of cases present after the age of 1 year.

2. Nearly two-thirds of cases are bilateral, but typically the degree of contracture is not equal between hands. Although the flexion contracture may worsen (particularly during growth spurts), progression after the teen years is rare.

3. The results of surgical treatment are often disappointing. PIP fusion offers the most reliable outcome for patients in whom surgery is warranted. Prolonged splinting should always precede surgical intervention.

4. Reasonable surgical results can be expected when an anomalous insertion or attachment of the lumbrical to the FDS can be diagnosed. In these patients, release of the lumbrical (with or without reattachment to the lateral band) will restore normal mobility of the digit.

REFERENCES

1. Courtemanche AD: Camptodactyly: Etiology and management. Plast Reconstr Surg 44:451–454, 1969.
2. McFarlane RM, Classen DA, Porte AM, Botz JS: The anatomy and treatment of camptodactyly of the small finger. J Hand Surg 17:35–44, 1992.
3. Siegert JJ, Cooney WP, Dobyns JH: Management of simple camptodactyly. J Hand Surg 15:181–189, 1990.
4. Wood VE: Camptodactyly. In Green DP, Hotchkiss R, Pederson WC (eds): Green's Operative Hand Surgery, 4th ed. New York, Churchill Livingstone, 1999.

Hand Therapy Pearls

1. Serial static casting has proven successful for correcting difficult PIP joint flexion contractures. However, this technique requires close follow-up, with return visits to the clinic for progression.

2. Splinting to restore joint motion must be of sufficient duration to permit soft tissue growth in length and magnitude that does not cause skin ischemia.

3. Preconditioning periarticular soft tissues, including the skin, using heat, joint mobilization, and gentle passive stretching is advisable prior to casting.

4. Assuming that the patient's PIP can be modified, a custom, static, volar gutter splint, worn at bedtime, may be used to maintain the extension gained through serial static casting. The splint should clear the DIP and MCP joints.

5. Motion gains *must* be reinforced through active and passive PIP extension exercises performed through the augmented range.

REFERENCES

1. Colditz JC: Modification of the digital serial plaster casting technique. Hand Ther 8:215–216, 1995.
2. Colditz JC: Therapist's management of the stiff hand. In Hunter JM, Mackin EJ, Callahan AD (eds): Rehabilitation of the Hand: Surgery and Therapy, 4th ed. St. Louis, Mosby, 1995, pp 1141–1159.

PATIENT 44

A 19-year-old man with a swollen, painful thumb

A 19-year-old basketball player presents to the emergency department with a swollen and painful left thumb after injuring it during the regional finals. His trainer thought that he had simply "jammed" it, and had tried for approximately 20 minutes to pull it out to reduce it, but was unsuccessful. He complains of pain mostly around the IP joint of his dominant thumb, and does not volunteer any other symptoms or complaints.

Physical Examination: General: thumb significantly swollen; other digits uninjured. Palpation: majority of tenderness at IP joint, on both volar and dorsal aspects, as well as radially and ulnarly. Musculoskeletal: marked decreased range of motion at IP joint; active and passive extension and flexion of finger not possible. Neurologic: decreased subjective sensation distally, with moving two-point discrimination approximately 9 mm at distal tip (4–5 mm on contralateral, uninjured side).

Laboratory Findings: Radiograph: see figure.

Questions: What is the diagnosis? What are his treatment options?

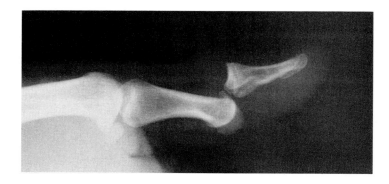

Answers: Dorsal IP joint dislocation. Since closed reduction failed, surgical exploration and relocation is required.

Discussion: Dorsal dislocations of the PIP and DIP joints are relatively common injuries, particularly among athletes. Due to its position in the hand and the lever-type forces that it can be subjected to, the PIP joint is the most commonly dislocated joint in the hand. It is a hinged-type joint that is extremely stable to external stresses.

The DIP and PIP joints are supported by three major ligamentous structures: the collateral ligaments on the radial and ulnar sides of the joint, and the volar plate. By virtue of its position, the volar plate prevents hyperextension of the joint. The collateral ligaments support the joint on either side of the finger, and prevent radial and ulnar deviation of the finger. Typically, any dislocation of the either the PIP or DIP joint involves disruption of the volar plate (usually from its distal attachment) and at least one of the collateral ligaments, if not both.

Since in this case the distal phalanx is dislocated *dorsal* to the proximal phalanx, it is termed a dorsal dislocation. This is the most common type of dislocation at the IP joints. Occurring much more rarely is the volar dislocation (in which the middle phalanx is dislocated volar to the proximal phalanx).

Reduction of dorsal dislocations is usually straightforward, accomplished by applying gentle, outward traction on the distal finger. If the digit is unable to be relocated after *a maximum of two* attempts at reduction, no further attempts should be made, and the patient should be taken to the operating room for exploration and repair. In this situation, there is typically an anatomic structure that is blocking the reduction (such as the volar plate or flexor tendon) and *making closed reduction impossible*. Further attempts at closed reduction are counterproductive, as they will only increase soft tissue damage and edema.

For example (see figure), the flexor pollicis longus (*white arrow*) may be entrapped between the proximal and distal phalanges (the articular surface of the proximal phalanx is demonstrated by the *black arrow*), thereby physically blocking closed reduction. This illustrates how an anatomic structure can make closed reduction impossible in certain circumstances, mandating surgical intervention.

Post-reduction care revolves around prevention of re-dislocating the joint, and reducing ultimate stiffness. Patients should be warned that persistent stiffness and edema may be present for 6 or more months after treatment (and may be permanent). Immediately after reducing the joint and confirming the reduction with radiographs, a carefully supervised program of progressive splinting and protected range of motion (see Perspectives For Therapy) is appropriate.

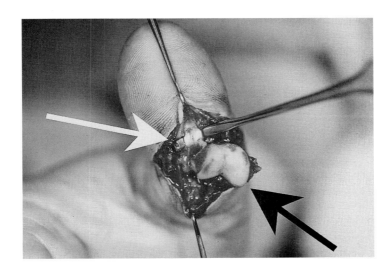

Clinical Pearls

1. The most common complication of dorsal PIP dislocation is stiffness secondary to prolonged immobilization. Prolonged immobilization with the PIP in flexion can also produce a flexion joint contracture ("pseudoboutonnière deformity").

2. Left untreated or unprotected, persistent hyperextension of the PIP joint can lead to recurvatum (swan neck deformity) secondary to dorsal migration of the lateral bands, or can result in chronic dislocation.

3. Fracture-dislocations of the PIP joint can be very difficult to treat. The distal head of the proximal phalanx fractures the lip of the middle phalanx, producing a comminuted articular fracture that can involve most of the articular surface. This situation is best addressed by reduction (preferably closed, if possible) and the application of dynamic traction.

REFERENCES

1. Bowers WH: The proximal interphalangeal joint volar plate. II: A clinical study of hyperextension injury. J Hand Surg 6:77–81, 1981.
2. Dawson WJ: The spectrum of sports-related interphalangeal joint injuries. Hand Clin 10:315–326, 1994.
3. Glickel SZ, Barron A, Eaton RG: Dislocations and ligament injuries in the digits. In Green DP, Hotchkiss R, Pederson WC (eds): Green's Operative Hand Surgery, 4th ed. New York, Churchill Livingstone, 1999.
4. Kasparyan NG, Hotchkiss RN: Dynamic skeletal fixation in the upper extremity. Hand Clin 13:643–663, 1997.

Perspectives For Therapy

Conservative hand therapy management of the patient with stable reduction of a dorsally dislocated PIP joint involves fabrication of a custom, dorsal-block splint that immobilizes the involved joint in 30–40° flexion and the DIP joint at 0°. The proximal margin of the splint base clears the MCP. A 1/16-inch, perforated, thermoplastic material is ideally suited for fabrication of finger-based splints, and two narrow Velcro straps are used to secure the splint.

From 6–8 times daily, the patient releases the distal splint strap and performs active composite finger flexion to the mid-palm, followed by active extension to the limit of the dorsal block splint. This exercise is repeated 10 times, and the splint is then resecured.

Cohesive dressings are appropriate for edema management, and splint fabrication should proceed *after* the finger is wrapped, since addition of a circumferential dressing will tend to *increase* the dimensions of the splint. In other words, secure the compression dressing first, then fabricate the patient's splint.

The patient is seen for follow-up visits in hand therapy once/week for 3–4 weeks. Edema is reassessed and, providing that the fracture remains reduced and is stable, the dorsal block splint is revised into extension 10°/week. The patient continues to perform active composite finger flexion exercises, followed by active extension to the new limit of the dorsal block splint. When the patient's PIP joint is at 0°, it is recommended that they wear the splint for 1 additional week for protection, and discontinue splint use thereafter (total of 4–5 weeks of splint use depending upon the initial flexion angle of immobilization).

For some patients, the use of a buddy-strap may be of benefit following discontinuation of use of their dorsal block splint. For example, in the athlete returning to sports, a buddy-strap may be indicated to provide additional joint support.

In the acute setting, if there is any question regarding the appropriate position of PIP joint immobilization, it is useful to remember: "The proximal phalanx points the way." Thus, in a dorsally dislocated PIP joint, the base of the middle phalanx is *dorsal* to the head of the proximal phalanx, and the palmarly directed proximal phalanx recalls PIP immobilization in flexion.

Hand Therapy Pearls

1. Conservative management of a dorsally dislocated PIP joint involves fabrication of a custom, dorsal-block splint that immobilizes the involved joint in 30–40° of flexion, and the DIP joint at 0°.

2. The patient performs active composite finger flexion to the mid-palm, followed by active extension to the limit of the dorsal block splint.

3. The patient is seen for follow-up visits in hand therapy once/week for 3–4 weeks. Providing that the fracture remains reduced and is stable, the dorsal block splint is revised into extension 10°/week.

4. Cohesive dressings are appropriate for edema management. The splint is fabricated *after* the finger is wrapped since addition of a circumferential dressing tends to *increase* the dimensions of the splint.

5. In the athlete returning to sports, a buddy-strap may be indicated to provide additional joint support once the dorsal block splint is discontinued.

6. In the acute setting, if there is any question regarding the appropriate position of PIP immobilization, it is useful to remember: "The proximal phalanx points the way."

REFERENCE
Blue C, Harris K, Hurov J, et al: Treatment guidelines for volar plate injuries. In Treatment Guidelines for the Upper Extremity, 2nd ed. The Hand Center, Winston-Salem, Bowman Gray/Baptist Hospital Medical Center, 1995, p 4.

PATIENT 45

A 17-year-old boy with hand pain after a fight

A 17-year-old, intoxicated boy presents to the emergency department at 2:30 AM complaining of several lacerations. He evidently was involved in a fistfight the evening before and complains of persistent pain in his dominant hand. He does remember hitting his opponent in the mouth.

Physical Examination: General: patient is lethargic, but responsive and mostly cooperative. Skin: small puncture wound over dorsal aspect of ring metacarpophalangeal joint (see figure); no active bleeding from wound. Musculoskeletal: active full extension and flexion of index finger.

Laboratory Findings: Radiographs: no fractures or dislocations; normal joint spacing.

Question: What is your treatment recommendation?

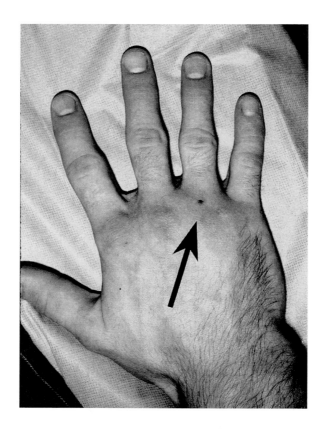

Answer: Exploration and irrigation of the MCP joint

Discussion: Human bites are among the most contaminated encountered in medical practice. In this situation the patient is at a very high risk of developing a septic joint. An important point in the diagnosis and management of this patient is the recognition of the wound as a *human bite* rather than a simple laceration. The skin laceration may only present as a small puncture wound that appears quite innocuous; typically the damage to the underlying structures is more severe. It is not unusual for early infections to have no systemic and minimal local symptoms, and so the physician needs to maintain a high level of suspicion in evaluating dorsal MCP wounds that may indeed be human bite wounds.

The possible late consequences of this injury (assuming there has been inoculation of the joint space) include arthritis with ultimate joint stiffness, osteomyelitis, and even toxic shock syndrome. These consequences are more likely if there has been a significant delay in diagnosis and treatment.

Human saliva has been estimated to contain $> 10^9$ colony-forming units per cc. The most commonly encountered organisms in human bite wounds are *Staphylococcus aureus, Streptococcus* species, and *Eikenella corrodens.* However, other organisms can be found including *Bacteroides* sp., *Neisseria* sp., *Clostridia* sp., spirochetes, *Micrococcus,* and/or *Actinomyces.* If the MCP joint (or *any* joint) is inoculated with these bacteria, septic arthritis can be a devastating consequence, with rapid loss of articular cartilage re-sulting in late joint stiffness and arthritis. Antibiotic therapy needs to be directed toward coverage of both common gram-positive as well as gram-negative anaerobic organisms.

When this history—a laceration over the dorsal MCP joint after a fight—has been obtained, aggressive treatment is warranted. Exploration with copious irrigation of the joint and debridement of all nonviable tissue is indicated in an attempt to reduce the bacterial count. During the course of the exploration, the joint needs to be opened and directly inspected: very often there will be visible defect in the cartilage from the tooth. Any purulence encountered (see figure) should be sent for culture and gram stain. Closure of the skin laceration is *not* indicated, to allow drainage and prevent abscess formation.

The hand should be splinted in a safe position and antibiotics administered (usually parenterally at the onset of therapy). A first-generation cephalosporin (such as cefazolin) *in combination with* penicillin (the latter to provide coverage of the anaerobic bacteria) is currently adequate coverage. In patients that are penicillin allergic, cefoxitin can be used as a replacement. The wound must be closely followed the first 4–5 days after the injury and re-explored and re-irrigated if necessary.

In the present patient, the laceration sustained was technically a human bite since it was created by someone's tooth. After copious irrigation of the wound, which was left open, dressing changes were instituted, and the patient was closely observed.

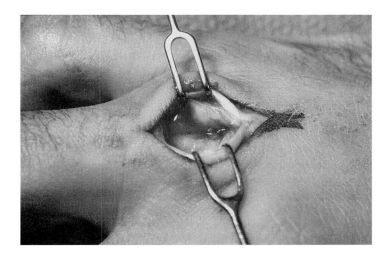

Clinical Pearls

1. Early diagnosis and aggressive treatment are the keys to minimizing the morbidity of septic arthritis in these injuries.

2. The examiner should maintain a high level of suspicion when wounds resulting from altercations are located on the dorsal aspect of the hand near the MCP joint. These are, in effect, human bite wounds, and articular inoculation is possible.

3. *Eikenella corrodens,* a facultative anaerobe and a component of normal human oral flora, is identified in approximately one-third of these injuries.

4. Antibiotic therapy requires coverage of both gram-positive organisms and gram-negative anaerobes.

REFERENCES

1. Goldstein EJ, Barones MF, Miller TA: *Eikenella corrodens* in hand infections. J Hand Surg 8:563–567, 1983.
2. Goldstein EJ, Miller TA, Citron DM, Finegold SM: Infections following clenched-fist injury: A new perspective. J Hand Surg 3:455–457, 1978.
3. Goldstein EJC: Infections following human bites. Infect Surg 1985;4:849.
4. Mann RJ, Hoffeld TA, Farmer CB: Human bites of the hand: Twenty years of experience. J Hand Surg 2:97–104, 1977.

Perspectives For Therapy

For dorsal hand wounds, therapy consists of fabrication of a static, volar, resting hand splint that provides 60–70° MCP joint flexion and 0° at the IP joints of the medial four fingers. Palmar wounds require that the splint be dorsally based with the hand postured similarly. If a forearm-based splint is requested by the hand surgeon, the wrist should be positioned in 0–30° extension. During the early stages of wound care it is desirable to splint the uninvolved joints of the hand.

There is some disagreement as to the appropriateness of initiating early active motion exercises in these patients. Activity potentially risks spreading micro-organisms to uninvolved tissues, while failure to begin exercise may result in tissue fibrosis and joint contractures, particularly when articular cartilage injury has occurred. In these cases, it is suggested that 3–5 days of immobilization, while wounds are closely managed by the medical team, may be acceptable, followed by supervised, active exercise.

The hand therapist should be poised to provide follow-up care, including extensor tendon rehabilitation, since hand wounds caused by fist-to-mouth contact usually occur over the dorsal aspects of the third, fourth, and fifth metacarpals.

Hand Therapy Pearls

1. Hand infections caused by bites represent one of the few instances when uninvolved joints may require immobilization in a resting splint.

2. Excellent communication between the hand surgeon and hand therapist is mandatory to establish the timing of an exercise program for the patient.

3. Once the patient is discharged from the hospital, the hand therapist should be prepared to provide follow-up care, such as extensor tendon rehabilitation. Discharge planning can include the transition to out-patient hand therapy services.

REFERENCE

Nathan R, Taras JS: Common hand infections. In Hunter JM, Mackin EJ, Callahan AD (eds): Rehabilitation of the Hand: Surgery and Therapy, 4th ed. St. Louis, Mosby, 1995, pp 251–260.

PATIENT 46

A 38-year-old tennis pro with dorsal wrist pain

An active and otherwise healthy tennis pro at the local country club presents to you for evaluation of dorsal wrist pain in his dominant hand. He has been experiencing the pain for 6–8 months. The hand has been extensively studied and evaluated by his friend and family physician, who has been unable to positively identify a cause. He has been splinted (using a prefabricated wrist cock-up splint) and also given nonsteroidal anti-inflammatory agents for 5 months without success. He is now referred to you for a second opinion.

Physical Examination: Neurologic: moving two-point discrimination 4–5 mm throughout hand in median, ulnar, and radial nerve distributions; no numbness or paresthesias; radial and ulnar arteries both intact. Vascular: adequate perfusion of hand and fingers. Musculoskeletal: full active and passive ROM of digits; strong flexion and extension; extreme wrist flexion and extension difficult and reproduces symptoms most reliably. Palpation: minimally tender at dorsal wrist just proximal to third metacarpal; nontender at anatomic snuff box.

Laboratory Findings: Electrodiagnostic diagnostic studies (obtained and forwarded by patient's primary physician): no evidence of nerve compression. Plain films and wrist MRI (also obtained by primary physician): see figures.

Questions: What is your diagnosis? What is your treatment recommendation?

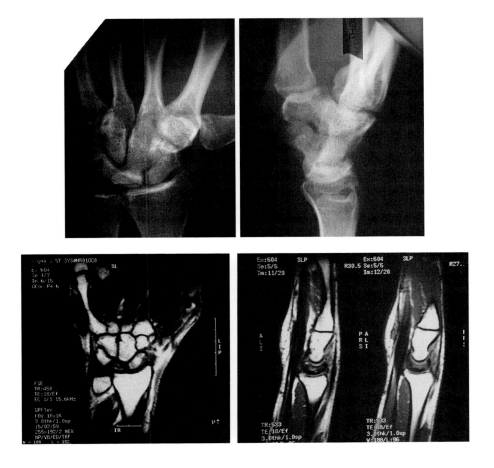

Answers: Kienbock's disease. Recommend radial shortening.

Discussion: Kienbock's disease is a progressive degenerative process involving avascular necrosis of the lunate. It is usually diagnosed between the ages of 15 and 40. A significant risk factor is the presence of negative ulnar variance, which gives credence to one popular theory concerning the etiology of this process: that it results from increased physical loading on the lunate.

Negative ulnar variance (see figure, *next page*) is measured on a PA zero rotation view radiograph (pronation artificially increases the variance measurement, while supination decreases it). A line is drawn from the level of the lunate fossa; a second line is drawn at the ulnar head. The amount of variance is the distance between these two lines. The mean ulnar variance is approximately 1 mm.

Symptoms of Kienbock's disease are quite variable and may include wrist pain and swelling. The pain may radiate proximally up the forearm. Passive extension of the middle finger is commonly uncomfortable for these patients. Patients may complain of limitation in wrist mobility, especially extension, and of grip weakness.

Diagnosis is assisted greatly by radiographic evaluation. X-rays in the early disease process may be normal, except for ulnar negative variance. Later, sclerotic changes can be seen within the lunate itself. As the disease progresses, compression, fragmentation, and flattening of the lunate can be seen. Finally, arthritic changes of the radiocarpal and intercarpal joints are evident.

There are several classification schemes (based on the radiographic findings) to stratify the severity of Kienbock's disease; this is of value when deciding what treatment option is best for the patient. The modified Stahl's classification is as follows:
Stage 1: Lunate structurally appears normal, but there may be a radiodense or radiolucent line across it (compression fracture)
Stage 2: Rarification (demineralization, the bone appears less dense than the normal adjacent bone) along the previously noted compression fracture line
Stage 3: Sclerosis of the proximal pole of the lunate
Stage 4: Progressive flattening or fragmentation of the lunate bone
Stage 5: Secondary arthritic changes notable at the radiocarpal and intercarpal joints.

There are multiple treatment options, which is usually an indication to the clinician that there is not a single reliable method that is successful in dealing with these patients. In general, the overall goal involves decreasing the axial loading on the lunate. Once this is accomplished, spontaneous revascularization may occur. In patients with a negative ulnar variance, radial shortening, ulnar lengthening, or capitate shortening will decrease axial loading on the lunate, (placing more stress on the scaphoid).

Of these options, radial shortening is perhaps the most popular and reliable. It has the same theoretical outcome as ulnar lengthening, without the added morbidity of the bone graft that is required in the lengthening procedure. Interestingly, only about 2 mm of radius needs to be removed to successfully unload the lunate, regardless of the degree of ulnar variance preoperatively. Capitate shortening (performed in conjunction with capitohamate fusion) can also unload the lunate, increasing the scaphoid loading by about 20%. However, this option has been criticized as being ineffective in transferring load to the ulnar wrist; it also requires the additional morbidity of bone grafting.

Another option in the treatment of early Kienbock's disease (up to stage 3) is scaphotrapezial-trapezoid fusion. This procedure can also unload the lunate, but is not as effective when the hand is placed in ulnar deviation. Care must be taken when performing this procedure to place the scaphoid in neutral or at most slight dorsiflexion to effectively unload the lunate (too much dorsiflexion will limit wrist mobility).

Since the pathologic process of Kienbock's is avascular necrosis of the lunate, some investigators have also focused their efforts on actively revascularizing the lunate bone. One method involves harvesting the 2nd or 3rd metacarpal artery, and implanting it into a drilled hole in the lunate (which is also filled with cancellous bone graft, after removing all necrotic bone from within the lunate).

In those patients with more advanced disease (stages 4 or 5), in whom essentially irreversible arthritic changes have occurred, treatment options consist of proximal row carpectomy or total wrist fusion. Prior to proceeding with the former option, both the proximal capitate and lunate fossa articular surfaces need to be evaluated and confirmed to be disease free.

In the past, some authors had advocated excision of the lunate and replacement with an implant. However, there is a very high rate of silicone synovitis with these implants in this position, and few surgeons currently advocate this option.

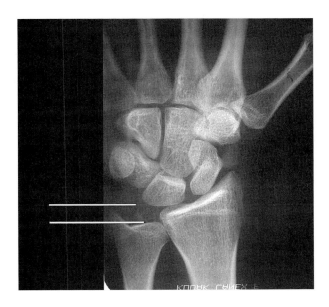

Clinical Pearls

1. While the treatment of Kienbock's remains controversial, radial shortening appears to now be the most commonly performed surgical treatment for this disease process. It has several advantages, including the fact that it does not require the harvest of bone graft. Additionally, it does not interfere with salvage procedures (such as proximal row carpectomy) if required later.

2. Due to the very high incidence of silicone synovitis, excision of the lunate and replacement with a silicone spacer is no longer advocated.

3. Most patients treated with radial shortening for Kienbock's report an improvement in symptoms within 6 months postoperatively. Interestingly, the radiographs typically do not improve, despite the clinical improvement in the patient.

REFERENCES

1. Armistead RB, Linscheid RL, Dobyns JH, Beckenbaugh RD: Ulnar lengthening in the treatment of Kienbock's disease. J Bone Joint Surg 64:170–8, 1982.
2. Murray PM, Wood MB. The results of treatment of synovitis of the wrist induced by particles of silicone debris. J Bone Joint Surg 80:397–406, 1998.
3. Viola RW, Kiser PK, Bach AW, et al: Biomechanical analysis of capitate shortening with captiate hamate fusion in the treatment of Kienbock's disease. J Hand Surg 23:395–401, 1998.
4. Watson HK, Monacelli DM, Milford RS, Ashmead D IV: Treatment of Kienbock's disease with scaphotrapezio-trapezoid arthrodesis. Hand Surg 21:9–15, 1996.
5. Weiss AP, Weiland AJ, Moore JR, Wilgis EF: Radial shortening for Kienbock disease. J Bone Joint Surg 73:384–91, 1991.
6. Yajima H, Ono H, Tamai S: Temporary internal fixation of the scaphotrapezio-trapezoidal joint for the treatment of Kienbock's disease: A preliminary study. J Hand Surg 23:402–410, 1998.

Perspectives For Therapy

The presence of negative ulnar variance, as seen on standard x-rays, represents an anatomical, or structural, predisposing factor associated with Kienbock's disease. More importantly however, is what might be termed **dynamic ulnar variance,** where minor structural variations in ulnar length are dramatically amplified by wrist and forearm motion and by gripping. Accordingly, those functional demands that require forearm supination and wrist radial deviation, in combination with a forceful, sustained grasp, result in local force concentration upon the radiolunate joint.

A *dynamic* decrease in ulnar length of as little as 1 mm therefore increases the load borne by the radiolunate joint by almost 10%.

Following radial shortening, the patient's wrist may be immobilized in neutral for up to 10 days to facilitate uneventful wound healing. However, the patient will benefit from early referral to hand therapy for instruction in edema management and active motion of the involved hand, elbow, and shoulder.

With creation of a stable construct, through plating of the shortened radius, active wrist exercises may be initiated 2–3 weeks postoperatively. When surgical wounds are well-healed and su-tures have been removed, scar management, compression, and massage are appropriate to help minimize soft-tissue adherence. Wrist splinting for comfort and support during performance of vigorous ADLs may be indicated for up to 3 months following surgery.

In a review of 16 patients who had undergone radial shortening osteotomy for treatment of Kienbock's disease, 10 experienced increased wrist motion and grip strength, compared to their preoperative measurements. Thirteen patients returned to their occupations and were essentially pain-free, as judged by verbal report, following full recovery from surgery.

Hand Therapy Pearls

1. The concept of dynamic ulnar variance is important for understanding the natural history of Kienbock's disease. Minor structural variations in ulnar length are dramatically amplified by wrist and forearm motion, and by gripping. Dynamic length changes of the ulna, of as little as 1 mm, can increase radiolunate joint loading by 10%.

2. Following radial shortening, the patient's wrist may be immobilized in neutral for up to 10 days to facilitate uneventful wound healing. The patient will benefit from early referral to hand therapy for instruction in edema management and active motion of hand, elbow, and shoulder.

3. With creation of a stable construct, through plating of the shortened radius, active wrist exercises may be initiated 2–3 weeks postoperatively.

REFERENCES

1. Palmer AK, Werner FW: Biomechanics of the distal radioulnar joint. Clin Orthop Rel Res 187:26–35, 1984.
2. Rock MG, Roth JH, Martin L: Radial shortening osteotomy for treatment of Kienbock's disease. J Hand Surg 16A:454–460, 1991.

PATIENT 47

A 46-year-old college professor with elbow pain

A 46-year-old college professor presents to your office complaining of elbow pain of 4-month duration. Approximately 6 months ago she joined a health club and has successfully undergone a 25-pound weight loss program. In addition to diet modification, she now routinely exercises (aerobics and weight training). She is right-handed and has been troubled with right elbow pain especially while working out. She locates the pain over the entire left side of her elbow.

Physical Examination: Palpation: tender at lateral aspect of elbow (see figure, *arrow*); not particularly tender over extensor and flexor muscle groups. Musculoskeletal: full and strong active flexion and extension of wrist and digits; pain reproduced upon resistance of active finger extension; simultaneous elbow extension, forearm pronation, and wrist flexion reproduces discomfort most reliably; no evidence of ligamentous instability at elbow; full active and passive ROM at elbow. Neurologic: median, ulnar, and radial nerve sensation intact; no symptoms of numbness or paresthesia; Tinel's sign negative at both cubital tunnel and carpal tunnel.

Questions: What is your diagnosis? What are your treatment recommendations?

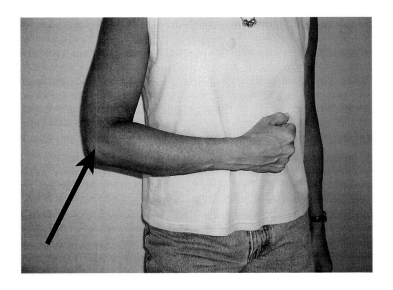

Answers: Lateral epicondylitis. Recommend conservative management (steroid injection, nonsteroidal anti-inflammatory agents, and directed therapy involving strengthening exercises).

Discussion: Lateral epicondylitis (tennis elbow) is an inflammatory process involving the common extensor origin at the lateral epicondyle. In lateral epicondylitis, the greatest amount of tenderness can be elicited with the elbow extended, forearm pronated, and the wrist flexed (see figure, *below*).

of lidocaine can also guide the clinician to the correct diagnosis: resolution of symptoms and radial nerve motor deficit after infiltration of 1% lidocaine can confirm radial tunnel syndrome.

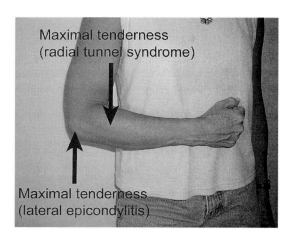

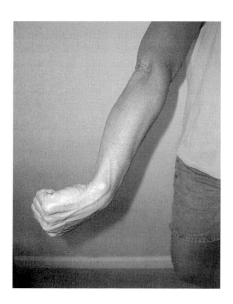

The differential diagnosis of proximal dorsal forearm pain or lateral elbow pain includes radial tunnel syndrome, which occurs approximately 1/10th as frequently as lateral epicondylitis (see table). The points of maximal tenderness differ in these two disorders (see figure, *right*). Radial tunnel syndrome has maximal tenderness approximately 5 cm distal to the lateral epicondyle. In particularly puzzling cases, electrodiagnosistic studies can confirm the presence of radial nerve entrapment. Provocative testing with infiltration

Ninety percent of patients diagnosed with lateral epicondylitis respond to conservative management. This involves referral to a hand therapist for specific rehabilitation and strengthening protocols. In the 10% of patients that do not completely respond to conservative management, operative intervention is indicated. Surgical management involves resection of the affected extensor origin and direct repair.

The etiology of this disease process is believed to involve a small tear at the extensor origin, although the clinical presentation at surgery is quite variable: a tear may not be apparent at exploration. Postoperatively, the patient is maintained in an above-elbow cast for 3 weeks, after which he or she is referred to hand therapy for range of motion and strengthening exercises.

Findings on Examination

	Lateral Epicondylitis	Radial Tunnel Syndrome
Maximal tenderness	Lateral epicondyle	5 cm distal to lateral epicondyle
Middle finger test	Negative	Positive
Xylocaine block	Infiltration at the lateral epicondyle resolves symptoms	Infiltration 5 cm distal to lateral epicondyle: relieves pain and produces radial nerve palsy
Electrodiagnostic studies	Negative	Evidence of radial nerve compression

Clinical Pearls

1. The treatment for lateral epicondylitis is conservative. Surgery is reserved for the 10% of patients who are nonresponsive to therapy.
2. In patients who do require surgical repair, specific postoperative therapy is required to regain range of motion (particularly at the elbow) and strength.
3. Overaggressive resection of the extensor mechanism at the lateral epicondyle risks posteriolateral elbow instability, due to disruption or resection of the lateral collateral and annular ligaments of the elbow.

REFERENCES

1. Froimson AI: Tenosynovitis and tennis elbow. In Green DP, Hotchkiss R, Pederson WC (eds): Green's Operative Hand Surgery, 4th ed. New York, Churchill Livingstone, 1999.
2. Lister GD, Belsole RB, Kleinert HE: The radial tunnel syndrome. J Hand Surg 4:52–59, 1979.
3. Nirschl RP, Pettrone FA: Tennis elbow: The surgical treatment of lateral epicondylitis. J Bone Joint Surg 61:832–839, 1979.

Perspectives For Therapy

The pathophysiology of lateral epicondylitis (tennis elbow) can be most easily understood from the standpoint of muscle performance. Simply stated, when functional demands significantly outpace the metabolic and structural adaptability of the muscle-tendon unit, a series of pathologic changes occur, including fibrosis, avascularity, edema, and tissue breakdown. High local strains appear to be concentrated at the elbow, a fact explained by the relatively inextensible common extensor aponeurosis. While these changes can affect any of the extrinsic extensors, they overwhelmingly involve the extensor carpi radialis brevis (ECRB), and this finding is confirmed at surgery. The ECRB is the "workhorse" muscle among the extrinsic extensors, a conclusion supported by anatomical studies demonstrating that the ECRB has a large physiologic cross-section and is capable of producing tension over a relatively limited excursion.

The majority of patients with lateral epicondylitis respond favorably to conservative treatment, which includes dexamethasone iontophoresis administered over the lateral epicondyle. The manufacture's recommendations and patient comfort dictate current settings. Six to nine treatments may be employed, depending upon symptom relief. The role of phonophoresis in transdermal drug delivery remains controversial. Carefully controlled studies on humans using therapeutic frequencies and durations are needed to determine skin penetration. Until additional scientific support for the use of phonophoresis becomes available, dexamethasone iontophoresis may be a better choice.

Use of a counter-force brace or tennis elbow strap is also indicated. The patient should be issued the strap on the first therapy visit, or told where to purchase one and instructed about use.

While the precise biomechanical mechanism of action is controversial, the strap decreases the (1) duration of extensor muscle activity, and (2) angular acceleration of the elbow. Both factors may serve to limit internal forces concentrated at the common origin of the extrinsic extensors.

To provide an interval of *relative rest* for the extrinsic extensors, a custom-fabricated, forearm-based, dorsal block splint may be worn for 3–6 weeks. The splint immobilizes the patient's wrist in neutral, limiting extension and lateral plane motion.

The patient is educated about modifying home and work activities, adjusting work stations, and evaluating and adjusting work tools as practical. The patient is also instructed in the Mill's stretch, to be performed before participating in racquet sports and each hour during the workday. Stretches consist of extending the elbow and, with the forearm pronated, flexing and ulnarly deviating the wrist—gentle overpressure may be added at the dorsum of the hand. The stretch is held for up to 10 seconds and repeated 5–7 times.

As pain symptoms resolve, the patient is instructed in a home exercise program. Currently, emphasis is shifting away from the classic home programs consisting of isolated wrist exercises using free weights, or weights suspended from a coil of rope. These activities may not be well-tolerated for two reasons. First, they have the potential to overload the numerous small joints in the wrist, and second, they fatigue the extrinsic extensors.

A much more desirable home program is now emerging, designed to improve the strength and condition of the large *proximal* upper extremity muscles, and it progresses to the *distal* muscles. Exercises that are well-tolerated rely on graded rubber bands or tubes and emphasize shoulder abduction, diagonal patterns, extension, external/internal rotation, flexion, and horizontal abduction/adduction. Elbow extension/flexion and forearm rotation are added later, and there appears to be a sufficient carry-over effect to recondition the extrinsic wrist extensors. Patients are instructed in achieving and sustaining neutral wrist mechanics during submaximal exercise. The home program is performed once daily, with up to 10 repetitions of each exercise. As fatigability improves, the intensity of exercise is gradually increased. In this case, the patient's avocational weight-training program at her health club must also be reviewed with an eye toward discontinuing provocative exercises and encouraging neutral wrist mechanics.

Patients who wish to return to racquet sports are encouraged to work with a qualified trainer to help improve technique. It is critical that the patient use a racquet of appropriate size, shape, and weight, with regard also given to handle diameter. String tension must be adjusted to minimize risk of reinjury. On court use of ice may help control pain symptoms.

Depending upon the extent of surgery to manage lateral epicondylitis, there may be variation in postoperative treatment, per the referring hand surgeon's discretion. In this case, discontinuation of the above-elbow cast at 3 weeks is followed by fabrication of a custom, forearm-based, thermoplastic splint. The splint immobilizes the patient's wrist in 20–30° extension and may be designed for either dorsal or volar placement.

The wrist splint is worn for up to 3 weeks, and the patient is instructed in active elbow and forearm exercises while wearing it. It is absolutely essential that the patient regain full active elbow extension and flexion within a very few days following discontinuation of the cast. Joint mobilization, contract-relax techniques, and gentle, passive-motion exercises may be initiated to regain full active elbow motion.

The patient is also instructed in active wrist exercises performed with the elbow positioned in full flexion. Exercises may be performed 6–8 times daily with up to 10 repetitions. The rationale for reciprocal wrist and elbow position during exercise is to protect the operated common extensor origin and lateral epicondyle.

With discontinuation of the wrist splint, the patient is instructed in general upper extremity strengthening and conditioning exercises as described above.

Hand Therapy Pearls

1. The etiology of lateral epicondylitis may be understood in terms of muscle performance. When functional demand significantly outpaces the metabolic and structural adaptability of muscle, a series of pathological changes occur, and these overwhelmingly involve the ECRB.

2. Dexamethasone iontophoresis, counterforce bracing, and an interval of *relative* rest, offered by a custom splint, remain the mainstays of conservative treatment.

3. Emerging home programs include strengthening and conditioning exercises that emphasize large *proximal* muscles and progress to *distal* groups.

4. Avocational activities, such as participation in racquet sports and health programs, must be carefully monitored to ensure proper technique and high-quality equipment.

5. Postoperative management may vary according to the extent of surgery and hand surgeon's discretion. Protected active elbow, forearm, and wrist motion are encouraged, and it is essential that the patient recover full active elbow motion within a very short time following discontinuation of the postoperative cast.

REFERENCES

1. Blue C, Harris K, Hurov J, et al: Treatment guidelines for post-operative management of lateral epicondylitis. In Treatment Guidelines for the Upper Extremity, 2nd ed. Winston-Salem, Bowman Gray/Baptist Medical Center, 1995, pp 10–12.
2. Cannon NM: Tendinitis/Tenosynovitis. In Diagnosis and Treatment Manual for Physicians and Therapists, 3rd ed. Indianapolis, The Hand Rehabilitation Center of Indiana, 1991, p 176.
3. Ellenbecker TS: Rehabilitation of humeral epicondylitis. In Surgery and Rehabilitation of the Hand with Emphasis on the Elbow. Philadelphia, Hand Rehabilitation Foundation, 2001, pp 140–142.
4. Gellman H: Tennis elbow (lateral epicondylitis). Orthop Clin North Am 23:75–82, 1992.
5. Groppel JL, Nirschl RP: A mechanical and electromyographical analysis of the effects of various joint counterforce braces on the tennis player. Am J Sports Med 14:195–200, 1986.
6. Lieber RL, Fazeli BM, Botte MJ: Architecture of selected wrist flexor and extensor muscles. J Hand Surg 15A:244–250, 1990.
7. Lieber RL, Jacobson MD Fazeli BM, et al: Architecture of selected muscles of the arm and forearm: Anatomy and implications for tendon transfer. J Hand Surg 17A:787–798, 1992.

PATIENT 48

A 35-year-old man with a painful hand lesion

A 35-year-old man is referred to you for evaluation and a second opinion: his primary care physician has been treating him for the past 8 weeks without success. Your patient owns a pet store, and cannot recall any specific injury. He does admit to occasional occupational scratches from dogs when he is grooming them at work, and also minor cuts when collecting coral or changing the layout of one of his reef tank aquariums on display at his store. His main complaint is of pain and swelling around a non-healing wound; he also complains of a modestly decreased range of motion. He originally did not think much of, nor particularly notice, the sore on his dorsal hand, but after 2 weeks (when it had become progressively more tender and still had not healed) he presented to his primary care physician. Cultures were negative; he has been treated with various antibiotics (cephazolin, cephotetan, ciprofloxacin).

Physical Examination: General: afebrile; denies any fevers. Musculoskeletal: unclear whether decreased ROM is due to physical blocking by swelling, or pain (or both). Skin: small, open wound on dorsal aspect of hand between index and long MCP joints (see figure); swelling and soft-tissue fullness, but no erythema. Palpation: epitrochlear lymphadenopathy, but no axillary adenopathy.

Laboratory Findings: WBC 8400/μl, ESR 8 (both normal).

Questions: What is your presumptive diagnosis? What diagnostic testing do you recommend? What treatment do you recommend?

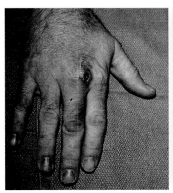 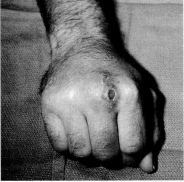

Answers: Presumptive diagnosis is *Mycobacterium marinum* infection. Recommend biopsy of proliferative synovium for histologic analysis and AFB culture. If strong clinical suspicion, start anti-tuberculosis antibiotic therapy.

Discussion: Mycobacterial infections of the hand are usually caused by *M. marinum*, although *M. kansasii, M. avium, M. bovis, M. tuberculosis,* and *M. intracellulare* can also be cultured in hand infections. *M. marinum* is associated with saltwater or marine environments, and thus is commonly associated with swimming or fish handling. The infection is usually slow and insidious; it rarely causes systemic complaints such as fever, and it rarely produces an elevation in white cell count or ESR. The most common symptom is painful swelling, representing the proliferation of synovium. Quite often this synovial proliferation will require surgical debridement in conjunction with antituberculosis agents to clear the infection.

The diagnosis is suggested by histologic examination of the synovium, which will show dermal and subdermal granulomas and/or Langerhans-type giant cells. The diagnosis can be confirmed with proper culture. These cultures need to be incubated at 30–32° C (standard cultures are at 37°) and incubated on Lowenstein-Jensen medium; they often take up to 6 weeks to become positive.

Synovectomy and debridement are often required in addition to prolonged antituberculosis antibiotic therapy (up to a year). Current protocols include various combinations of isoniazid, ethambutol, and rifampin for 9 to 12 months. Infectious disease consultation should be obtained to assist in guiding that aspect of the therapy.

Clinical Pearls

1. *M. marinum* is the most commonly encountered atypical bacterial infection in the hand. Commonly associated with marine environments, people far from the ocean may still come in contact via hobbyist aquarium exposure.

2. Strong clinical suspicion is the key to making the diagnosis: routine cultures and lab work typically do not provide any clues. Histologic analysis of the synovium and affected skin will show the characteristic granulomas of this disease process. Special AFB cultures will confirm the diagnosis.

REFERENCES
1. Gunther SF, Elliott RC, Brand RL, Adams JP: Experience with atypical mycobacterial infection in the deep structures of the hand. J Hand Surg 2:90–96, 1977.
2. Gunther SF, Levy CS: Mycobacterial infections. Hand Clin 5:591–598, 1989.
3. Hurst LC, Amadio PC, Badalamente MA, et al: *Mycobacterium marinum* infections of the hand. J Hand Surg 12:428–435, 1987.
4. Wagner RF, Tawil AB, Colletta AJ, et al: *Mycobacterium marinum* tenosynovitis in a Long Island fisherman. N Y State J Med 81:1091–1094, 1981.

Hand Therapy Pearls

1. Hand therapy includes fabrication of a custom, hand-based, volar splint to rest the patient's hand in the intrinsic-plus position. The thumb can be omitted from the splint design, and the splint is worn between exercise sessions and at bedtime.

2. Unless contraindicated, due to concern about risk of spreading infection, tendon gliding exercises are beneficial. The intrinsic-minus position, for differential recruitment of ED, is prioritized.

3. Following surgery, edema management, including elevation and cohesive dressings, is mandatory. Wound care may also be indicated, following the hand surgeon's guidelines.

Continues on next page.

4. Once surgical wounds are healed and sutures removed, particular attention needs to be paid to scar management, to minimize adherence of the extensor mechanism in Zone 5.

5. The hand therapist should be poised to initiate extensor tendon treatment, following Zone 5 guidelines, should it be necessitated by synovectomy and debridement.

REFERENCE

Nathan R, Taras JS: Common infections in the hand. In Hunter JM, Mackin EJ, Callahan AD (eds). Rehabilitation of the Hand: Surgery and Therapy, 4th ed. St. Louis, Mosby, 1995, pp 251–260.

PATIENT 49

A 26-year-old man with acute onset of wrist pain after a fall

A 26-year-old, male carpenter fell headfirst approximately 12 feet from scaffolding at work. He landed on his outstretched hands. He has been brought into the emergency department complaining of significant right hand pain and swelling. Other than his hand symptoms, he has no other complaints or injuries (he has been evaluated and discharged by the trauma service).

Physical Examination: Skin: diffusely edematous and tender at right hand and wrist; no lacerations, but superficial abrasions both volarly and dorsally. Neurologic: markedly decreased sensation at volar right thumb, index, and long fingers; sensation normal on ring and fifth fingers. Musculoskeletal: no abnormalities of flexor and extensor tendons; FDP, FDS, FPL, EDC, and EPL all intact; no bony or ligamentous instability of digits; wrist ROM significantly limited by pain.

Laboratory Findings: Radiographs: see figures.

Questions: What is your diagnosis? What are your treatment recommendations?

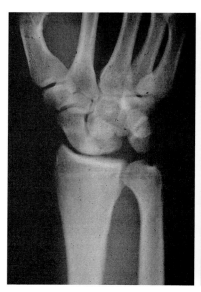 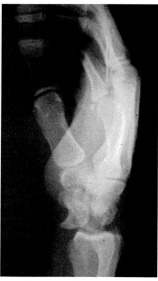

Answers: Acute perilunate dislocation with median nerve impingement. Recommend emergent exploration and operative fixation to decompress the median nerve.

Discussion: Perilunate dislocation is the most common dislocation pattern at the wrist level. This is most likely due to the very strong attachment of the lunate to the radius in combination with its relatively weak attachment to the carpus: with sufficient force, the weaker distal ligamentous support is disrupted, allowing bony displacement. The scaphoid often fractures in injuries of this type (transcaphoid perilunate fracture-dislocation). The transosseous fracture dislocations are also termed "greater arc injuries," while the ligament-only perilunate injuries are termed "lesser arc injuries." This nomenclature simply reflects the path of the forces that have acted on and disrupted the carpus.

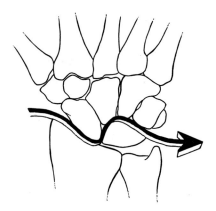

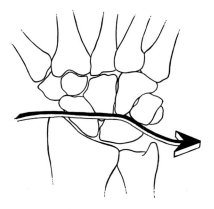

In greater arc injuries, the force travels radially through the midportion of the scaphoid and continues just distal to the lunate (see figure, *above*). In lesser arc injuries, the disruption pathway travels through the scapholunate interval (see figure, *right*). In both injuries, the force is then transmitted through the space of Poirier (the lunate-capitate articulation) and travels through (possibly disrupting) the lunate-triquetral articulation.

In more severe cases (such as in the present patient), the lunate can be displaced volarly into the carpal tunnel. When this occurs, the lunate typically remains attached volarly, and is "tipped"

down into the carpal tunnel (since the volar ligaments are typically much stronger than the dorsal ones, they are the last to be disrupted in injuries like this). Volar rotation of the lunate can cause significant impingement on the median nerve, and if this is symptomatic, urgent decompression is indicated to minimize the possibility of permanent nerve injury.

These injuries do reflect a significant amount of force: it requires a great deal of energy to detach the lunate from the distal carpus. The common mechanism is the same as for a Colles' fracture (fall on an outstretched hand, hyperdorsiflexion). Radiographs of the injury typically are dramatic because the linear alignment of the capitate, lunate, and radius is disrupted; the capitate is often located dorsal to the lunate (see figure, *next page*).

The surgical approach may be dorsal, volar, or both, depending on the type and severity of the injury as well as surgeon preference. Clearly, when neurologic impairment is occurring due to lunate compression on the median nerve (as in the present patient), a volar component is required. The volar approach also facilitates operative repair in patients with scaphoid fractures. This author (MC) often uses both a dorsal and volar approach to these injuries, to facilitate anatomic reduction and optimize surgical efforts at repair.

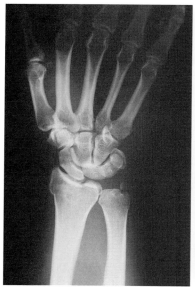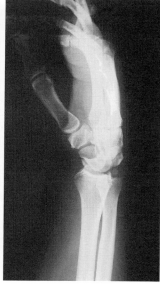

Clinical Pearls

1. Symptoms of median nerve compression (via impingement by the lunate) are an indication for urgent surgical decompression.

2. Quite often in transosseous injuries, the fractured segment of the scaphoid or the capitate is devascularized. There is a higher risk of nonunion and avascular necrosis in these individuals.

3. A tremendous amount of force is required to disrupt the carpus in perilunate dislocations, and the injury to the soft tissue and osseous structures of the carpus can be devastating. Warn patients that some late loss of motion in wrist mobility is likely, and they are at significant risk (nearly 60%) of developing arthritic degeneration requiring further surgical intervention.

4. Transcaphoid perilunate fracture-dislocations are twice as common as lesser arc injuries (with no bony fractures) and carry a higher than usual risk for avascular necrosis of the proximal scaphoid fragment.

REFERENCES
1. Cooney WP, Bussey R, Dobyns JH, Linscheid RL: Difficult wrist fractures: Perilunate fracture-dislocations of the wrist. Clin Orthop 214:136–147, 1987.
2. Herzberg G, Comtet JJ, Linscheid RL, et al: Perilunate dislocations and fracture-dislocations: A multicenter study. J Hand Surg 18:768–779, 1993.
3. Mayfield JK, Johnson RP, Kilcoyne RK: Carpal dislocations: Pathomechanics and progressive perilunar instability. J Hand Surg 5:226–241, 1980.
4. Panting AL, Lamb DW, Noble J, Haw CS: Dislocations of the lunate with and without fracture of the scaphoid. J Bone Joint Surg Br 66:391–395, 1984.

Perspectives For Therapy

The initial presentation of perilunate dislocation may be underestimated or missed because of multitrauma. Note that delay in treatment has a uniformly negative impact on outcome measures, including pain, motion, strength, and return to pre-injury level of activity.

Perilunate dislocation represents a high-energy injury. There is considerable soft-tissue disruption, which predisposes the patient to significant edema, scar formation, and adhesions. Therefore, early postoperative referral to hand therapy for instruction in active exercise for the *uninvolved* joints of the upper extremity—hand, elbow, and shoulder—is highly beneficial.

Following discontinuation of closed reduction, 4–6 weeks postoperatively, a volar, forearm-based, thumb spica splint with a radial gutter component is fabricated for patient use for up to 8 weeks. The patient's wrist is supported in neutral to minimize pressure on the median nerve, and the thumb IP joint is left free. Active exercises for wrist and forearm are added at this time, with continued splint use between exercise sessions and at bedtime.

It is important to evaluate sensory status on an ongoing basis, particularly with documented paresthesia in the median nerve distribution, and educate the patient accordingly. Intrinsic thenar muscle function should also be tested.

With complete healing of an associated scaphoid fracture, usually at 14 weeks postoperatively, splint use may be discontinued, and general upper extremity strengthening and conditioning exercises initiated.

Hand Therapy Pearls

1. Delay in treatment of perilunate dislocation has a uniformly negative impact on outcome measures.
2. Early postoperative referral to hand therapy is crucial.
3. Four to six weeks postoperatively, treatment comprises splint use and active exercises for the wrist and forearm.

REFERENCES

1. Herzberg G, Comtet JJ, Linscheid RL, et al: Perilunate dislocations and fracture-dislocations: A multicenter study. J Hand Surg 18A:768–779, 1993.
2. Inoue G, Imaeda T: Management of trans-scaphoid perilunate dislocations. Herbert screw fixation, ligamentous repair and early wrist mobilization. Arch Orthop Trauma Surg 116:338–340, 1997.
3. Levine WR: Rehabilitation techniques for ligament injuries of the wrist. Hand Clin 8:669–681, 1992.
4. Prosser R, Herbert T: The management of carpal fractures and dislocations. J Hand Ther 9:139–147, 1996.

PATIENT 50

A 30-year-old surgery resident with wrist pain after a fall

A 30-year-old man was rollerblading on his day off, when he tripped and fell forward onto his hands. He was wearing wrist and knee protectors and a helmet. He presented to the emergency department (ED) primarily for treatment of multiple abrasions. On evaluation, he did complain of some right wrist and hand pain, prompting the ED physician to obtain radiographs. Although he cannot detect any injuries, he consults you to definitively rule out any hand injury.

Physical Examination: Neurologic: sensation intact over median, radial, and ulnar nerve distributions of both hands. Musculoskeletal: full active and passive range of motion of all fingers and both wrists; soreness on extreme wrist flexion and extension. Palpation: no tenderness except at radial right wrist over 2nd extensor compartment (see figure, *top*).

Laboratory Findings: Radiographs (obtained by ED physician): see figure, *bottom*.

Questions: What is your recommendation? What is your presumptive diagnosis?

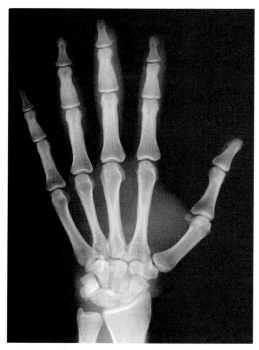

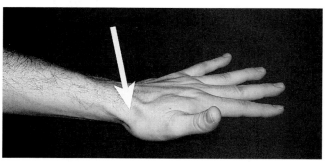

Answers: Long-arm thumb spica cast; repeat examination and radiographs in 7–10 days. Presumptive diagnosis is possible scaphoid fracture.

Discussion: In your evaluation, the radiograph shows no evidence of any bony injury or fracture. However, your patient is tender at the anatomic snuffbox, which is one of the symptoms of scaphoid injury. It is quite common for scaphoid fractures to be invisible on initial x-rays. Therefore, if a patient presents with an injury in which a significant amount of force has been transferred to the wrist (i.e., falling on an outstretched hand, perhaps the most common etiology for scaphoid and distal radius fractures) and has anatomic snuffbox tenderness, the presumptive diagnosis should be of scaphoid fracture (until proven otherwise). It is better to err on the side of caution (overtreat) than to potentially miss a fracture and allow it to progress to nonunion.

Scaphoid fractures are commonly classified based on the location of the fracture within the bone: distal, middle, and proximal thirds. The location of the fracture has some impact on prognosis of bony healing. The blood supply to the scaphoid enters at the *distal dorsal* aspect of the bone, and therefore distal fractures (the rarest of the scaphoid fractures) usually heal well because they are so well vascularized. Middle-third fractures (the most common location of fractures within the scaphoid) also usually heal with immobilization alone, as long as they are not displaced. Proximal-third fractures (see figure, *right*) have the highest incidence of avascular necrosis and nonunion because of the scaphoid vascular pattern and the propensity for loss of the blood supply at the time of injury. In these higher-risk fractures, open reduction and internal fixation (ORIF)—with a cannulated screw, see figure *next page*—is indicated to hopefully improve chance of bony union.

Surgical fixation of scaphoid fractures has been made more efficacious by the development of cannulated screws. The Herbert screw is a specialized device that was quite widely used for the open treatment of these fractures; it has a differential pitch on the screw, which helps provide compression of the two bone fragments. While it remains available today, its use is limited because it is technically challenging to properly place, and requires

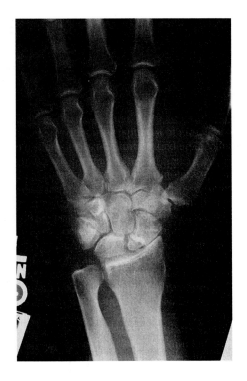

resection of a portion of the trapezium for the specialized jig placement. Currently, cannulated screw systems are available that allow direct or percutaneous placement of a K-wire across the scaphoid fracture, and then placement of the screw over this guide. Compression of the fracture can be easily accomplished with these systems as well.

Scaphoid healing may take a protracted length of time; 4–6 months of immobilization (or longer) has been advocated if necessary. If scaphoid nonunion does occur, bone grafting (such as corticocancellous graft from the distal radius or iliac crest) or vascularized graft is indicated to attempt to promote bone healing. If arthritic changes begin to occur (the late sequelae of scaphoid nonunion and scapholunate dissociation is dorsal intercalated segment instability), salvage procedures such as proximal row carpectomy or four-corner fusion may be required.

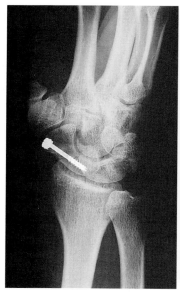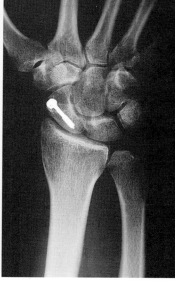

Clinical Pearls

1. Any patient with a history of a fall on an outstretched hand should be checked for anatomic snuffbox tenderness. If this is present, treat presumptively for a scaphoid fracture.

2. Fractures of the proximal pole should be surgically fixed to decrease the risk of nonunion. All displaced fractures should be surgically reduced and fixed. Remember during surgery that the blood supply enters the scaphoid distally and dorsally: do not disrupt this supply in the course of the surgical procedure.

3. If the plain films are nonconclusive, a CT scan or MRI should be done after prolonged immobilization if the patient complains of persistent pain.

REFERENCES
1. Amadio PC, Berquist TH, Smith DK, et al: Scaphoid malunion. J Hand Surg 14:679–687, 1989.
2. Cooney WP, Dobyns JH, Linscheid RL: Fractures of the scaphoid: A rational approach to management. Clin Orthop 149:90–97, 1980.
3. Cooney WP III, Dobyns JH, Linscheid RL: Nonunion of the scaphoid: Analysis of the results from bone grafting. J Hand Surg 5:343–354, 1980.
4. Herbert TJ, Fisher WE: Management of the fractured scaphoid using a new screw. J Bone Joint Surg 66:114–123, 1984.
5. Mack GR, Bosse MJ, Gelberman RH, Yu E: The natural history of scaphoid non-union. J Bone Joint Surg 66:504–509, 1984.

Perspectives For Therapy

In some clinical settings, the hand therapist may be called upon to provide evidence that confirms or disconfirms suspected scaphoid injuries. It is therefore important that the hand therapist have an appreciation for the locations and contents of the various wrist compartments and be capable of performing a thorough wrist evaluation. This requires a palpatory examination and provocative testing, including, for example, the scaphoid shift test. Of course, the hand therapist must also be able to interpret and communicate the results of the examination, and understand its implications and limitations.

Scaphoid fractures are second in frequency among wrist injuries, after distal radius fractures, and they are first in frequency, up to 79%, among carpal fractures. Conservative treatment options include immobilization with the Muenster, thumb spica, or Philadelphia splint, and the choice of splint is based on the degree to which immobilization of the patient's forearm and wrist is needed. Regardless of design, custom splints are indicated for patients with acute scaphoid fractures, malunions, and nonunions, and they are worn at all times, with the exception of during hygiene tasks.

The **Meunster splint** is a one-piece, radial gutter, forearm-based orthosis that positions the patient's elbow in 90° flexion and forearm and wrist in neutral (see figure *A*, next page). The Meunster splint provides the most stability of the three aforementioned splints, limiting forearm rotation and wrist motion.

A **volar forearm–based, thumb spica splint,** that includes a radial gutter component, offers support of the wrist and thumb to the level of the MCP joint. This splint is also a one-piece design, and permits forearm rotation (see *B* and *C*).

The **Philadelphia splint** is a two-piece, custom orthosis comprising a dorsal hand–based, thumb spica component and a dorsal forearm–based component. These two components are united at the wrist at both the radial and ulnar borders using flexible polypropylene rods (see *D*). The articulated design of the Philadelphia splint permits up to 30° each of active wrist extension and flexion, while limiting radial and ulnar deviation. Forearm rotation is also permitted by the Philadelphia splint.

Open reduction and internal fixation of scaphoid fracture has the potential to provide a stable construct permitting early active wrist, forearm, and elbow motion at 7–14 days postoperatively. Active exercise is the mainstay of treatment through 6 weeks, when passive motion and joint mobilization techniques may be initiated. Custom splints such as the Philadelphia and thumb spica may be worn between exercise sessions and at bedtime for protection.

Progressive resisted exercise, using graded rubber band or tubes, may be initiated at 8–12 weeks postoperatively. Emphasis in therapy is placed on general upper extremity strengthening and conditioning, rather than on isolated wrist strengthening exercises and forceful gripping—both of which may jeopardize fracture fixation.

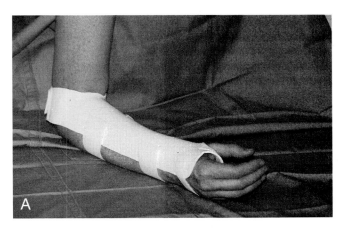

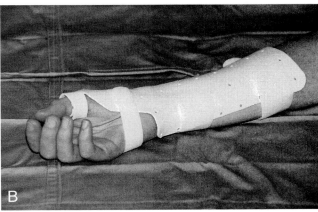

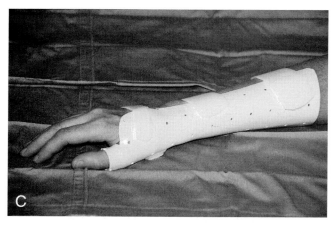

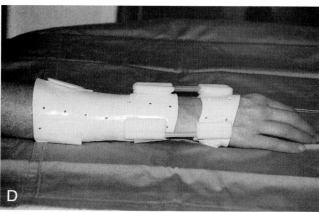

Hand Therapy Pearls

1. In some clinical settings, the hand therapist may be called upon to provide evidence that confirms or disconfirms suspected scaphoid injuries. He or she must also be able to interpret and communicate the results of the examination, and understand its implications and limitations.

2. Conservative treatment options include the Muenster, thumb spica, and Philadelphia splints. Splint choice depends upon the need to immobilize the patient's forearm and wrist.

3. Early active wrist motion is indicated following ORIF of scaphoid fracture, providing the construct is stable.

REFERENCES
1. Amadio PC, Taleisnik J: Fractures of the carpal bones. In Green DP, Hotchkiss RN, Pederson WC (eds): Green's Operative Hand Surgery 4th ed. Philadelphia, Churchill Livingstone, 1999, pp 809–864.
2. Bora WF, Culp RW, Osterman AL, et al: A flexible wrist splint. J Hand Surg 14A:574–575, 1989.
3. Jeter E, Degnan GG, Lichtman DM: Postoperative wrist rehabilitation. In Lichtman DM, Alexander AH (eds): The Wrist and its Disorders 2nd ed. Philadelphia, Saunders, 1997, pp 709–714.
4. LaStayo P, Howell J: Clinical provocative tests used in evaluating wrist pain: A descriptive study. J Hand Ther 8:10–17, 1995.
5. Skirven T: Clinical examination of the wrist. J Hand Ther 9:96–107, 1996.

PATIENT 51

A 45-year-old surgeon with thumb avulsion

A 45-year-old cardiothoracic surgeon who is on staff with you at the local hospital is rushed to the emergency department (ED) after having his dominant thumb amputated in an avulsion injury while working at his brother's farm. According to the patient, he was wearing work gloves and helping his brother with various chores around the farm, when he inadvertently became entangled at the power takeoff on the back of the tractor they were using. His glove (containing his thumb) was pulled from his hand. The two men immediately retrieved the digit and came directly to the ED.

Your patient is a nonsmoker, and he has no other hand injuries. His only other medical conditions include hypertension (he is on Lopressor) and a history of attention deficit disorder. He drinks 6 to 8 cups of coffee a day.

Physical Examination: Thumb avulsed at the MCP joint; tendons and nerves avulsed from forearm and attached to thumb. No other hand injuries.

Laboratory Findings: Radiographs: no other fractures or dislocations.

Question: Should replantation be attempted, or should he be counseled to have a thumb reconstruction?

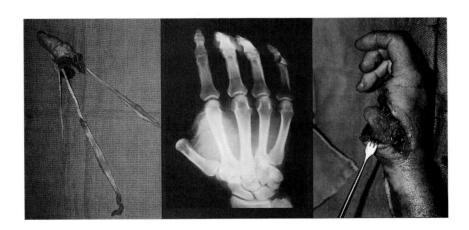

Answer: Although he does have a relative contraindication to replantation (avulsion type injury), he also has a relative indication (thumb amputation). Assuming he desires attempted replantation, he is a candidate.

Discussion: The relative indications and contraindications for replantation have been discussed extensively in Case 39. Recall that these are all *relative;* there is no easy, cookbook formula as to who is and who is not a candidate for attempted replantation. Preoperatively, this patient should be warned that the procedure has a higher risk of failure secondary to arterial intimal damage and risk of late thrombosis.

In this scenario, the prognosis is grim due to the mechanism of injury: the avulsive mechanism destroys the intima layer of the arteries proximal and distal to the actual site of amputation. The surgeon needs to be aware of this and plan to resect all damaged vessel (to be replaced with vein graft). The damaged segment of artery can be identified under magnification. Vessel walls may be ecchymotic, and the intima may appear physically separated from the media (creating two concentric lumens, one within the other, when looking down the vessel). The situation may be that after resecting the entire damaged portion of the artery, there is insufficient vessel distally to revascularize. In such a case, replantation is simply not possible.

When it has been decided that the patient is a replantation candidate, the surgeon should proceed immediately to the operating room (OR) with the amputated part to begin exploration. It may take an hour or so for the patient to be brought to the OR (while awaiting lab tests, anesthesiology evaluation, etc.). During that time, the digital structures (arteries, veins, nerves, tendons) can be identified and tagged with suture. The flexor tendons can be tagged with braided nonabsorbable suture using the Tajima technique: repair then is simply a matter of tying the proximal to the distal Tajima repairs.

When performing thumb replantation, particularly in an avulsion situation, there may not be enough uninjured veins present on the thumb for primary venous repair. In that case, consider taking the large dorsal vein (see figure above, *arrows*) from the radial aspect of the index finger. This vessel can be dissected reliably as far distally as the PIP joint, and then mobilized to the dorsal thumb. This can give greater vessel length to reach uninjured vessels on the amputated thumb.

Access to the volar thumb structures is difficult (i.e., if attempting to repair the digital artery). During revascularization, consider connecting a vein graft from the proximal radial artery at the

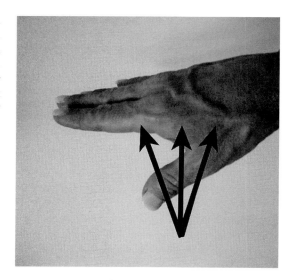

anatomic snuffbox to the ulnar digital artery of the thumb (see figure below, *black line*). This allows direct access to both microvascular anastomoses and has the added advantage of using a larger-caliber inflow vessel that is outside of the zone of injury.

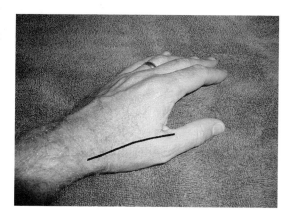

If the replantation is successful, there is still a higher risk of postoperative thrombosis and digit loss in avulsion injuries (see figure, *next page*). This risk of thrombosis can be reduced by the continuous infusion of heparin at a low dose just proximal to the proximal vein graft anastamosis. The infusion can be at 500 units an hour, small enough to not have a significant effect on systemic coagulation, but enough to protect the anastomosis until repair of the endothelium has occurred.

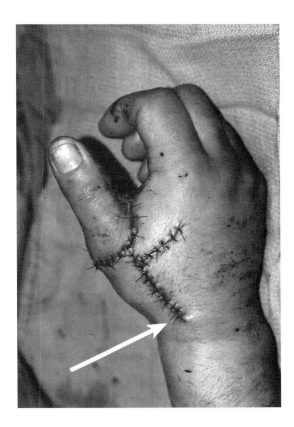

Clinical Pearls

1. When performing thumb replantation, there may be difficulty finding adequate venous outflow to reconnect. Consider using the nearly constant vein that lies on the radial aspect of the index finger.

2. Access to the volar thumb structures is difficult. Consider taking the vein graft from the proximal radial artery at the anatomic snuffbox to the ulnar digital artery of the thumb.

REFERENCES
1. Dellon AL: Sensory recovery in replanted digits and transplanted toes: A review. J Reconstr Microsurg 2:123–129, 1986.
2. Gould JS, Gould SH, Caudill-Babkes EL: Interpositional microvascular vein grafting. Hand 11:332–336, 1979.
3. Merle M, Dautel G: Advances in digital replantation. Clin Plast Surg 24:87–105, 1997.
4. Tseng OF, Tsai YC, Wei FC, Staffenberg DA: Replantation of ring avulsion of index, long, and ring fingers. Ann Plast Surg 36:625–628, 1996.

Perspectives For Therapy

Postoperative rehabilitation of the patient with replantation of an amputated upper extremity part is highly challenging both from technical and personal standpoints. The cornerstone of a well-planned postoperative therapy program is establishment of realistic goals for the patient, and this requires excellent communication among the patient, family members, hand surgeon, and hand therapist.

A replanted upper extremity part requires consideration of skeletal connective tissues, muscle tissue, neurovascular tissues, and integumentary tissues. Treating all of these tissues, regardless of the level of injury, necessitates an understanding of basic priniciples of wound care and edema management, splinting, and protected motion to restore upper extremity function and appearance.

The guidelines presented here are intended as a general framework that can be used for patient treatment during early rehabilitation, i.e., from 1 week to 5 weeks postoperatively. Of course, in the hand clinic, treatment will be individualized to meet the specific demands of each patient.

Wound care and edema management. Replantation of an amputated upper extremity part involves multiple tissue types that heal at different rates. Epithelialization and contraction of uncomplicated, sutured integumentary wounds may be complete in several days to several weeks. On the other hand, clinical bone healing (stability of a fracture site) may take 6–8 weeks. The goal of hand therapy is to ensure uncomplicated wound healing within this variable milieu. This goal is accomplished by minimizing the exposure of healing tissues to physical stress. Physical stress in healing tissues (1) prolongs inflammation and edema, (2) decreases oxygen perfusion within the wound environment, and (3) contributes to increased scar tissue formation. Remember that "fibroblasts follow macrophages." Thus, the prolonged appearance of inflammatory cells and their products in the wound environment heralds fibroblast recruitment, collagen synthesis, and a predictable increase in scar tissue formation.

Continuous elevation of the operated extemity at heart level is the mainstay of early edema management, and the skin must be monitored for signs of vascular insufficiency. Decreased arterial flow is indicated by pale, cool skin; cyanotic or violaceous skin may indicate venous congestion and decreased outflow. While upper extremity elevation is an assist to venous and lymphatic return to the heart, it can impede vascular inflow, particularly in repaired arteries that may be prone to vasospasm. Many patients believe that by maintaining their elbow in flexion with their hand postioned at the level of the heart, they are practicing upper extremity elevation. This posture can actually impede circulation to the replanted part, and patients must be educated to elevate their entire upper extremity to the level of the heart *with the elbow in extension.*

Cohesive dressings, applied distal-to-proximal in a circumferential manner are recommended for edema control once revascularization has occurred. Cotton dressings are desirable for use against sutured wounds because they permit air circulation. With suture removal, non-cotton cohesive dressings can be substituted. Cohesive dressings are economical to use because they can be reused.

Regardless of the specific wound dressings employed, they should be changed when they become soiled or struck through with serosanguinous drainage; even petrolatum-gauze dressings can become adherent to wounds. Although it is time con-

suming in a fast-moving clinic, adherent dressings should be removed, causing as little trauma to underlying healing tissues as possible. Trauma can be avoided by applying a saline drizzle to the dressing. One tablespoon of salt dissolved in one quart of ordinary tapwater can be prepared for home use, and is very cost-effective.

Application of chemical agents including alcohol, peroxide, or peroxide:saline solutions for removing dressings and wound cleansing are to be condemned due to their cytotoxic effects on granulation tissue. Patients and family members must be educated about dressing removal and wound cleansing. Occasionally, healthcare workers also require tactful reminders. The price to be paid for violating the wound environment with careless removal of dressings and/or application of cytotoxic agents is prolonged wound healing and treatment time, increased scar tissue formation, and diminishment of patient rapport.

Carefully monitor ambient air temperature to avoid ischemia and vasoconstriction to the replanted part. The patient's diet should exclude caffeine, chocolate, and cheese; all are potent vasoconstrictors. Similarly, smoking and smoke exposure are prohibited due to the vasoconstrictive effects of nicotine.

Splinting. The goals of splinting during early postoperative rehabilitation of the patient with a replanted upper extremity part are: (1) to provide protection for the replanted part during tissue healing, and (2) to ensure optimum joint positioning. Optimal splinting, whether dorsal or volar-based, places ligaments at their elongated lengths. For example, the forearm is splinted in neutral rotation, wrist in 20° extension to 20° flexion, depending upon the location of repairs, finger MCP joints flexed 60–90°, and IP joints fully extended. The thumb is positioned in abduction, maintaining the dimension of the first webspace. Because the thumb accounts for approximately 80% of hand function, it is critical to ensure mobility of the first CMC joint.

With adequate skeletal fixation and intact motors, uninvolved joints are omitted from splint design, and unless contraindicated, these joints are permitted protected active motion.

Protected motion. The hand therapist member of the replantation team will review surgery reports, look at x-rays, and discuss precautions with the attending hand surgeon(s). The hand therapist will be familiar with those structures that were repaired, including the type(s) of skeletal fixation and joint(s) crossed, neurovascular and musculotendinous repairs, and wound appearance, including coverage and tissue condition. This information is used in an ongoing manner to educate the patient and family members, plan/modify treatment, and stage realistic goals.

Early protected motion begins approximately 1 week after replantation (range 4–14 days) and is directed toward mobilizing repaired tendons to minimize adhesion formation. Active-assist tenodesis exercises, consisting of wrist flexion and finger (or thumb) extension and wrist extension to neutral and finger (or thumb) flexion, are initially carried out under hand therapist supervision, and the patient is returned to the splint between exercise sessions. These exercises are taught to the patient so that he or she may actively participate in the rehabilitation.

At 7–21 days after replantation, tendon gliding exercises, consisting of intrinsic-plus and -minus hand positions, are initiated with the wrist in neutral. For the thumb, reciprocal motions consist of MCP and IP flexion with the CMC extended and, conversely, MCP and IP extension with the CMC flexed. Over the course of 2 weeks, exercises are progressed from passive positioning, to place-hold, to active-assist and active motion, and it is important to ensure full IP extension during and between exercise sessions. Finger-walking exercises, both "forward" and "back," improves reciprocal motion, coordination, and individuation. Opposition is an excellent means of actively engaging the thumb and fingers simultaneously, and enhances motion of the first CMC.

Whenever the hand therapist uses early protected motion to prioritize repaired tendons, external support must be provided to more slowly healing repaired fractures. This can be accomplished using manual support and through the use of gutter splints.

Wrist extension beyond neutral, combined with active thumb and finger flexion, may begin 4 weeks after replantation. This is followed by active composite thumb and finger extension as the wrist is brought into 20° flexion. These tenodesis exercises minimize passive tension in the antagonists during muscle activity. The compositely flexed fingers provide an ideal motion "stop" for the replanted thumb, and active thumb flexion can be progressed to the palm as the patient maintains the fingers in extension.

Joint-blocking exercises promote differential tendon gliding and are initiated 5 weeks after surgery. The patient should be encouraged to perform light ADLs, such as hand-writing (if the dominant hand was involved), dressing, grooming, and feeding, with the involved upper extremity.

Grade I and II oscillatory mobilization techniques may be applied early on one joint proximal to, or distal to, a fracture site. Involved joints are mobilized following removal of skeletal fixation. For example, early mobilization of the DIP joint and wrist are indicated following repair of a P1 fracture. If replantation of a disarticulated finger was effected through soft tissue reconstruction only (e.g., replantation of a finger at the MCP level), early Grade I mobilization of the MPJ may also performed.

Intermediate and late treatment guidelines. Starting 4–6 weeks after surgery, when sutures have been removed and skin grafts are revascularized, wound care consisting of desensitization, scar massage, and compression using elastomer putty or silicone gel sheeting is appropriate.

Active, active-assist, passive range of motion, and progressive resistive exercises are implemented. Dynamic, serial static, and static progressive splinting may be required to help increase motion, or to substitute for functional imbalance produced by motor nerve injury. However, fractures *must* be clinically healed prior to initiating passive motion exercises and applying any member of this family of splints.

Neuromuscular electric stimulation can also be used to recruit flexors and extensors. Tetanic tension can be achieved at 30 pps, and electrodes may be placed to achieve reciprocal activation. A 5-minute treatment interval using 10 seconds "on" and 20–30 seconds "off" is recommended to initiate reciprocal recruitment.

Despite the fact that peripheral nerve regeneration is limited to 1–4 mm/day, the hand therapist must evaluate sensory (and motor) nerve recovery. Significantly diminished protective sensation (threshold $\geq$ 4.31 Semmes-Weinstein monofilament, or 2.04 gmf), requires patient instruction in methods of compensation to protect soft tissues. Diminished protective sensation is a relative contraindication for the use of thermal modalities in the clinic much greater than 100° F due to an insensate replant. Moreover, the venous, lymphatic, and integumentary systems cannot dissipate heat effectively. Those patients in whom protective sensation is returning (thresholds less than the 4.31 Semmes-Weinstein monofilament), are candidates for discriminative sensory reeducation. Return of nerve function is highly predictive of functional use of the replanted part.

Hand Therapy Pearls

1. The specifics of each replantation case—wound coverage, neurovascular repairs, and extent and stability of musculoskeletal fixation—determine the hand therapist's treatment objectives.

2. Strict upper extremity elevation at the level of the heart, monitoring revascularization, and protection of the wound environment during dressing changes are critical for successful replantation of an upper extremity part.

3. Early splinting of the upper extremity with a replanted part should maintain ligaments in their lengthened positions at rest. Intermediate and late splinting are indicated to increase motion and substitute for muscle function.

4. Early protected motion prioritizes repaired tendons and is designed to minimized adhesions during interval healing. While skeletal fixation maintains alignment of fracture fragments, external manual support and that provided by gutter splints is also used during exercise. Progressive motion and strengthening are instituted as soon as tissue healing permits.

5. Return of nerve function will dictate patient candidacy for instruction in methods of compensation to protect soft tissues and for discriminative sensory reeducation.

REFERENCES

1. Buncke, HJ, Jackson RL, Buncke GM, et al. The surgical and rehabilitative aspects of replantation and revascularization of the hand. In Hunter JM, Mackin EJ, Callahan AD (eds): Rehabilitation of the Hand: Surgery and Therapy, 4th ed. St. Louis, Mosby, 1995, pp 1075–1100.
2. Burkhalter WE. Mutilating injuries of the hand. In Hunter JM, Mackin EJ, Callahan AD (eds): Rehabilitation of the Hand: Surgery and Therapy, 4th ed. St. Louis, Mosby, 1995, pp 1037–1056.
3. Silverman PM, Willette-Green V, Petrilli J. Early protected motion in digital revascularization and replantation. J Hand Ther 1989;2:84–101.
4. Stewart KM. Therapist's management of the complex injury. In Hunter JM, Mackin EJ, Callahan AD (eds): Rehabilitation of the Hand: Surgery and Therapy, 4th ed. St. Louis, Mosby, 1995, pp 1057–1073.

PATIENT 52

A 60-year-old gentleman with longstanding rheumatoid arthritis

A 60-year-old man is referred to you by his rheumatologist. He has longstanding rheumatoid arthritis and has been increasingly troubled with hand pain and a corresponding decrease in hand function. He has been reluctant to proceed with surgical options, preferring to get by with medical management alone. However, he has now reached the point where he is so symptomatic and has lost function to such a degree that he is willing to consider surgical intervention (if you recommend it).

Physical Examination: General: fingers ulnarly deviated at MCP joints; boggy soft tissue and fullness at dorsal MCP and PIP joints (see figure). Musculoskeletal: limited flexion of fingers, particularly at MCP joints; hyperflexion at thumb MCP joint; some resistance to flexion of index and long fingers (pain at volar proximal palmar crease with attempted flexion). Palpation: small nodules at this level move with finger flexion.

Laboratory Findings: Radiograph: see figure.

Question: What treatment modalities can you offer this patient that may decrease his pain and/or increase his function?

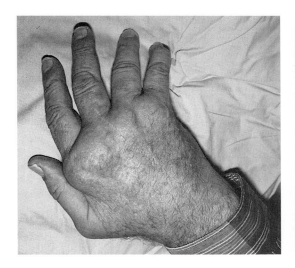 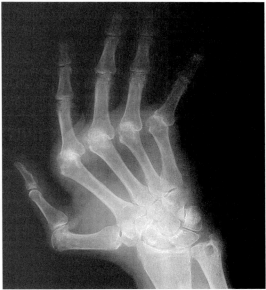

Answer: MCP joint replacement at the index, long, ring, and fifth fingers with silastic spacers; extensor tendon re-balancing; crossed intrinsic tendon transfer; extensive synovectomy; trigger finger release (index and long fingers); thumb exploration and possible MCP joint fusion.

Discussion: Entire texts have been devoted to the treatment of rheumatoid hand deformities. This discussion can only superficially address some of the major issues. This patient demonstrates several deformities typically seen in patients with severe hand involvement of rheumatoid disease. The diagnosis in this case includes proliferation of hypertrophic synovium (MCP and PIP levels); subluxation of the MCP joints with probable cartilaginous destruction; ulnar dislocation of the extensor mechanism at the MCP joints; shortening of the ulnar finger intrinsics; trigger finger (index and long); and boutonnière deformity (thumb).

Synovial proliferation is one of the earliest manifestations of this disease process in the hand. Microscopically, the synovium is infiltrated by inflammatory cells. It then becomes proliferative, invading bone, cartilage, and ligaments, and can displace normal anatomic structures (such as the ligaments supporting the joints or tendons). "Preemptive" synovectomy has been advocated as a preventative measure to prevent further deformity.

Subluxation of the MCP joints with extensor tendon displacement occurs secondary to synovial proliferation. Intrinsic contracture often follows. However, this intrinsic tightness may be idiopathic: if there is intrinsic tightness but the MCP joints have not subluxed, recurvatum will be present at that digit (swan neck deformity). In the usual case of longstanding MCP joint subluxation with ulnar deviation, the ulnar lateral bands are severely contracted.

A crossed intrinsic transfer, which is a useful method to maintain correction of ulnar deviation, can be done at the time of reconstruction. The contracted ulnar lateral band of the 5th finger is divided, allowing the 5th finger to assume its more radial (anatomic) position. The contracted ulnar lateral band to the **ring finger** is also divided, and sutured to the *radial* lateral band of the 5th finger, assisting in maintaining its normal position. Similarly, the ulnar lateral band to the long finger is divided, and sutured to the radial lateral band of

the ring finger. This procedure stabilizes the digits in the desired positions (in the correct radial-ulnar plane), preventing recurrence of ulnar deviation (see figure, *next page;* before and after MCP joint replacements with silicone spacers and crossed intrinsic transfers).

Treatment options at the MCP joint involve synovectomy, rebalancing of the extensor tendons, and release of the contracted intrinsics (with transfer to the adjacent ulnar digit, as discussed above). If there is a significant loss of or damage to the articular surface (noted intraoperatively) joint replacement is advocated. This is most commonly accomplished with silastic joint spacers such as the Swanson implants.

Stenosing tenosynovitis is common in rheumatoid patients, and is manifested in the present patient by triggering at the index and long fingers. Release of the A-1 pulley is sufficient to relieve these symptoms and improve mobility. It is important (after division of the pulley) to explore the tendons to make sure no further adhesions remain.

Derangements of the extensor mechanism are also common in patients with rheumatoid arthritis (RA). They may be manifest by a boutonnière deformity (as in this patient) or swan neck deformity. The boutonnière deformity is the most common **thumb** deformity in RA; it arises secondary to arthritis at the thumb MCP joint in combination with attrition of the extensor pollicis brevis tendon. Treatment of a boutonnière deformity at the thumb depends on the stage of disease. If both the MCP and IP joints are correctable passively, temporary fixation of the MCP joint in extension (with K-wires, for 4 weeks) may be all that is required. In later stages, if the MCP joint is more involved and has a fixed deformity (and the IP remains able to be passively flexed), then fusion of the MCP can halt further progression of the disease. If allowed to progress, treatment may require fusion of both the MCP and IP joints (if the CMC joint retains mobility). The EPL tendon may be contracted, in which case tendon lengthening may be required to allow full thumb IP flexion.

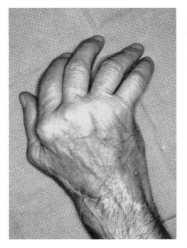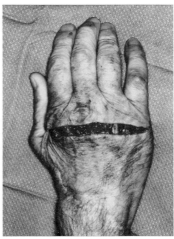

Clinical Pearls

1. Crossed intrinsic transfer corrects the ulnar deviation of the digits in the treatment of rheumatoid disease at the MCP joints.

2. The single most helpful surgical procedure for patients with rheumatoid arthritis (RA) is synovectomy *before* major derangements have been allowed to occur. Preventing joint subluxation and tendon ruptures is a much more successful approach than attempting to recover lost function after the fact.

3. The boutonnière deformity is the most common thumb deformity in patients with RA. The swan neck deformity is more common at the thumb in patients with osteoarthritis. Osteoarthritis originates at the CMC joint; RA primarily involves the MCP joint.

REFERENCES

1. El Gammal TA, Blair WF: Motion after metacarpophalangeal joint reconstruction in rheumatoid disease. J Hand Surg 18:504–511, 1993.
2. Harris ED: Rheumatoid arthritis. Pathophysiology and implications for therapy. N Engl J Med 322:1277–1289, 1990.
3. Nalebuff EA: The rheumatoid swan-neck deformity. Hand Clin 5:203–214, 1989.
4. Toledano B, Terrono AL, Millender LH: Reconstruction of the rheumatoid thumb. Hand Clin 8:121–129, 1992.
5. Wilson RL, Carlblom ER: The rheumatoid metacarpophalangeal joint. Hand Clin 5:223–237, 1989.

Perspectives For Therapy

Patient education, wound care, splinting, and early active exercise are the cornerstones of postoperative hand therapy for the patient having undergone MCP arthroplasty and reconstructive hand surgery.

Patients are provided basic information about the anatomy of their hands, the implants used to substitute for their MCP joints, and the surgical procedure. Joint protection also is an important aspect of postoperative care. Patients are instructed in ways they can perform ADLs that minimize the magnitude and duration of stresses acting upon their hands and wrists. ADLs can be safely performed by: (1) using the large proximal muscles groups in the upper extremities, (2) sharing the load between both hands, and (3) increasing the contact area by building up the handles of common household items. In particular, the patient must learn to recognize and attempt to avoid those activities and postures that cause ulnar deviation of the reconstructed MCP joints.

Postoperative wound care includes patient instruction in dressing changes and edema management effected through elevation of the operated extremity. The hand therapist should appreciate that delayed wound healing is a potential complication of steroid use necessitated by RA. Once sutures are removed, attention turns to scar massage and compression.

One objective that must be met during the first 3 weeks of postoperative hand therapy is uneventful tissue healing around the implants forming the longest possible MCP capsules. A static, forearm-based, volar resting hand splint, fabricated for the patient 1–2 days after surgery, helps meet this objective. This splint is used by the patient at all times, except during hygiene activities and dressing changes, until a dynamic splint is fabricated (see below). The static splint positions the patient's wrist in 15–20° extension, MCPs in 60–70° flexion, and IPs in neutral. In this manner, the resting hand splint maintains the lengths of the IP collateral ligaments and promotes adaptive lengthening of dorsal scar tissue during encapsulation of the MCP implants.

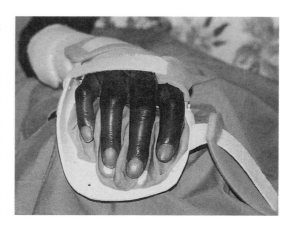

If the thumb has been operated, e.g., in the case of MCP fusion, a thumb component that promotes CMC abduction is added to the splint design (see figure, *above*). Elastomer finger spacers are galvanized to the hand component of the splint. These serve to align the patient's fingers in neutral, or slight radial deviation, with respect to the coronal plane. Addition of a distal MCP strap, secured in *radial-to-ulnar fashion,* also contributes a component of radial force to the fingers (see figure, *right*).

At the patient's next follow-up therapy visit, usually 3–5 days postoperatively, a forearm-based, dorsal dynamic MCP extension splint is fabricated. The patient's wrist is again postioned in 15–20° extension. An outrigger is galvanized to the splint base,

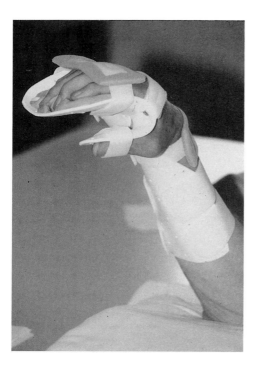

and finger-loops are led to the proximal phalanges of the operated fingers. Rubber-band traction is then applied to the finger loops to effect dynamic MCP extension, and a component of radial pull (5–10°) helps minimize MCP ulnar drift (see figure, *next page*) The rubber bands are adjusted to permit 70° of active MCP flexion with dynamic return to −20° extension. The dynamic splint therefore promotes adaptive lengthening of volar scar tissue during encapsulation of the MCP implants, encourages active MCP motion in the sagittal plane, and fulfills the need for extensor tendon gliding.

During the initial 3 weeks of therapy, the patient is instructed to apply the dynamic splint from 6–8 times daily and perform 10 repetitions of active composite finger flexion, followed by dynamically assisted MCP extension. The patient is also instructed in PRN range of motion exercises for the elbow and shoulder of the operated extremity. The wrist can be exercised between splint changes. Rubber bands are replaced as necessary.

Clinic activities consist of the application of heat followed by range-of-motion exercises for the MCPs and IPJs. The patient's goal is to consistently achieve 60–70° of active MCP flexion and at least −20° of active MCP extension. If PIP flexion is gained rapidly, at the expense of MCP flexion, the PIPs can be splinted in extension during exercise. This permits the flexion moment to be applied primarily to the MCPs.

Toward the end of the second or beginning of the third postoperative week, tendon gliding exercises are added to the patient's home program, and these are performed in the dynamic splint. At 4–6 weeks postoperatively, the dynamic splint is worn during waking hours, and the resting hand splint is reserved for bedtime wear. The patient is also encouraged to begin using the operated hand for "light" ADLs (e.g., handwriting, eating, dressing, grooming) outside of the dynamic splint. At 6–8 weeks postoperatively, the patient may begin weaning from the dynamic splint, wearing it 2 hours "on" and 2 hours "off." At 8–12 weeks postoperatively the dynamic splint is discontinued, and the patient is encouraged to continue use of the static splint for up to 6 months after surgery.

Impairment outcomes for MCP arthroplasty have been well documented. Reconstructive surgery and postoperative hand therapy improve finger alignment. By moving the extension/flexion arc of motion into a *sagittal* plane, functional grasping is accomplished. In the early postoperative period, patients achieve an average of 65° of active MCP flexion and demonstrate an active extension lag of −5°. Ulnar deviation is 0–10°. In long-term follow-up studies (5–20+ years), patients reliably experience 40–50° of active MCP flexion, with extension lags of −12° to −20°. Decreases in active MCP extension average 3°/year, within the first 5 years postoperatively.

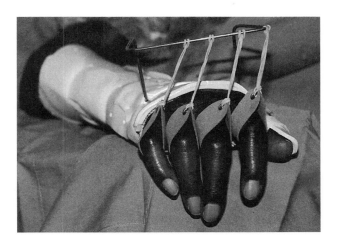

Hand Therapy Pearls

1. Patient education, wound care, splinting, and early active exercise are the cornerstones of postoperative hand therapy for the patient having undergone MCP arthroplasty and reconstructive hand surgery.

2. Patients are educated about principles of joint protection: avoiding motions and postures that invite joint deformity, using large proximal muscle groups, distributing forces between two hands, and increasing the contact area of handles of commonly used household items.

3. Static and dynamic splinting are necessary to promote adaptive lengthening of periarticular soft tissues during encapsulation of the MCP implants. Well-made splints contribute to improved finger posture and motion in the sagittal plane.

4. Early active and active-assist ROM exercises improve muscle performance and promote extensor tendon gliding.

5. Long-term impairment outcome studies of active motion indicate that patients may reliably expect 40–50° of active MCP flexion, with extension lags ranging from −12° to −20°. Decreases in active MCP extension average 3°/year, within the first 5 years postoperatively.

REFERENCES

1. Blue C, Harris K, Hurov J, et al: MP arthroplasty treatment guidelines. In Treatment Guidelines for the Upper Extremity, 2nd ed. Winston-Salem, Bowman Gray/Baptist Medical Center, 1995, pp 58–62.
2. Cannon NM: Arthroplasties. In Diagnosis and Treatment Manual for Physicians and Therapists, 3rd ed. Indianapolis, The Hand Rehabilitation Center of Indiana, 1991, pp 3–5.
3. El-Gammal TA, Blair WF: Motion after metacarpophalangeal joint reconstruction in rheumatoid disease. J Hand Surg 18A:504–511, 1993.
4. Stirrat CR: Metacarpophalangeal joints in rheumatoid arthritis of the hand. Hand Clin 12:515–529, 1996.
5. Swanson AB, de Groot Swanson G, Leonard JB: Postoperative rehabilitation programs in flexible implant arthroplasty of the digits. In Hunter JM, Mackin EJ, Callahan AD (eds): Rehabilitation of the Hand: Surgery and Therapy, 4th ed. St. Louis, Mosby, 1995, pp 1351–1375.

PATIENT 53

A 60-year-old man with failed thumb replantation

A 60-year-old man amputated his non-dominant thumb at the level of the MCP joint while working in his woodworking shop. Replantation was attempted, but the amputated part was too badly injured, and a revision amputation was performed. A large section of skin was lost from the thenar eminence; this was replaced with skin from the amputated thumb as a graft. Now that his wounds have healed (see figure), he is anxious to discuss methods to increase his hand function. He is interested in prosthetics, or any surgical revisions you may be able to offer. The patient is a nonsmoker, and is otherwise healthy; he has no other medical problems, and is on no medications.

Question: What thumb reconstruction option would you recommend for this gentleman?

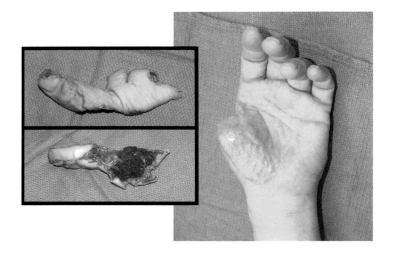

Answer: Pollicization of index finger, toe-to-thumb microsurgical transfer, or Matev first metacarpal lengthening

Discussion: The combination of the thumb's mobile carpometacarpal joint and stable metacarpophalangeal (MCP) and interphalangeal (IP) joints allows both precision pinch and grasp. The loss of the thumb can be devastating in regards to total hand function, and most patients faced with this situation are eager to attempt to recover that function.

Pollicization of the index finger is a popular and very successful method for thumb reconstruction in infants and children, particularly those that suffer from some variation of thumb hypoplasia or aplasia. In the adult, pollicization should be last on the list of options. Adults tend to have a much more difficult time with sensory and motor reeducation after this procedure than infants do.

Toe-to-thumb microsurgical transfer has been popularized nearly as long as microsurgical techniques have existed. The great toe is harvested and then used to reconstruct the thumb. It is vascularized based on the dorsalis pedis or first dorsal metatarsal artery. The flexor and extensor tendons are repaired to their corresponding donors, as are the toe digital nerves to the hand digital nerves. Successfully accomplished, the neo-thumb should have active flexion and extension, as well as near normal sensation. While both aesthetic and functional results can be excellent, care must be taken to select the proper candidate: adequate digital nerves need to be available at the hand to connect to the digital nerves of the thumb, or the neo-thumb is destined to be insensate (and

far less functional). Inadequacies of the tendons, artery, and vein on the donor (hand) side are easier to compensate for, because additional length can be taken with toe harvest. This is a very technically demanding procedure, and should be reserved for individuals and centers with adequate experience in this area.

Metacarpal lengthening is another option for thumb reconstruction. It is relatively easy to perform and does not require a great deal of specialized microsurgical experience. First described by Matev, it is reminiscent of the Ilizarov bone-lengthening technique used for the long bones. Matev lengthening is a reliable method for gaining thumb length (allowing grasp and pinch) when microsurgical toe-to-thumb transfer is not an option or desired.

Simply put, an osteotomy is created at the midportion of the first metacarpal. Several transversely oriented K-wires or pins are then placed both proximal and distal to the osteotomy, and secured to a specialized distraction device (see figure, *below*). This device has a small screw which, when turned, gradually distracts the proximal and distal metacarpal segments. The patient turns this screw several times a day, for a total of about 1 mm per 24 hours. Once the desired amount of lengthening has occurred, the bony defect is grafted and fixed with a plate.

Strongly consider performing a 1st webspace deepening procedure, as well, to allow the patient better grasp (see figure, *next page*).

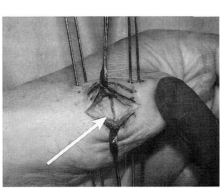

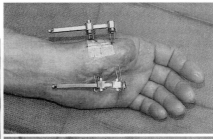

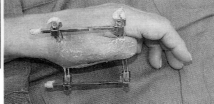

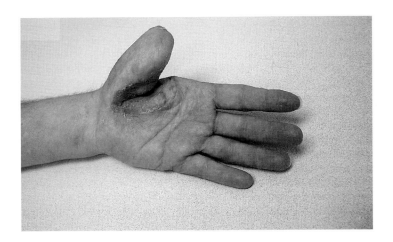

Clinical Pearls

1. Toe-to-thumb transfers are very sensitive to cooler temperatures in the early post-operative period, and may appear to be completely ischemic if allowed to become cold. Make every effort to keep the transfer digit warm (e.g., with an ambient warmer or external warm air blower).

2. Transferred great toes occasionally may appear too large (particularly too wide) on the patient's hand. If this is a concern, the deformity can be minimized 6–12 months after the transfer by making a lenticular excision (oriented parallel to the axis of the volar digit, at the midline of the thumb) of the excess tissue, with primary closure.

3. When making the osteotomy of the metacarpal for Matev lengthening, make the skin incision parallel to the axis of the metacarpal (not transversely oriented). Therefore, as the bone is distracted, the skin incision will not be forced open (refer again to figure, *top*).

4. In contrast to Ilizarov techniques, in the hand it is of little concern whether bone will form across the widening osteotomy site. It is difficult to predict in which patients adequate bone will form, although younger patients typically produce a significant amount. A bigger problem is consolidation of bone when the distraction has progressed too slowly. Consolidation limits further distraction.

REFERENCES

1. Lister G: The choice of procedure following thumb amputation. Clin Orthop 195:45–51, 1985.
2. Matev IB: Thumb reconstruction through metacarpal bone lengthening. J Hand Surg 5:482–487,1980.
3. May JW Jr, Daniel RK: Great toe to hand free tissue transfer. Clin Orthop 133:140–153, 1978.
4. Moy OJ, Peimer CA, Sherwin FS: Reconstruction of traumatic or congenital amputation of the thumb by distraction-lengthening. Hand Clin 8:57–62, 1992.
5. Poppen NK, Norris TR, Buncke HJ Jr: Evaluation of sensibility and function with microsurgical free tissue transfer of the great toe to the hand for thumb reconstruction. J Hand Surg 8: 516–531, 1983.

Perspectives For Therapy

Toe-to-thumb transfer. Postoperative care in toe-to-thumb transfer involves the same principles and priorities outlined for digit replantation (see Case 51). A forearm-based radial gutter splint that extends to the distal end of the new "thumb" is fabricated for the patient. The hand therapist must ensure that the splint straps place no pressure on the soft tissues of the first webspace that could interfere with vascular supply. The patient's wrist is supported in neutral and the thumb secured in the position of skeletal fixation.

In toe-to-thumb transfer, the proximal and distal motor nerves supplying the extrinsic and intrinsic thumb muscles are preserved. Therefore, these patients should be candidates for early active-assist exercises following guidelines recommended for thumb replantation.

Once the vascular supply of the new thumb is no longer in question, and the patient has been cleared to attempt walking, he or she may begin using a platform-walker and stand-by assist. The need to protect the vascular supply of the operated hand is paramount and will determine progression to unassisted walking.

Impairment outcomes are directly related to the duration of immobilization prior to initiating hand therapy. Within a sample of five patients who underwent toe-to-hand transfer for isolated thumb loss at the MCP level, or distally, abduction at the thumb CMC was 30–55° and extension was 30–60°. Average MCP motion was $-15/30°$, indicating a 15° flexed posture of the MCP at rest and 15° of active flexion (range 23° hyperextension to 61° flexion). Similarly, average IP motion was $-15/40°$, indicating a 15° flexed posture of the IP at rest and 25° of active flexion (range 30° hyperextension to 55° flexion).

Sensory evaluation using two-point discrimination was directly related to the patient's age at the time of surgery. On average, patients returned results in the 14–15 mm range.

Grip strength was 80–109%, lateral (key) pinch 65–169%, three-point pinch 50–178%, and tip pinch 62–138% of the uninvolved hand.

Clearly, strength, sensory status, mobility, ability to control thumb position, thumb length, and pain combine in unique ways to determine the patient's abilities to return to functional activities. In terms of functional and cosmetic assessment, all patients either returned to work or school following surgery. None reported being limited by pain symptoms; however, cold intolerance was a consistent finding. No patient reported a barrier to social acceptance due to the appearance of the hand, although the operated hand was frequently a topic of conversation.

Pollicization. Simply stated, pollicization involves transfer of a finger to substitute for the thumb. The neurovascular bundles and extrinsic tendons are preserved within the transferred finger. The hand therapist should appreciate the manner in which pollicization has been carried out by the hand surgery team. For example, how were the intrinsic muscles of the thumb connected with the intrinsic tendons of the transferred finger? How was skeletal fixation achieved between the metacarpal of the transferred finger and that of the residual thumb? Were skin grafts required to accomplish a satisfactory webspace and to effect wound closure?

All of the extrinsic and intrinsic hand muscles are innervated *proximal* to the site of transfer, and the thumb CMC is intact. Therefore, early active motion beginning 3–5 days postoperatively has been advocated. Vascular status, stability of skeletal fixation, and skin integrity are three factors contributing to the decision to initiate early active motion.

Priniciples of wound care, edema management, and sensorimotor reeducation have been outlined previously and are applicable to adult pollicization (see Cases 11 and 51). Static splinting, to protect the pollicized finger between exercise sessions and at bedtime, may also be indicated.

Distraction lengthening. Reconstruction of the thumb by distraction lengthening involves surgical division of the thumb metacarpal and placement of an external frame by which adjustment increases the length of the supporting soft-tissues of the thumb. This technique does not enhance thumb motion. Rather, the length that is gained improves the patient's ability to perform motor skills such as opposition, grasp, and pinch.

Gradual lengthening of soft-tissues is under patient control. Once the desired length is achieved, bone graft is inserted between the ends of the divided thumb metacarpal, and this construct is fixed using hardware. Deepening of the patient's first webspace may also be conducted in surgery.

Providing that adequate skeletal fixation has been achieved, the patient may begin active thumb opposition exercises 7–14 days postoperatively. Static gutter splints applied to the thumb will provide distal support during exercise sessions, and a spica splint can be worn between exercise sessions and at bedtime to protect the patient's thumb. As discussed previously, skeletal fixation is a relative contraindication to passive motion secondary to risk of failure of fixation and fracture (see Cases 16 and 30).

Hand Therapy Pearls

1. In order to provide optimal postoperative care for the patient, the hand therapist must understand the manner in which thumb reconstruction surgery is performed.

2. The basic trio of vascular status, skeletal fixation, and skin integrity dictate the timing of hand therapy treatment following thumb reconstruction. In most cases, sensorimotor function is preserved, but must remain subservient to these three factors.

3. Retrospective studies of thumb function support early referral to hand therapy for instruction in protected active motion. Simply stated, early motion translates into superior functional outcomes.

REFERENCES

1. Brunelli GA, Brunelli GR: Reconstruction of traumatic absence of the thumb in the adult by pollicization. Hand Clin 8:41–55, 1992.
2. Buncke HJ, Jackson RL, Buncke GM, et al: The surgical and rehabilitative aspects of replantation and revascularization of the hand. In Hunter JM, Mackin EJ, Callahan AD (eds): Rehabilitation of the Hand: Surgery and Therapy, 4th ed. St. Louis, Mosby, 1995, pp 1075–1100.
3. Ma H-S, El-Gammal TA, Wei F-C: Current concepts of toe-to-hand transfer: Surgery and rehabilitation. J Hand Ther 9:41–46, 1996.
4. Moy OW, Peimer CA, Sherwin FS: Reconstruction of traumatic or congenital amputation of the thumb by distraction-lengthening. Hand Clin 8:57–62, 1992.
5. Poppen NK, Norris TR, Buncke HJ: Evaluation of sensibility and function with microsurgical free tissue transfer of the great toe to the hand for thumb reconstruction. J Hand Surg 8A:516–531, 1983.

PATIENT 54

A 22-year-old man with metacarpophalangeal pain after punching a wall

You are called to see a patient that presented to the emergency department approximately 2 days after punching a wall, angry over his recent breakup with his girlfriend. He complains of persistent hand pain (particularly over the 5th MCP joint), hand swelling, and decreased mobility of his fingers (most marked on the 5th finger). He has no other complaints or injuries.

Physical Examination: Skin: edematous; intact. Palpation: tender right dorsal hand, especially just proximal to 5th MCP joint; remainder of hand nontender. Musculoskeletal: decreased range of motion at 5th MCP joint; no rotational deformity of 5th finger; all other digits normal. Neurologic: intact throughout.

Laboratory Findings: Radiograph: see figure.

Question: What is your diagnosis?

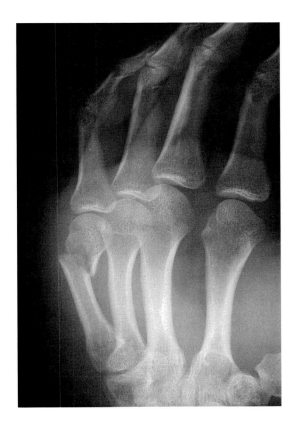

Answer: Boxer's fracture (fracture of the distal 5th metacarpal)

Discussion: The term "boxer's fracture" is reserved for the situation of a distal neck fracture of the 5th metacarpal, with the etiology being an axial blow. Distal fractures of the other metacarpals and more proximal fractures of the 5th metacarpal are not called boxer's fractures.

Physical examination of the patient with a boxer's fracture should include analysis of any rotational deformity with flexion and extension of the finger. The presence of any scissoring with flexion requires reduction and maintenance of the reduction: this may be accomplished with casting or splinting alone, but sometimes requires internal fixation.

Besides persistent scissoring, another finding that may suggest operative intervention is the presence of volar angulation > 45 degrees on lateral radiograph. It is important to ensure that the radiograph is a true lateral. The reason that up to 45 degrees of angulation is acceptable in this metacarpal fracture (but *not* in fractures of the other metacarpals) is due to the degree of hyperextension that is possible at the MCP joint of this digit. In most individuals, full extension of the finger is still possible even with this degree of angulation: if an individual cannot fully extend, a corrective osteotomy of the 5th metacarpal may be required to regain this motion.

Patients should be warned to expect loss of prominence of their 5th "knuckle" (i.e., MCP joint) with conservative (casting) management. Volar displacement of the metacarpal head can produce a clawing deformity; this is a cosmetic problem, but good function remains.

In the acute setting, attempted closed reduction (using a hematoma block for anesthesia) to minimize volar angulation is appropriate. The reduction can be held using either a volar cast or an ulnar gutter splint. It is often helpful to buddy tape the 5th finger to the ring finger, to assist in minimizing any angular or rotational deformity (note that such taping is rarely a good idea if motion is to be allowed, e.g., a PIP dislocation). Because the MCP collateral ligaments are the only remaining attachment to the metacarpal head, it is important to place these in a "tightened" position (i.e., MCP flexed) to help control the distal fracture fragment and maintain the reduction. If immobilization is the only treatment, the splint can be converted to a more secure plaster cast at about 1 week post injury, after most of the soft tissue edema has resolved.

If reduction is not successful, or cannot be held with the splint, or if angulation remains on the AP view (representing rotational deformity), then arrangements need to be made for surgical fixation. Procedures include percutaneous K-wire fixation, and ORIF with fixation maintained by either a K-wire (see figure, *next page;* note significant volar displacement of distal fragment prior to surgical fixation) or tension band. The advantage of tension band placement is earlier return of mobility and, hopefully, decreased incidence of stiffness at the MCP joint.

If K-wire fixation is required, use the K-wire as a "joystick." Introduce it percutaneously at the distal fragment, *pointed dorsally.* After securing the K-wire through the proximal cortex of the distal metacarpal, redirect the distal tip *volarly,* pulling the distal fragment dorsally into position. In particularly difficult cases, there is little morbidity to placing a 1.5- to 2.0-cm, longitudinally oriented incision directly over the fracture: this allows direct visualization of the fracture, and anatomic reduction can be rapidly gained and confirmed.

The best indicator that bony healing has occurred is the lack of tenderness at the fracture site; this usually occurs 4–6 weeks after the injury, depending on age of the patient, immobilization, etc. After the patient has become nontender, it is appropriate to discontinue the immobilization and begin a supervised program of hand therapy, focused on regaining range of motion and minimizing stiffness. Heavy activities are best deferred for an additional 2 to 3 weeks after immobilization has been discontinued.

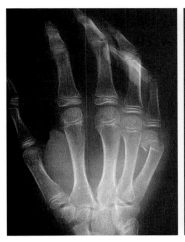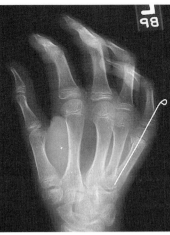

Clinical Pearls

1. Buddy taping the ring finger to the injured 5th finger greatly assists in minimizing rotational or angular deformities.

2. "Boxer's fracture" refers *only* to distal neck fractures of the 5th metacarpal. Fractures of the more proximal 5th metacarpal and those of adjacent metacarpals do not share this name.

REFERENCES
1. Ali A, Hamman J, Mass DP: The biomechanical effects of angulated boxer's fractures. J Hand Surg 24:835–844, 1999.
2. Ford DJ, Ali MS, Steel WM: Fractures of the 5th metacarpal neck: Is reduction or immobilization necessary? J Hand Surg Br 14:165–167, 1989.
3. Porter ML, Hodgkinson JP, Hirst P, et al: The boxers' fracture: A prospective study of functional recovery. Arch Emerg Med 5:212–215, 1988.
4. Vaccaro AR, Kupcha PC, Salvo JP: Accurate reduction and splinting of the common boxer's fracture. Orthop Rev 19:994–996, 1990.

Perspectives For Therapy

Metacarpal fractures comprise up to one-third of hand fractures, and of these, about one-half involve the 5th metacarpal. Depending upon the hand surgeon's preferred method of treatment, there are several options for managing the patient with a nonarticular metacarpal fracture. The hand therapist must appreciate the type and location of the patient's fracture(s), type(s) of operative intervention, if any, and associated soft tissue injuries—because these are primary determinants of treatment. This discussion will be divided into nonoperative and postoperative hand therapy management.

Nonoperative management. Following discontinuation of closed reduction, it is desirable to fabricate a thermoplastic hand-based splint for the patient. This may be a volar resting, ulnar gutter, or radial gutter design. It is advisable to splint one adjacent digit to support the injured digit. Thus, if the long and ring metacarpals are injured, the index and small fingers are incorporated into the splint design.

The primary considerations for hand splinting are to *position the MCP joints of interest in at least 50–60° flexion and permit unrestricted active motion of the IP joints.* The thermoplastic splint is worn between exercise sessions and at bedtime for approximately 3 weeks.

Treatment activities include edema management (elevation, retrograde massage, and contrast baths) and active motion emphasizing isolated MCP extension (recruits ED and encourages differential gliding of extrinsic flexors, FDS, and FDP), composite finger extension (recruits ED and hand intrinsics), and composite finger flexion (recruits extrinsic flexors and interossei). Mobilization techniques, performed at end-range MCP flexion, and intermetacarpal joint mobilization are used to enhance finger flexion.

There is some disagreement regarding wrist immobilization by splinting. Unless it is recommended, perhaps due to the proximity of a metacarpal fracture to the CMC joint, it is preferable to free the wrist from the splint design.

Patients with minimally displaced, stable metacarpal fractures that do not require casting can be treated with early referral to hand therapy and splinting for 3–4 weeks. Metacarpal fractures tend to be inherently stable for several reasons. First, the intermetacarpal ligaments and intrinsic muscles (interossei) unite the adjacent metacarpals and provide "internal splinting." Second, as the fingers are flexed, the MCP collateral ligaments are maximally lengthened. At end-range flexion, the MCPs are in their close-pack and most stable positions.

Functional fracture bracing is the treatment method of choice in the above scenario. A thermoplastic splint is designed for the patient that provides circumferential compression of soft tissues that *passively* stabilize and support the metacarpal fracture. This technique also calls for early active IP motion. Internal tension developed by active muscle is constrained by the splint and returned to support and stabilize the fracture.

Guidelines for functional bracing of a metacarpal fracture consist of fabricating a thermoplastic hand-based ulnar (ring and small) or radial gutter splint (index and long fingers) that positions the MCPs in at least 50–60° flexion and permits early active IP motion. The advantages of early active IP motion include fluid circulation to help manage edema and tendon gliding exercises to minimize risk of tendon adherence.

For isolated metacarpal neck fractures (i.e., those involving the distal metaphysis), it is sufficient to immobilize two adjacent fingers. For isolated metacarpal shaft fractures, it is desirable to support all four metacarpals. With clinical fracture healing, hand therapy is progressed to active motion and joint mobilization as outlined above.

Postoperative management. Surgical treatment for metacarpal fracture that yields a stable construct, for example ORIF, permits early active motion 24–72 hours postoperatively. Following surgery, extensor tendon gliding exercises are particularly desirable to minimize scar adherence. Scar management, including massage and compression, is initiated after sutures are removed.

A thermoplastic splint is fabricated for patient use between exercise sessions and at bedtime for approximately 4–6 weeks. It is sufficient to immobilize the injured digit in a volar, hand-based resting splint that maintains a minimum of 50–60°

MCP flexion. However, as a practical matter, due to the intermetacarpal ligaments, the adjacent finger(s) will tend to passively flex at the MCPs.

Following interval fracture healing and discontinuation of protective splinting, the patient may be instructed in general upper extremity strengthening and conditioning exercises using graded rubber-bands or tubes. Putty use may also be initiated at this time.

Splinting for protection may be required for an additional 6–8 weeks with return to sports activities. Note that vigorous grasping should be delayed until 12 weeks following surgery. The athlete must be familiar with and adhere to sport-specific rules of conduct governing on-field use of hard orthoses.

Complications. In a retrospective study of complications following ORIF of 66 metacarpal fractures, problems involving soft tissues were twice as prevalent as those involving skeletal fixation or infection. The most frequent occurrences were active MCP extension lags and decreased total active flexion ($\leq 195°$).

One of the most troublesome problems in hand rehabilitation is a fixed MCP extension contracture (see figure). This mechanical fault evolves from not respecting the requirement to position the MCPs in at least 50–60° flexion, which maintains the lengths of the collateral ligaments and dorsal joint capsule. Accordingly, these MCP soft tissues undergo adaptive shortening, and the patient demonstrates an "intrinsic-minus" finger posture characterized by MCP extension. The MCP can be actively and passively flexed only with difficulty, and the patient is unable to achieve composite finger flexion with impaired grasping.

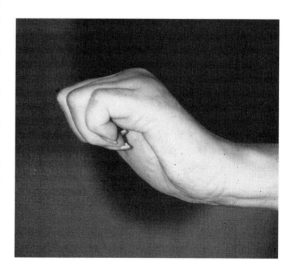

Persistent dorsal edema also promotes intrinsic-minus hand positioning. The resultant fibrosis and adaptive shortening of the MCP collateral ligaments and dorsal capsule will lead to MCP extension contracture. Additional problems include scar adherence in zones 5 and 6 that may limit gliding of extrinsic extensor tendons. Adherence of the extensor tendons to adjacent fracture callus or hardware also has the potential to adversely affect tendon gliding.

Splinting for joint mobilization may include dynamic and static progressive designs. The best chance for improving *passive* MCP motion exists when the joint has a springy end-feel; however, the patient *must* be encouraged to exercise actively through his or her augmented range. The splint-wearing schedule is based on progress in gaining motion and tolerance for splint use. A useful starting point is to bring the patient to the end-range of MCP flexion, using the minimal amount of force necessary, and to recommend splint wear for 1–2 hours followed by a similar duration without the splint; this is repeated 6–8 times daily. A static, resting hand splint can be used at bedtime, but use must be revised on an ongoing basis to match increases in MCP flexion achieved through dynamic or static progressive splinting.

Hand Therapy Pearls

1. The primary considerations for splinting the patient with a metacarpal fracture are to position the MCP joints of interest in at least 50–60° flexion and permit unrestricted active motion of the IP joints.

2. There is some disagreement regarding wrist immobilization by splinting. Unless it is recommended, perhaps due to the proximity of a metacarpal fracture to the CMC joint, it is preferable to free the wrist from the splint design.

3. Functional fracture bracing offers an alternative to cast immobilization for selected stable, minimally displaced metacarpal fractures. The thermoplastic splint provides circumferential compression of soft tissues that *passively* stabilize and support the metacarpal fracture. Internal tension, developed by early active motion, is constrained by the splint and returned to also support and stabilize the fracture.

4. One of the most troublesome problems in hand rehabilitation is a fixed MCP extension contracture.

REFERENCES

1. Cannon N: Metacarpal fractures. In Diagnosis and Treatment Manual for Physicians and Therapists, 3rd ed. Indianapolis, Hand Rehabilitation Center of Indiana, 1991, p 98.
2. Colditz JC: Functional fracture bracing. In Hunter JM, Mackin EJ, Callahan AD (eds): Rehabilitation of the Hand: Surgery and Therapy, 4th ed. St. Louis, Mosby, 1995, pp 395–406.
3. Colditz JC: Therapist's management of the stiff hand. In Hunter JM, Mackin EJ, Callahan AD (eds): Rehabilitation of the Hand: Surgery and Therapy, 4th ed. St. Louis, Mosby, 1995, pp 1141–1159.
4. Lee S-G, Jupiter JB: Phalangeal and metacarpal fractures of the hand. Hand Clin 16:323–332, 2000.
5. Meyer FN, Wilson RL: Managment of nonarticular fractures of the hand. In Hunter JM, Mackin EJ, Callahan AD (eds): Rehabilitation of the Hand: Surgery and Therapy, 4th ed. St. Louis, Mosby, 1995, pp 353–375.
6. Page SM, Stern PJ: Complications and range of motion following plate fixation of metacarpal and phalangeal fractures. J Hand Surg 23A:827–832, 1998.

PATIENT 55

A 36-year-old man with limited motion of his right index finger

A 36-year-old man reports falling through a glass door and cutting his right hand. He was seen emergently at a local medical center, where his hand wounds were closed primarily, and he went on to delayed primary repair of tendon lacerations approximately 1 week later. The patient is now referred to your clinic for evaluation and treatment, 6 weeks following his surgical repair and interval hand therapy.

Physical Examination: Skin: well-healed, 60-mm, dorsal scar passing obliquely within second intermetacarpal interval (proximomedial to distolateral); 30-mm, dorsal scar, concave distally, crossing perpendicular to second metacarpal (figure, *top*). Musculoskeletal: active motion right index finger—MCP 15/75° (0° passive extension), PIP 0/95°, DIP 0/45° (figures, *bottom*). Special tests: active index finger extension to 0° in intrinsic minus position (figure, *next page*).

Question: What are the affected anatomic structures?

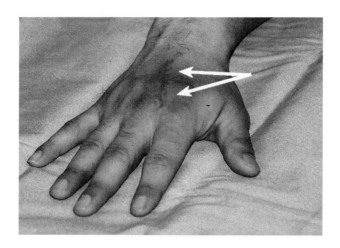

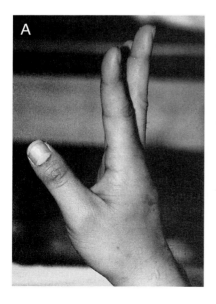

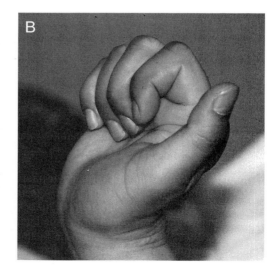

Answer: Extensor digitorum and extensor indicis proprius

Discussion: When a patient is referred from an outside hand surgeon, the hand therapist may not have immediate access to operative reports, and must rely instead on the patient's verbal report of the injury, visual appraisal, ROM, and special tests. The positions and lengths of the present patient's scars are consistent with lacerations of the ED and EIP in zones 5 and 6. Remember that the EIP is *parallel* and *medial* to the ED in zone 6, and passes within the second intermetacarpal interval.

The extrinsic extensors are primarily extensors of the MCPs. They contribute to extension of the PIPs through the central tendons, and of the DIPs through fibrous connections with the intrinsic extensors, lumbricals, and interossei, forming the terminal tendons.

Scar that adheres to the extensor tendons in zones 5 and 6 results in predictable patterns of motion restriction. In this patient, the extensor moment was sufficient to produce 0° MCP extension in the intrinsic minus position, indicative that the ED and EIP were intact (see figure, *right*). When the extrinsic extensors were challenged to contribute to *composite* MCP and IP extension, however, an active MCP extension lag was appreciated. Note that the intrinsic extensors were capable of fully extending the IPs (see figure *A, previous page*).

Scar adherence in zones 5 and 6 limits distal glide of the extensor expansion, and this also restricts composite flexion of the index finger MCP and IPs (see figure *B, previous page*). The fact that the flexion limitation occurred with the wrist *extended* helped identify a pattern of restriction caused primarily by scar adherence, rather than

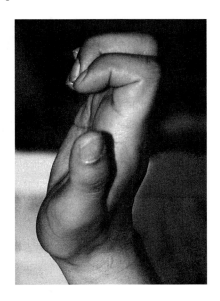

extrinsic shortness, *per se*. However, extrinsic extensor shortness cannot be unequivocally ruled out, particularly if the hand surgeon was required to revise an untidy laceration or resect devitalized extensor tendon prior to repair.

Treatment for this patient emphasized scar mobilization and isolated active extension of the index finger in a gravity-lessened position—that is, with the forearm in neutral rotation. Progress was made to an antigravity position, with the forearm prone. Composite index finger flexion was also performed, varying the patient's wrist position from full extension to full flexion.

Hand Therapy Pearls

1. The presence of scar provides important clues about pathology location and affected anatomic structures. Visual appraisal, ROM, and special tests are prerequisite components of the hand therapist's evaluation; however, they are made more vital when the patient's surgical report is not readily available.

2. Adherent scar results in predictable patterns of motion restriction. Challenging the extrinsic extensors of the index finger reveals active insufficiency during composite extension and passive restraint during flexion, even with the patient's wrist extended.

REFERENCE
Rosenthal EA: The extensor tendons: Anatomy and management. In Hunter JM, Mackin EJ, Callahan AD (eds): Rehabilitation of the Hand: Surgery and Therapy, 4th ed. St. Louis, Mosby, 1995, pp 519–564.

PATIENT 56

A 39-year-old woman with interphalangeal joint flexion contractures

A 39-year-old woman fell onto her outstretched right hand and sustained a distal radius fracture. It was managed with open reduction and internal fixation using Kirschner wires, and with an external fixator. She is now referred to hand therapy for fabrication of an anti-claw splint 4 weeks status-post surgery. The patient complains of numbness involving her right ring and small fingers and hypothenar eminence.

Physical Examination: General: hypothenar flattening. Position of external fixation: right wrist 10° flexion and 35° ulnar deviation. Musculoskeletal: active ROM—ring MCP hyperextension 30°, PIP 50/90°, DIP 15/65°; small MCP hyperextension 20°, PIP 45/75°, DIP 25/55° (see figure). Passive ROM—IP joint extension 0°. Neurologic: diminished protective sensation at volar surfaces of both right small finger and medial aspect of right ring finger (Semmes-Weinstein 4.31 monofilament equivalent to 2.04 gmf); normal sensation dorsal surfaces of both fingers (2.83 monofilament equivalent to 68 mgf).

Question: Where is the pathology located?

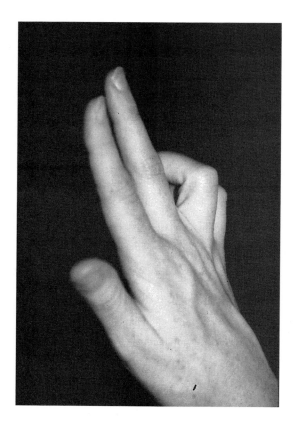

Answer: Guyon's canal

Discussion: Normally, active extension of the IP joints of the ring and small fingers is brought about by activity of the dorsal and palmar interossei and the ulnar two lumbricals. These muscles are supplied by motor branches of the ulnar nerve. In patients with ulnar nerve entrapment, these intrinsic hand muscles are unable to contribute to the extension moment acting over the IP joints. Activity of the extensor digitorum and extensor digiti minimi, which are supplied by motor branches of the radial nerve, results in hyperextension of the MCPs, and this causes passive tenodesis with flexion of the IP joints of the ring and small fingers. The index and long fingers tend to be spared due to the fact that their lumbrical muscles are supplied by motor branches of the median nerve. These small hand intrinsic muscles are often sufficient to contribute to the extensor moment acting over the index and long finger IP joints.

The primary purpose of an anti-claw splint is to correct the imbalance between activity in the extrinsic extensors and the passive tension developed in the tendons of the flexor digitorum profundus and superficialis. This is accomplished by using a hand-based, dorsal orthosis; ulnar gutter splint; or figure-of-eight strap (see figure, *below*). The orthosis is created from a length of 1/8-inch Aquaplast. The material is cut to approximately 1/4-inch width and bonded to itself to create a figure-of-eight strap. The splint is lined with moleskin where it is in contact with the dorsum of the patient's hand.

Positioning the MCPs in as little as 10–20° of flexion reduces passive tension in the extrinsic flexors and enables the extrinsic extensors to contribute an extension moment acting over the IP joints. Tension is transmitted from the central slip to the terminal extensor tendon, via the lateral bands (see figure, *below*).

Active PIP extension also contributes to DIP extension in an indirect fashion as follows: because the ORL passes *volar* to the PIP and *dorsal* to the DIP, active extension of the PIP results in passive extension of the DIP as the ORL becomes taut.

In the present patient, entrapment of the ulnar nerve within Guyon's canal is consistent with the symptoms and objective clinical findings of sensory deficits, atrophy of ulnar-innervated intrinsic hand muscles, and muscle weakness.

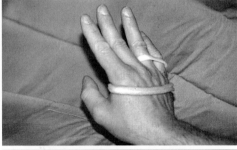

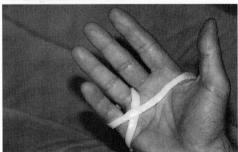

Hand Therapy Pearls

1. Injury to the ulnar nerve at wrist level can result in sensory deficits, muscle atrophy, and motor weakness in the territory supplied by the nerve.

2. The term "ulnar claw hand" is used to describe a mechanical fault characterized by MCP hyperextension coupled with passive IP flexion of the ring and small fingers.

3. A hand-based anti-claw splint is used to correct the imbalance between the extrinsic extensors and extrinsic flexors. By positioning the MCPs in as little as 10–20° of flexion, passive tension in the extrinsic flexors is minimized, permitting the extrinsic extensors to transmit active and passive tension to the IP joints.

REFERENCES

1. Bell-Krotowski JA: Sensibility testing: Current concepts. In Hunter JM, Mackin EJ, Callahan AD (eds): Rehabilitation of the Hand: Surgery and Therapy, 4th ed. St. Louis, Mosby, 1995, pp 109–128.
2. Lindsey JT, Watumull D: Anatomic study of the ulnar nerve and related vascular anatomy at Guyon's canal: A practical classification system. J Hand Surg 21A:626–633, 1996.
3. Tubiana R: Architecture and functions of the hand. In Tubiana R (ed): The Hand, Vol 1. Philadelphia, WB Saunders, 1981, pp 19–93.
4. Valentin P: The interossei and the lumbricals. In Tubiana R (ed): The Hand, Vol 1. Philadelphia, WB Saunders, 1981, pp 244–254.
5. Valentin P: Physiology of extension of the fingers. In Tubiana R (ed): The Hand, Vol 1. Philadelphia, WB Saunders, 1981, pp 389–398.

PATIENT 57

A 39-year-old man with motion restriction of his left index finger

A 39-year-old man presents with a history of laceration to the dorsum of the left index finger. He was able to control the hemorrhage, and he applied a bandage and a home-made splint that maintained his index finger in extension. The splint was worn for 10 days. He was referred to an orthopedic surgeon for evaluation and is now referred to hand therapy 2 weeks following onset of injury.

Physical Examination: Skin: well-healed, 15-mm, C-shaped scar (concave proximally) at dorsum of left index finger, over base of middle phalanx; edema at PIP, circumference 7.2 cm (7.1 cm right). Palpation: scar tender; contour of middle phalanx raised, approximating shape of scar. Musculoskeletal: at rest—PIP 35° flexed attitude, DIP hyperextended; active motion—MCP 0/55°, PIP 10/80° (0° passive extension), DIP HYP/HYP. Muscle testing: left index FDS and FDP intact; 30° isolated, active DIP flexion. Positive oblique retinacular ligament test: 45° passive DIP flexion with PIP flexed, versus 30° with PIP extended.

Question: Based on the patient's history, what disorder do you suspect?

Answer: A zone III extensor tendon laceration

Discussion: The hallmark of an isolated central slip laceration is a boutonniére mechanical fault characterized by flexion of the PIP joint and hyperextension of the DIP (see figure, *below*). Tendon injury at the dorsum of the base of the middle phalanx releases the mechanical restraint provided by the extensor mechanism and permits the PIP joint to flex, passively protruding through the extensor mechanism. The lateral bands concentrate their active and passive extension force distally, resulting in DIP joint hyperextension. The oblique retinacular ligament passes *volar* to the PIP joint and *dorsal* to the DIP. Thus, a positive test is one in which passive DIP flexion is limited when the examiner maintains the PIP joint in extension. Adaptive shortening of the oblique retinacular ligament reinforces the posture of the finger—PIP flexion and DIP hyperextension.

of the central slip over the PIP joint. With the MCP of the index finger positioned near 0°, active PIP joint extension was performed from a position of full flexion. This exercise permits the extensor digitorum to transmit tension to the central slip of the extensor mechanism. The intrinsic extensors of the index finger, interossei and lumbrical, are also recruited for PIP joint extension. Isolated DIP flexion of the index finger, while maintaining the PIP joint in extension (blocked or braced DIP flexion), permits the FDP to act independently across the DIP, and achieves passive lengthening of the oblique retinacular ligament (ORL; see figure, *below*).

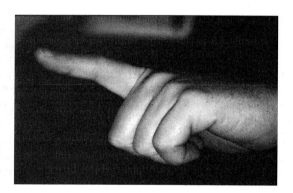

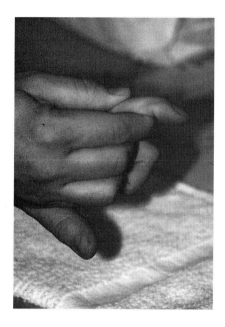

It was fortuitous that the patient splinted his injured finger in extension, thus permitting approximation of the ends of the central slip. The fact that the patient demonstrates 0° passive PIP joint extension suggests that full active extension may be attainable. Although the oblique retinacular ligament test is positive, considerable active flexion of the DIP remains.

This patient was treated with scar mobilization and exercise to enhance the mechanical efficiency

Dynamic extension of the PIP joint, using a finger-based splint, may also be indicated to achieve adaptive lengthening of the ORL and volar soft tissues (see figure, *next page*). However, the patient must be encouraged to actively extend the PIP joint through the augmented range of extension achieved through dynamic splint use.

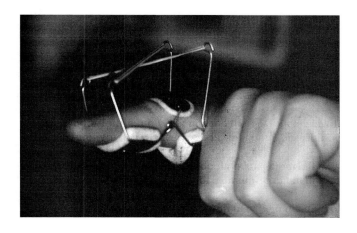

Hand Therapy Pearls

1. Left unrepaired, a zone III extensor tendon laceration can evolve into a Boutonniére mechanical fault, characterized by PIP flexion and DIP hyperextension.

2. Passive mobility of the IP joints reveals the favorability of prognosis following a zone III extensor tendon laceration.

3. An active PIP joint extension lag that is passively correctable to neutral, and the capability for isolated active DIP flexion, suggest that active PIP extension may be regained, and that the oblique retinacular ligament may be elongated through exercise and splinting.

REFERENCES

1. Rosenthal EA: The extensor tendons: Anatomy and management. In Hunter JM, Mackin EJ, Callahan AD (eds): Rehabilitation of the Hand: Surgery and Therapy, 4th ed. St. Louis, Mosby, 1995, pp 519–564.
2. Valentin P: The interossei and the lumbricals. In Tubiana R (ed): The Hand, Vol 1. Philadelphia, WB Saunders, 1981, pp 244–254.
3. Valentin P: Physiology of extension of the fingers. In Tubiana R (ed): The Hand, Vol 1. Philadelphia, WB Saunders, 1981, pp 389–398.

PATIENT 58

A 31-year-old man with shoulder pain and limited motion

A 31-year-old electrician was carrying equipment up a ladder and transferring it onto an overhead shelf when he experienced an intense, sharp pain in his right shoulder. Over the next 7 months, he continued to complain of right shoulder discomfort, and he received five cortisone injections with minimal pain symptom relief. Thereafter, he underwent arthroscopic debridement and right rotator cuff repair, and he has been released from work following this initial surgical procedure. Three months later, a second procedure involving right shoulder manipulation under anesthesia was performed, and the patient is now referred to therapy for evaluation and treatment. He complains of severely restricted activities of daily living (ADLs) caused by right shoulder discomfort and limited motion.

Physical Examination: General: standing at rest, right shoulder girdle elevated and upper arm internally rotated; right scapula relatively protracted, elbow flexed, forearm in neutral rotation, and wrist and fingers flexed; muscle contours normal. Soft tissue: no localized atrophy nor edema; tissue texture and color normal. Active ROM right shoulder: abduction 0–70° (100° passive), flexion 0–125° (125° passive), external rotation 0–20° (25° passive), internal rotation 0–25° (45° passive). Musculoskeletal: during abduction, limited external rotation; patient side-bent trunk to left (see figure, *left*); during flexion, limited external rotation; patient extended trunk (see figure, *right*).

Question: What is the diagnosis for upper extremity therapy?

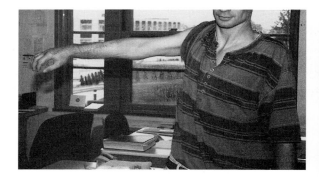
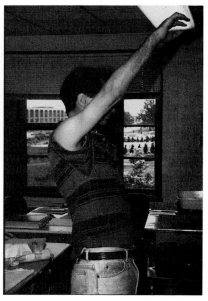

Diagnosis: Glenohumeral joint restriction in a capsular pattern

Discussion: Glenohumeral joint capsular syndrome or, more descriptively, "frozen shoulder" is characterized by significant motion restrictions in multiple directions. Normally, specific regions of the glenohumeral joint capsule as well as its associated ligaments are responsible for limiting end-range motion. In glenohumeral joint restriction, all regions of the capsule are affected, resulting in a global capsular constraint on shoulder motion. The so-called protected position of the upper extremity represents the neutral isometric position of relaxed tension for the glenohumeral joint caspule, and is characterized by elevation of the shoulder girdle, internal rotation of the upper arm, and scapular protraction.

Whether the stiff shoulder is brought about by processes intrinsic to the glenohumeral joint capsule (idiopathic) or initiated by trauma, the final common pathway is identical. The patient presents to therapy with a history of relative or absolute inactivity that results in limited motion of the shoulder joint complex. Motion restriction manifests itself in a *capsular pattern,* defined as follows: loss of both active and passive motion are proportionally greatest for external rotation, followed by abduction, and lastly internal rotation. For example, the patient may exhibit as little as 0–10° active external rotation and 45° active abduction, where 90° and 180° are normal, respectively. Interestingly, glenohumeral joint flexion appears to be least affected by chronic inactivity.

When reaching overhead, motion occurs at the glenohumeral and scapulothoracic joints, with lesser contributions made by the acromioclavicular and sternoclavicular joints. The humeral head normally translates inferiorly on the slope of the glenoid fossa, and this motion is brought about by three muscles: subscapularis, infraspinatus, and teres minor. Of 180°, approximately 120° are contributed by glenohumeral joint motion, while the remaining 60° are contributed by scapular and clavicular rotations. A 2:1 ratio, reflective of the differential contributions of the glenohumeral and scapulothoracic joints, is frequently used to describe this "scapulohumeral rhythm."

The inferior component of the glenohumeral joint capsule is normally redundant when the arm is resting by the side. It is this redundancy that permits inferior translation of the humeral head during overhead reaching, and it is normally taken up as the humeral head translates down the glenoid slope. Thus, the inferior joint capsule constrains inferior translation of the humeral head and defines the end-ranges of overhead motion.

The pathologic anatomy of adhesive capsulitis is characterized by capsular thickening (fibroplasia), capsular shortening with the presence of myofibroblasts, obliterated redundancies of the inferior joint capsule, inflammation with fibrosis (scarring), decreased capsular volume and synovial fluid, and adhesions affecting the joint surfaces.

From a pathophysiologic viewpoint, motion of the humeral head is always severely constrained, and clinically, a 1:1 scapulohumeral rhythm emerges. Thus, if the patient is able to abduct the shoulder 60°, 30° will be contributed by the glenohumeral joint and 30° by the scapulothoracic joint. Moreover, reaching overhead is characterized by antalgic trunk motion, with compensatory elevation of the shoulder girdle. Patients with glenohumeral joint restriction complain of pain symptoms interfering with the performance of ADLs and of an inability to find a position of comfort at bedtime; lying on the affected shoulder is not well tolerated.

Joint motion is crucial to provide synovial lubrication of articular cartilage, decrease hypersensitivity, and lengthen periarticular soft tissues. Therefore, from the standpoint of functional rehabilitation, the goals of therapy are to restore pain-free motion of the shoulder joint complex and return the patient to his or her normal ADLs.

Initial treatment efforts for this patient were directed at increasing isolated glenohumeral joint motion, particularly external rotation and abduction, and realigning the scapula posteriorly and inferiorly on the thorax. These treatment goals were accomplished through: (1) progressive joint mobilization, (2) exercises designed to increase inferior humeral gliding upon the glenoid fossa and decrease the recruitment of the upper trapezius muscle, and (3) postural retraining. Compliance with selected home exercises by the patient ensured carry-over of clinic activities. Mobility and transfer training were also used, to help minimize stresses acting upon the shoulder joint complex and restore a more normal sleep pattern.

A therapeutic pool proved invaluable for achieving pain-free, isolated glenohumeral joint motion. End-ranges were always defined by appropriate scapular and humeral mechanics, and quality of motion was emphasized; amplitude of motion was secondary. The resistance offered by the water also prepared the scapulothoracic and scapulohumeral muscles for reaching horizontally and overhead.

Treatment was progressed to land-based strengthening exercises using free weights and graded rubber-bands targeting specific upper extremity muscle groups. Progression to work conditioning and simulation was also used for this patient, and practical suggestions were offered to modify work tasks, tools, and the work environment.

Hand Therapy Pearls

1. Glenohumeral joint capsular (GJC) syndrome, or "frozen shoulder," is characterized by global motion restriction in a capsular pattern, with external rotation loss > abduction loss > internal rotation loss.

2. Whether due to idiopathic factors or to trauma, the final common pathway leading to GJC syndrome is prolonged immobility. Adhesions obliterate the normal redundancies in the inferior glenohumeral joint capsule, preventing inferior gliding of the humeral head, which is a biomechanical prerequisite for overhead reaching.

3. Rehabilitation efforts must emphasize exercises that restore isolated motion of the glenohumeral joint and reposition the scapula inferiorly and posteriorly on the dorsal thorax. In the early stages of therapy, motion quality is primary; motion amplitude is secondary.

4. When patients have been released from work for an extended interval, excellent communication among the patient, referring physician, case manager, and therapist is vital for case resolution. It is important to address the patient's return-to-work concerns, such as duration of work and duties. In some cases, vocational rehabilitation may be appropriate.

REFERENCES

1. Burkart SL, Post WR: A functionally based neuromechanical approach to shoulder rehabilitation. In Hunter JM, Mackin EJ, Callahan AD (eds): Rehabilitation of the Hand: Surgery and Therapy, 4th ed. St. Louis, Mosby, 1995, pp 1655–1698.
2. Harryman DT, Lazarus MD, Rozencwaig R: The stiff shoulder. In Rockwood CA, Matsen FA, Wirth MA, Harryman DT (eds): The Shoulder, 2nd ed. Philadelphia, WB Saunders, 1998, pp 1064–1112.
3. Inman VT, Saunders M, Abbott LC: Observations on the function of the shoulder joint. J Bone Joint Surg 26A:1–30,1944.
4. MacConaill MA, Basmajian JV: Muscles and Movements: A Basis for Human Kinesiology, 2nd ed. Huntington, RE Krieger, 1977, pp 31–44.
5. Norkin CC, White DJ: Measurement of Joint Motion: A Guide to Goniometry. Philadelphia, FA Davis, 1985, p 138.

PATIENT 59

A 22-year-old woman with wrist pain and paresthesia

A 22-year-old woman entering her seventh month of pregnancy complains of a 1-month history of bilateral wrist pain, hand clumsiness, and night pain and numbness involving her index and long fingers. She has been referred to hand therapy for evaluation and treatment, including issuance of custom-fabricated, 0° wrist support splints.

Physical Examination: General: hand appearance unremarkable bilaterally; wrist and distal forearm contours conspicuously enlarged (see figure). Musculoskeletal: active motion normal, pain-free, unlabored; thumb opposition strength 5/5 bilaterally, pain-free to resisted testing. Neurologic: diminished light touch in median nerve distribution of index and long fingers (Semmes Weinstein 3.61 monofilament equivalent to 407 mgf); Tinel's test positive bilaterally over median nerve at wrist level; Phalen's compression test positive bilaterally.

Questions: What are the affected anatomic structures? What is accomplished using 0° wrist support splints?

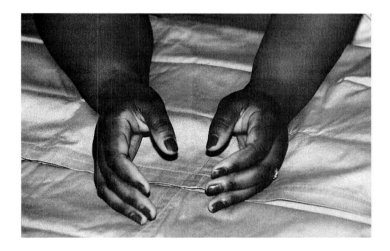

Answers: The median nerve within the carpal tunnel is affected. Neutral splinting minimizes extremes of wrist position and provides relative rest for the extrinsic flexor tendons.

Discussion: The carpal tunnel is quadrilateral in section, with a floor formed dorsally by the carpal bones, a medial wall provided by the hook of the hamate, and a lateral wall created by the tubercles of the scaphoid and trapezium. The transverse carpal ligament, which inserts into the triquetrum, pisiform, hook of the hamate, and tubercles of the scaphoid and trapezium, forms the roof of the carpal tunnel. The free edges of the transverse carpal ligament mark the openings of the carpal tunnel proximally, at the level of the wrist crease, and distally, over the base of the third metacarpal. Nine digital flexor tendons—flexor pollicis longus, flexor digitorum superficialis (4), and flexor digitorum profundus (4)—their synovial sheaths, and the median nerve occupy the carpal tunnel.

Normal weight gain during pregnancy, partially accounted for by fluid, results in systemic elevation of tissue pressures. Because the skeletal boundaries and transverse carpal ligament are inelastic, hydrostatic pressure compresses the microvasculature of the median nerve, causing ischemia. Carpal tunnel pressures may be further increased, as much as 10-fold, during wrist flexion and extension.

Under ischemic conditions, there is decreased O_2 available to nerve cells and edema results, further contributing to elevated tissue fluid pressure. The development of edema, coupled with O_2 deficiency, impairs the oxygen-dependent ion pumps that maintain the electrochemical gradients across the neuron plasma membrane, and neurotransmission fails.

This patient was treated with custom-fabricated splints that maintained the wrists in a neutral position. Neutral wrist positioning minimizes pressure on the median nerve caused by extremes of wrist position, and provides a period of relative rest for the extrinsic flexor tendons. The patient was advised to wear splints during sleep to lessen nocturnal pain and paresthesia. Splint wear during waking hours was also recommended, to address activity-induced paresthesia. Perforated thermoplastic materials of ³⁄₃₂-inch thickness are highly desirable for custom splint fabrication because they are light-weight, permit air circulation, and possess sufficient rigidity to limit extremes of wrist motion. The patient reported symptom relief during late-term pregnancy while using the splints, and discontinued their use 1–2 months following delivery, with complete symptom resolution.

Hand Therapy Pearls

1. The cardinal signs and objective symptoms of carpal tunnel syndrome include a positive Tinel's sign elicited over the median nerve at wrist level, positive Phalen's test, and nocturnal pain and paresthesia in the median nerve distribution of the hand.

2. Systemic elevation of tissue pressure during pregnancy, as a function of normal maternal weight gain, may increase hydrostatic pressure within the carpal tunnel and cause compression of the median nerve microvasculature. Extremes of wrist position may exacerbate these conditions.

3. Conservative care, consisting of custom-fabricated splints that support the wrists in neutral, is effective for minimizing increases in carpal tunnel pressure due to extremes of wrist position.

REFERENCES

1. Concannon MJ, Gainor B, Petroski GF, et al: The predictive value of electrodiagnostic studies in carpal tunnel syndrome. Plast Reconstr Surg 100:1452–1458, 1997.
2. Flynn CJ, Farooqui, AA, Horrocks LA: Ischemia and hypoxia. In Siegel GJ, Agranoff BW, Albers RW, et al (eds): Basic Neurochemistry, 4th ed. New York, Raven Press 1989, pp 783–795.
3. Gelberman RH, Hergenroeder PT, Hargens AR, et al: The carpal tunnel syndrome: A study of carpal canal pressures. J Bone Joint Surg 63A:380–383, 1981.
4. Guyton AC: Pregnancy and lactation. In Guyton AC: Textbook of Medical Physiology, 5th ed. Philadelphia, WB Saunders 1976, pp 1104–1121.
5. Sailer SM: The role of splinting and rehabilitation in the treatment of carpal and cubital tunnel syndromes. Hand Clin 12:223–241, 1996.
6. von Schroeder HP, Botte MJ: Carpal tunnel syndrome. Hand Clin 12:643–655, 1996.

PATIENT 60

A 42-year-old woman with a finger fracture after a fall

A 42-year-old woman employed in the construction trade fell from scaffolding at work and sustained an injury to her left hand. She was seen emergently, and x-rays revealed a closed transverse fracture of the proximal metaphysis of the left small finger proximal phalanx (see figure, *left*). Comminution, shortening, and ulnar angulation, with involvement of the MCP joint, were also appreciated. Upon open exploration, the fracture was deemed inappropriate for open reduction and internal fixation, and management by dynamic traction was elected. A Kirschner wire was placed transversely through the proximal phalanx (see figure, *right*), and the fracture was manually reduced. Once the patient was able to leave the recovery department following surgery, she was immediately referred to hand therapy.

Physical Examination: Skin: sutured, linear surgical incision over distal aspect of left small finger metacarpal crossing MCP joint.

Questions: Describe your treatment approach. What combined method is appropriate for this disorder?

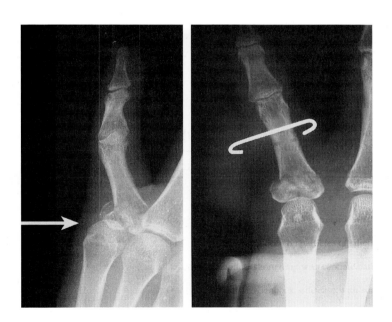

Answers: Dynamic traction splint, which combines distraction force with joint motion

Discussion: Dynamic traction combined with early motion is indicated for use in patients with phalangeal fractures when the physician believes other available methods are inadequate for treatment. This decision is based on the percentage of articular surface involvement, comminution, extent of subluxation/dislocation, and degree of fracture fragment displacement.

The method of dynamic traction to manage intra-articular fractures of the phalanges combines distraction force with joint motion. Distraction reduces the fracture fragments and realigns the joint surfaces through ligamentotaxis. Interval traction, during skeletal connective tissue healing, minimizes the risk of collapse of the fracture fragments and lessens contracture of periarticular soft tissues. Joint motion contributes to cartilage repair and articular congruity.

The dynamic traction splint comprises four components: a splint base, an attached circular outrigger, rubber bands providing traction, and a movable key, or tab, that rides on the outrigger and permits the rubber bands to occupy different positions on the outrigger. The splint components are custom-fabricated by the hand therapist from low-temperature thermoplastic (see figure).

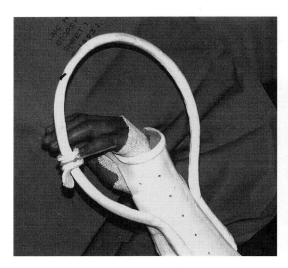

When fabricating a dynamic traction splint, the outrigger must align with the extension-flexion plane of the finger of interest. This arrangement optimizes the alignment of the fracture fragments, promotes a physiological arc of motion of the involved finger, and minimize varus and valgus stresses.

Dynamic traction is effected through the application of suitable rubber bands, attached in serial fashion to one end of the transosseous K-wire, passed over the outrigger and movable key, and attached to the other end of the K-wire (see figures,

next page). The desired magnitude of traction force is empirically determined by the radiographic appearance of the joint. Apply only the amount of traction force that meets the requirement to obtain and maintain alignment of the fracture fragments while restoring articular congruity. These forces are about 100–150 gmf for a small finger MCP joint, to 300 gmf for an index finger PIP joint, and are confirmed using a commercially available tension gauge. The linearity of applied tension in the rubber bands is verified in a minimum of three positions along the outrigger: full extension, full flexion, and rest position of the joint of interest, and fatigued rubber bands are replaced when indicated.

The duration of dynamic traction is 5 to 8 weeks. The decision to discontinue dynamic traction is made by the hand surgeon and is empirically based on the extent of osteosynthesis, as judged radiographically; tenderness to palpation; pain with motion; and maintenance of joint architecture.

The present patient was treated with interval dynamic traction and early active motion for 5.5 weeks. Active ROM at discharge from therapy was MCP 0/65° (85° passive flexion), PIP 20/80 (5/90 passively), and DIP 0/50 (65° passive flexion). Active motion was pain-free and unlabored, and x-rays taken at 22 weeks postoperatively showed acceptable articular congruity with restoration of alignment of P1 (see x-ray; note preservation of MCP joint space). The patient made a full return to construction work.

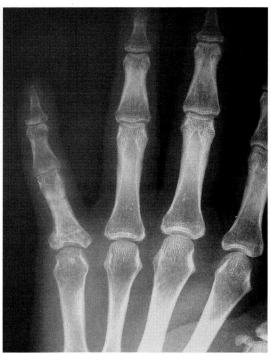

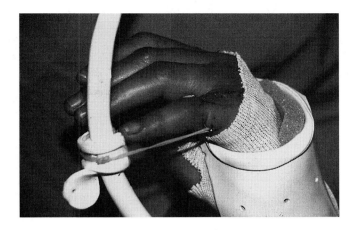

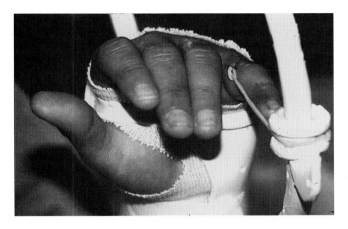

Hand Therapy Pearls

1. If sufficient lead time is available, the outrigger component of the dynamic traction splint should be fabricated. The outrigger should be aligned with the injured finger and permit full extension of the MCP and IP joints. The center of the outrigger should approximate the center of rotation of the joint of interest.

2. The magnitude of applied traction force, determined empirically by radiographic assessment, should be sufficient to obtain and maintain joint space and align the fracture fragments.

3. Rubber-band tension should be assessed in a minimum of three positions along the outrigger: full extension, full flexion, and rest.

4. The duration of dynamic traction is determined empirically through radiographic assessment, tenderness to palpation, pain with motion, and maintenance of joint architecture.

REFERENCES

1. Hurov JR, Concannon MJ: Management of a metacarpophalangeal joint fracture using a dynamic traction splint and early motion. J Hand Ther 12:219–227, 1999.
2. Kearney LM, Brown KK: The therapist's management of intra-articular fractures. Hand Clin 10:199–209, 1994.
3. Schenck RR: The dynamic traction method. Hand Clin 10:187–198, 1994.

PATIENT 61

A 38-year-old man with a laceration on his left long finger

A 38-year-old man was placing his left arm into his coat, and as his hand emerged from the end of the sleeve, he struck and broke a glass light fixture suspended from a ceiling fan. At the emergency department, he complained of inability to straighten his left long finger, and primary skin closure of multiple lacerations was performed. The patient was then seen by his primary care physician, who made a referral to a hand surgeon for definitive evaluation. The patient underwent delayed primary repair of complex extensor digitorum (ED) tendon lacerations, involving the left long finger at the level of the PIP joint and, separately, at the proximal phalangeal level. Now, on the third postoperative day, the patient is referred to hand therapy for evaluation and treatment.

Physical Examination: Skin: two surgical wounds at dorsal surface of left long finger. View from above, with fingers in adduction, reveals PIP surgical wound passing transversely; oblique wound over P1 passing mediolaterally in proximal to distal fashion.

Question: What is the most likely zone of extensor tendon injury?

Answer: The history and locations of the surgical wounds are most consistent with lacerations of the ED in zones III and IV of the long finger.

Discussion: The extensor tendons of the hand and wrist are divided into eight zones. By convention, the numbering system begins with zone I at the level of the DIPs and concludes with zone VIII, proximal to the carpal bones. These zones reflect the structural and insertional variation of the extensor tendons. Within any given zone, however, the extensor tendons reveal their kinematic identity and structural equivalence, and this leads to preferred methods of treatment of tendon injuries within each zone of the extensor tendon system.

Zone III is dorsal to the PIP joints of the medial four digits and includes the central slip and conjoined lateral bands. The central slip inserts onto the dorsum of the base of P2 and contributes to PIP extension. The lateral bands continue distally and converge to form the terminal extensor tendon that inserts on the dorsum of the base of P3. The lateral bands therefore contribute to DIP extension.

Zone IV represents the extensor mechanism between the MCP joints (zone V) and PIP joints (zone III) and is closely associated with the proximal phalanges. Structurally, zone IV comprises five conjoined tendons; those of the interossei and lumbricals on each side of the finger (the so-called lateral bands—note the abductor digiti minimi on the medial aspect of the small finger), the dorsal ED, and the interosseous hood. The interosseous hood represents the distal continuation of the sagittal bands and unites the lateral bands and ED tendon. Together, these five conjoined tendons form a broad connective tissue sheet disposed about the proximal phalanx of each digit. Functionally, zone IV coordinates and transmits extensor force to the IP joints.

As with any tendon injury, the rehabilitative prognosis is influenced by the timing of repair, wound tidiness, involvement of adjacent skeletal and soft tissues, and neurovascular injury. In this case, management is potentially complicated by the relative delay in definitive diagnosis and extensor tendon repair. However, the hand therapist should be familiar with this scenario, as it is being played out with increasing frequency in the managed healthcare environment.

The hand therapist should appreciate the suture techniques used to repair extensor tendon lacerations, and their biomechanical characteristics. In zone IV, Bunnell, Kessler, or modifications of these techniques yield repairs that are approximately two-fold stronger than a simple mattress suture, as judged by mechanical testing to produce a 2-mm gap and failure of the repair.

Extensor tendon repairs in zone IV are at special risk for adhesion formation due to their broad tendon-bone interface. The likelihood of adhesion formation also increases with the complexity of injury. Adhesion formation literally "spot welds" the extensor tendon to underlying bone, resulting in decreased tendon gliding, *distal to the adhesion.* Insufficient excursion results in extensor tendon lag and limited flexion. Moreover, when treated with the traditional 4–6 weeks of immobilization, in which the healing tendon is deprived of early controlled stress, extensor tendons repaired in zones III and IV suffer from limited joint motion precisely because of adhesion formation. Therefore, a high percentage of poor results are to be expected.

There are three basic approaches to extensor tendon management: immobilization, passive mobilization using rubber-band traction, and short-arc mobilization in which the patient produces active motion through a prescribed arc. The overall objective of rehabilitation is to ensure a strong repair that glides freely. The gold standard for postoperative tendon excursion that accomplishes functional gliding is 3–5 mm. To obtain this in zones III and IV, the PIP joint of interest is moved through a precise arc of motion. Model calculations support the use of 30° active PIP motion, and calculated internal tendon tension < 300 g is well within the tensile strength of the repaired ED, even when simple mattress or figure-of-eight repair techniques have been used.

In the present patient, the extensor tendons repaired in zones III and IV were treated similarly during the initial 2 weeks of postoperative therapy. Between exercise sessions, the IPs of the involved finger were immobilized at 0° in a custom-fabricated, thermoplastic splint of a volar, finger-based design.

Two volar, finger-based exercise templates were also created. The first template (no. 1) was molded to permit 30° of active PIP flexion and 20–25° of active DIP flexion. The second template (no. 2) was molded to maintain the PIP at 0° extension and permit full active DIP flexion (had the lateral bands been repaired, active DIP flexion using template splint no. 2 would have been limited to 30–35°).

Each waking hour, the patient removed his immobilization splint. Using the uninvolved hand, the patient placed exercise template no. 1 against the volar surface of his long finger and performed up to 20 repetitions of slow, active composite IP extension (see figure, *A*) and flexion (*B*). He then placed exercise template no. 2 against the volar surface of his long finger, stabilized the PIP at 0° with his uninvolved hand, and performed up to 20 repetitions of isolated active DIP extension (see figure, C) and flexion (D). Independent flexion of the DIP, with the PIP stabilized at 0° extension, creates 3–5 mm of extensor tendon glide effected through the conjoined attachment of the lateral bands to the ED in zone IV.

The uninvolved joints of the hand and wrist were permitted unrestricted motion, and tenodesis exercises supplemented the patient's controlled mobilization exercises. With the IPs splinted in extension, active motion of the wrist and tenodesis of the MCPs engenders minimal tension at the repair sites in zones III and IV.

The IP joint exercises were done by the patient with his involved wrist positioned in 30° flexion and the MCP near 0°. Positioning the wrist in 30° flexion minimizes passive tension in the antagonist extrinsic flexors, and this reduces the work of the repaired ED. Positioning the MCPs near 0° allows the repaired ED to transmit tension to the extensor mechanism in zones III/IV. Together with intrinsic muscle activity (interossei and lumbricals), the ED facilitates PIP extension.

At the beginning of the third and fourth postoperative weeks, exercise template no. 1 was remolded to permit an additional 10° of active flexion at each IP joint (with lateral band repair, exercise template no. 2 would also have been modified to permit 45° and 55° of isolated active DIP flexion during the third and fourth postoperative weeks, respectively). At beginning of the fifth postoperative week, 70–80° of active PIP flexion was permitted while using exercise template no. 1. Also at this time, the patient was instructed in gentle putty exercises for grip and pinch strengthening.

Static extension splinting was discontinued at the end of the sixth postoperative week, with liberalization of left hand use for activities of daily living. The patient was also instructed in a home exercise program designed for general left upper extremity strengthening and conditioning using rubber bands.

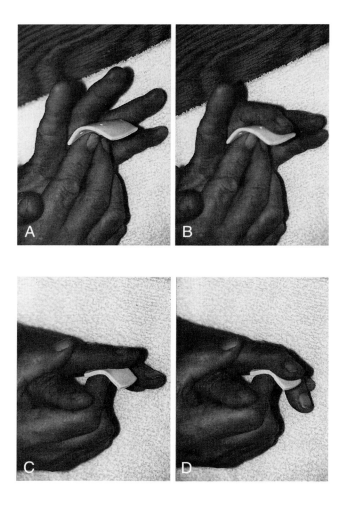

Hand Therapy Pearls

1. Extensor tendon repairs in zones III and IV, representing the PIP and P1 level, respectively, are especially prone to adhesion formation due to the presence of a broad tendon-bone interface.

2. Extensor tendon repairs in zones III and IV are particularly amenable to early active mobilization (within 3–5 days postoperatively) using treatment guidelines for short-arc motion.

3. Early active mobilization of extensor tendons repaired in zones III and IV produces internal tension that is within the safety margin of the tensile strength of the repaired tendon, even when simple mattress and figure-of-eight repair techniques have been employed.

4. Precise positioning of the wrist, MCPs, and IPs during early active motion results in 3–5 mm of extensor tendon gliding, which promotes strong repair, minimizes adhesion formation, and ensures the greatest likelihood of excellent IP joint motion.

REFERENCES

1. Duran RJ, Houser RG: Controlled passive motion following flexor tendon repair in zones 2 and 3. In The American Academy of Orthopaedic Surgeons: Symposium on tendon surgery in the hand. St. Louis, Mosby, 1975, pp 105–114.
2. Evans RB: An analysis of factors that support early active short-arc motion of the repaired central slip. J Hand Ther 5:187–201, 1992.
3. Evans RB: Immediate active short-arc motion following extensor tendon repair. Hand Clin 11:483–512, 1995.
4. Evans RB: An update on extensor tendon management. In Hunter JM, Mackin EJ, Callahan AD (eds): Rehabilitation of the Hand: Surgery and Therapy, 4th ed. St. Louis, Mosby, 1995, pp 565–606.
5. Newport ML, Pollack GR, Williams CD: Biomechanical characteristics of suture techniques in extensor zone IV. J Hand Surg 20A:650–656, 1995.
6. Rosenthal EA: The extensor tendons: Anatomy and management. In Hunter JM, Mackin EJ, Callahan AD (eds): Rehabilitation of the Hand: Surgery and Therapy, 4th ed. St. Louis, Mosby, 1995, pp 519–564.
7. Tubiana R: Architecture and functions of the hand. In Tubiana R (ed): The Hand, Vol. 1. Philadelphia, WB Saunders, 1981, pp 19–93.
8. Valentin P: Physiology of extension of the fingers. In Tubiana R (ed): The Hand, Vol. 1. Philadelphia, WB Saunders, 1981, pp 389–398.

PATIENT 62

A 49-year-old mechanic with lacerations of his fingers

A 49-year-old mechanic was using a hack-saw to perform repairs when the saw-blade jumped and struck the dorsum of his right hand. In the emergency department, he complained of inability to straighten his long and ring fingers, and the resident on call suspected disruption of the extensor tendons. The patient underwent open exploration and primary repair of the extensor digitorum (ED) tendons of the long and ring fingers, proximal to the juncturae. Now, 24 hours following surgery, he is referred to hand therapy for evaluation and treatment.

Physical Examination: Skin: 4-cm, oblique surgical wound at dorsum of right hand, over bases of long and ring finger metacarpals; abrasion at dorsum of index finger MCP.

Questions: What is the most likely zone of extensor tendon injury? What options are available to treat this patient?

Answers: Extensor zone VI. The three basic approaches to extensor tendon management are: immobilization, passive mobilization using rubber band traction, and early active mobilization.

Discussion: The extensor tendons of the hand and wrist are divided into eight zones; these are described in the previous case, Patient 61. The extensor tendons in zone VI are dorsal to the metacarpal shafts of the medial four digits of the hand and contribute to MCP extension. Zone VI also includes the juncturae tendinum—literally, "tendinous joints." The juncturae connect the ED tendons, and they are capable of transmitting force between adjacent ED tendons. Moreover, during finger flexion, the juncturae develop passive tension that stabilizes the transverse metacarpal arch and centralizes the ED tendons.

As with any tendon injury, the rehabilitative prognosis is influenced by the timing of repair, wound tidiness, involvement of adjacent skeletal and soft tissues, and neurovascular injury. Given the nature of this patient's job and the offending object, injury to the dorsum of the hand resulted in a relatively contaminated and untidy wound. The saw blade possessed sufficient energy to completely divide the extensor tendons, and their cut ends were ragged, requiring sharp revision in the operating room prior to co-apting the tendon ends. Shortening the extensor tendons, even by a few millimeters, may result in altered mechanics of the hand and prolong the rehabilitative program.

A consideration of the biomechanical characteristics of the suture techniques used to repair extensor tendon lacerations is critical when designing a hand therapy program. In the emergency department, a simple mattress or figure-of-eight suture technique is often used to repair a lacerated extensor tendon. Bunnell, Kessler, or a modification of these techniques is also used, and four-strand repair techniques have been developed. When used in extensor zone VI, mattress and figure-of-eight suture techniques possess approximately one-half to one-third the strength of their augmented counterparts. Therefore, confirmation of the suturing technique, the type of suture material used, and the number of suture strands crossing the repair are variables that must be appreciated to optimize the patient's plan of care.

As for Patient 61, the overall objective of rehabilitation is to ensure a strong repair that glides freely. The prerequisite 3–5 mm of linear excursion in extensor tendons repaired in zone VI can be obtained by moving the MCP through a precise arc of motion. The desired MCP motion for therapy is determined as follows:

$$\text{Desired MCP motion for therapy}$$
$$= 5\text{-mm tendon glide}$$
$$\times \frac{\text{Normal MCP motion (degrees)}}{\text{Extensor tendon excursion (mm)}}$$

Normal ranges of motion for the MCPs are: index 85°, long 88°, ring 90°, and small 92°. The extensor tendon excursions required to accomplish these angular rotations at the MCPs are: index 15 mm, long 16 mm, ring 11 mm, and small 12 mm. Thus, for the index and long fingers, approximately 30° of MCP motion is required to achieve the prerequisite 5 mm of linear tendon excursion. For the ring and small fingers, approximately 40° of MCP motion will yield the prerequisite 5 mm of linear tendon excursion.

The present patient was treated using early mobilization within a custom, forearm-based, dorsal dynamic splint (see figure, *next page*). The splint was molded to position the patient's left wrist in 45° extension, and the splint base ended proximal to the MCPs. Perforated material was chosen for splint fabrication to promote air circulation, resulting in improved splint comfort and compliance. A wire and thermoplastic outrigger was galvanized to the splint base centered over the proximal phalanges of the medial four fingers. In this patient, the uninvolved digits were included in the splint design, and the IP joints were permitted freedom of motion.

The dynamic component of the splint consisted of monofilament threads tied to finger loops that supported the proximal phalanges of the medial four fingers. The free ends of the threads were led through the outrigger and tied to rubber-bands. The rubber-bands, in turn, were secured to short lengths of Velcro hook, and these were positioned on a similar short segment of Velcro loop secured proximally to the splint base. Tension in the rubber-bands was adjusted to position the MCPs at 0° extension— this is critical to prevent extensor lag. Stop beads were fastened to the monofilaments *proximal to the outrigger* and adjusted to permit 30° and 40° MCP flexion of index/long fingers and ring/small fingers, respectively (see figure, page 231).

When extensor tendon repair is performed *proximal to the juncturae,* as in this patient, the uninvolved fingers must also be splinted in extension to minimize tension on the repairs. When extensor tendon repair is performed *distal to the juncturae,* the adjacent fingers need not be incorporated into the splint design; unrestricted MCP flexion of the adjacent finger(s) is actually desirable because it advances the *proximal* ends of the repaired extensor tendons, thereby minimizing tension on the repair site. Thus, it is important that the hand therapist appreciate the level of extensor tendon repair within zone VI and its relationship to the juncturae. In the present case, unprotected MCP flexion of the uninjured index and small fingers could, through the juncturae, advance the *distal* tendon ends, possibly resulting in gap formation at the repair sites.

While wearing his splint, the patient was instructed to perform 20 repetitions of active MCP flexion to the limits of the stop beads, followed by passive extension, effected by rubber band traction. The patient was also instructed in active composite IP motion for all fingers, while the MCPs are maintained in extension by the rubber bands. Isolated IP extension and flexion results in little ED excursion in zone VI.

At the beginning of postoperative week 2, the stop beads were adjusted proximally on each monofilament, permitting an additional 10° of active MCP flexion (40° index/long and 50° ring/small). At the beginning of the third postoperative week, the stop beads were again readjusted proximally on each monofilament allowing 60° and 70° of active MCP flexion, respectively, of the index/long and ring/small fingers. The stop beads were discontinued beginning on the fourth postoperative week, and the patient was permitted unrestricted MCP flexion within the splint, followed by dynamically assisted extension effected by rubber-band traction.

Clinic activities consisted of wound care, splint checks, and adjustments of the stop beads. Rubberbands were replaced when fatigued. During the initial postoperative week, under therapist guidance, the patient performed place-hold MCP extension of the long and ring fingers, using the minimum amount of muscle tension required to hold each joint at 0°. This exercise was performed outside of the splint, with the wrist positioned in 20° flexion. Positioning the involved wrist in flexion minimizes passive tension in the extrinsic flexors and reduces the work of the repaired ED. Then, with the wrist positioned in 45° extension, the patient was instructed to actively flex the long finger MCP 30°. Positioning the patient's wrist in extension minimizes passive tension on the repaired ED during active MCP flexion. The patient's wrist was then guided back into 20° flexion, and he actively extended his long finger MCP to neutral.

Wrist tenodesis exercises were repeated for the ring finger, allowing 40° of active MCP flexion followed by active extension to neutral. Tenodesis exercises during the second and third postoperative weeks permitted 40° and 60° of active MCP flexion of the long finger, and 50° and 70° of active MCP flexion of the ring finger, respectively, exactly matching those adjustments made to the stop beads. Beginning in postoperative week 4, again under therapist guidance, the patient initiated tenodesis exercises consisting of unrestricted MCP flexion, followed by active extension.

Dynamic traction was discontinued in postoperative week 5, and the patient performed tenodesis exercises outside of the splint independently. However, he continued splinting for 1 additional week, for protection, between exercise sessions.

Splinting was discontinued in postoperative week 6, and the patient was instructed in active composite wrist and finger flexion. Strengthening exercises using a light resistance putty were also initiated during week 6.

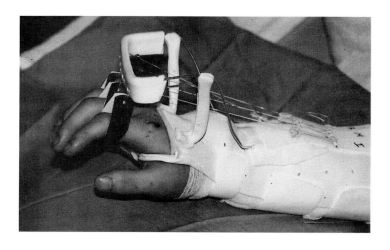

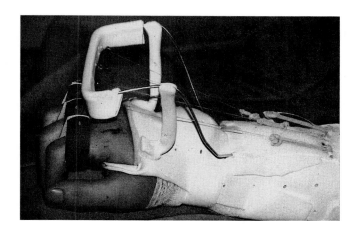

Hand Therapy Pearls

1. The extensor tendons are divided into eight zones which reflect their structural and functional characteristics.

2. Extensor tendon repairs in zone VI, at the dorsum of the metacarpals, require clarification with respect to the juncturae tendinum. When repaired *distal* to the juncturae, the adjacent MCPs may be omitted from splint design. When repaired *proximal* to the juncturae, the adjacent MCPs must be included in the splint design.

3. Three to five millimeters of excursion is necessary to promote a strong extensor tendon repair that glides freely. In zone VI, this is effected by 30–40° of MCP flexion, followed by extension to 0°.

4. Under therapist guidance, postoperative treatment includes early active motion consisting of place-hold and tenodesis exercises. These maneuvers generate minimal active muscle-tendon tension that appears to be well within the repair strength of the sutured extensor tendon.

REFERENCES

1. Boyes JH: The normal hand. In Bunnell's Surgery of the Hand. Philadelphia, Lippincott, 1964, p 14.
2. Duran RJ, Houser RG: Controlled passive motion following flexor tendon repair in zones 2 and 3. In The American Academy of Orthopaedic Surgeons: Symposium on tendon surgery in the hand. St. Louis, Mosby, 1975, pp 105–114.
3. Evans RB: An update on extensor tendon management. In Hunter JM, Mackin EJ, Callahan AD (eds): Rehabilitation of the Hand: Surgery and Therapy, 4th ed. St. Louis, Mosby, 1995, pp 565–606.
4. Howard RF, Ondrovic L, Greenwald DP: Biomechanical analysis of four-strand extensor tendon repair techniques. J Hand Surg 22A:838–842, 1997.
5. Newport ML, Williams CD: Biomechanical characteristics of extensor tendon suture techniques. J Hand Surg 17A:1117–1123, 1992.
6. Rosenthal EA: The extensor tendons: Anatomy and management. In Hunter JM, Mackin EJ, Callahan AD (eds): Rehabilitation of the Hand: Surgery and Therapy, 4th ed. St. Louis, Mosby, 1995, pp 519–564.

PATIENT 63

An 18-year-old woman with a laceration of her left small finger

An 18-year-old woman presented emergently with a history of laceration involving the palmar surface of the left small finger. The injury was caused by broken glass. She was seen by the resident on call, who suspected disruption of the flexor tendons. She underwent exploration and repair of the flexor digitorum profundus tendon of the left small finger, and she is referred to hand therapy for evaluation and treatment 48 hours following surgery.

Physical Examination: Skin: zig-zag surgical wound with sutures placed at palmar surface of left small finger, extending from the DIP joint flexion crease proximally to distal palmar crease; small finger edematous and erythematous. Musculoskeletal: PIP in 25° of flexion.

Questions: What is the most likely zone of flexor tendon injury? What options are available to treat this patient?

Answers: Zone II. The three basic approaches to flexor tendon management are: early passive mobilization with, and without, rubber-band traction; early active mobilization, and immobilization.

Discussion: To optimize this patient's care, the mechanism of injury, location of the injury on the patient's hand, and the timing of tendon repair should be determined by questioning the patient. The rehabilitative prognosis will be influenced by the timing of repair. Primary tendon repair usually occurs within 24 hours of injury. Delayed primary repair occurs between 24 hours and 10 days after injury; early secondary repair between 10 to 28 days after injury; and late secondary repair after 28 days. Often, factors outside the control of the treating hand therapist dictate not only the timing of repair, but also when referral to hand therapy is made. The longer tendon repair and referral to hand therapy are delayed, the more guarded the prognosis.

It is essential to determine which tendons were repaired, whether tendon laceration was partial or complete, the zone(s) of tendon injury, wound tidiness, whether the neurovascular bundles were repaired, and the integrity of the digital flexor sheath. Each of these factors also influences the prognosis and treatment options. For example, the A2 and A4 pulleys are biomechanically the most significant for determining finger motion and power, and significant loss of either may result in IP joint flexion contractures. On the other hand, a bulky repair that does not glide freely beneath a repaired pulley will result in decreased tendon excursion. Finally, surgical revision of even a few millimeters of devitalized flexor tendon has the potential to result in decreased IP extension.

Confirmation of the suturing technique, the type of suture material used, and the number of suture strands crossing the repair are variables that must also be appreciated in order to optimize the patient's care. For example, the new 4- and 6-strand suture methods are roughly two-to-three times stronger than 2-strand techniques, and may therefore permit early active motion during postoperative rehabilitation.

Discussion with the referring hand surgeon, thorough review of operative reports, when available, and the hand therapist's expertise will determine the postoperative treatment guidelines to be employed. The need for immobilization is justified in some circumstances — for example, in the young pediatric patient, those with cognitive impairments, and patients who, for any reason, may be noncompliant with postoperative rehabilitation. The alert, motivated patient who demonstrates understanding of the treatment guidelines and precautions is appropriate for early mobilization.

The present patient was treated using early passive mobilization performed within a custom-fabricated dorsal block splint. The splint immobilized the patient's left wrist in 30° flexion, MCPs of the medial four fingers in 50° flexion, and IPs at 0° (see figure). During the initial 3 weeks of rehabilitation, exercise consisted of *passive finger flexion* followed by *active extension* within the confines of the dorsal block splint, and 10 repetitions of each of the following exercises were performed each waking hour. The patient first unfastened one end of the top strap. The PIP was then exercised in isolation, followed by the DIP, and lastly, composite flexion of the IPs and MCP was performed. Clinic activities also included PIP mobilization to minimize the risk of flexion contracture. The uninvolved fingers were passively flexed and actively extended to minimize joint stiffness.

At 3 weeks postoperatively, the dorsal block splint was remolded to permit neutral wrist positioning. At this time also, the patient was instructed to remove the splint to perform place-hold composite flexion of the medial four fingers with the wrist positioned in 30° extension. Wrist flexion resulted in passive finger extension. At 4–5 weeks postoperatively, tendon gliding exercises were initiated, and at 6 weeks, the dorsal block splint was discontinued. At this time, joint blocking exercises were initiated. At 8 weeks, progressive resisted exercises were implemented, and at 12 weeks, the patient was released from therapy with unrestricted activity.

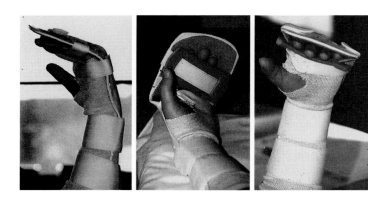

Hand Therapy Pearls

1. Successful postoperative management of the patient with a repaired flexor tendon depends upon excellent communication among hand therapist, hand surgeon, and patient.

2. Immobilization is indicated whenever there is a question regarding the patient's ability to understand and comply with the treatment regimen.

3. Early mobilization, or exercise, is desirable in the compliant patient with a repaired flexor tendon. The basic rehabilitation goal is to ensure a strong repair that glides easily.

4. The new 4- and 6-strand suture techniques for repairing flexor tendons are approximately two-to-three times stronger than 2-strand repairs and may permit early active mobilization.

5. The time frame for progression of treatment must remain flexible and patient-specific: scar tissue formation and the return of functional tendon gliding are two important factors dictating the timing and selection of exercises to be employed in rehabilitation of the patient with a repaired flexor tendon.

REFERENCES

1. Cash SL: Primary care of flexor tendon injuries. In Hunter JM, Schneider LH, Mackin EJ, Callahan AD (eds): Rehabilitation of the Hand: Surgery and Therapy, 3rd ed. St. Louis, Mosby, 1990, pp 379–389.
2. Duran RJ, Houser RG: Controlled passive motion following flexor tendon repair in zones 2 and 3. In The American Academy of Orthopaedic Surgeons: Symposium on tendon surgery in the hand. St. Louis, Mosby, 1975, pp 105–114.
3. Gelberman RH, Woo SL-Y: The physiological basis for application of controlled stress in the rehabilitation of flexor tendon injuries. J Hand Ther 2:66–70, 1989.
4. Kubota H, Manske PR, Aoki M, Pruitt DL, Larson BJ: Effect of motion and tension on injured flexor tendons in chickens. J Hand Surg 21A:456–463, 1996.
5. Stewart KM, van Strien G: Postoperative management of flexor tendon injuries. In Hunter JM, Mackin EJ, Callahan AD (eds): Rehabilitation of the Hand: Surgery and Therapy, 4th ed. St. Louis, Mosby, 1995, pp 433–462.
6. Strickland JW. Development of flexor tendon surgery: 25 years of progress. J Hand Surg 25A:214–235, 2000.

PATIENT 64

A 17-year-old boy with restricted proximal interphalangeal joint motion

A 17-year-old boy was playing basketball and described striking his right index finger on the knee of another player. He discontinued play and applied ice to his index finger, which had become noticeably swollen and discolored. He was seen in the hospital the following day, where x-rays demonstrated small avulsion chip fractures, both dorsally and volarly, involving the base of P2 (see figure). An alumifoam splint, immobilizing the index PIP joint in flexion, was used for 2 weeks, and the patient is now referred to hand therapy for evaluation and treatment.

Physical Examination: Musculoskeletal: active ROM right index finger MCP 0/90°, PIP 15/60° (15/75° passive), DIP 0/25° (50° passive flexion). Right index finger PIP joint circumference: 7.2 cm (left = 5 cm).

Question: What is the diagnosis for hand therapy?

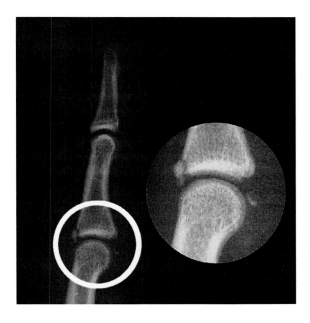

Answer: PIP joint motion restriction in a capsular pattern

Discussion: When the PIP is immobilized in flexion following dorsal dislocation, joint contracture can result. A fixed flexion contracture is confirmed by the inability of the examiner to passively extend the PIP to neutral, and this is known as motion restriction in a capsular pattern. The normal arc of physiologic motion at the PIP joint is approximately 100° and consists of flexion and extension about a transverse axis passing through the head of P1. It is important to appreciate that the osseous anatomy and articular soft tissues comprising the PIP constrain axial rotation, lateral bending, and hyperextension throughout this normal physiologic arc. Thus, the PIP is described as a uniaxial joint with 1° of freedom.

The bony configuration of the PIP consists of the bicondylar of head of P1 received by corresponding fossae at the base of P2. When viewed from the side, both the head of P1 and base of P2 appear compressed dorsoventrally. When viewed in transverse section, the PIP is trapezoidal in outline, i.e., the palmar aspect of the joint is approximately twice the width of the dorsal.

The soft tissues comprising the PIP and contributing to its stability include the volar plate and the radial and ulnar collateral ligaments. Each collateral ligament consists of two portions distinguishable from each other by attachment, fiber direction, and fiber density. The proper collateral ligament (PCL) is thick and attaches proximally to the lateral fossa of P1. PCL fibers pass distally and inferiorly, *dorsal* to the axis of joint rotation, and insert on the volar three-quarters of the lateral aspect of the base of P2. During flexion, PCL fibers are elongated as they pivot over the wide volar base of the PIP. PCL fibers are therefore under tension when the PIP is flexed, and these fibers are the primary lateral stabilizers of the joint beyond 30° of flexion.

The accessory collateral ligament (ACL) arises in common with the PCL, from the lateral fossa of P1. ACL fibers are relatively thin and pass *ventral* to the axis of joint rotation. Fanning out to insert into the palmar surface of the volar plate, ACL fibers form a transverse sling as they blend with ACL fibers from the opposite side of the joint. ACL fibers are elongated during PIP motion from approximately 10–15° flexion to terminal extension, and it is in this range that they contribute to lateral joint stability and prevent PIP hyperextension.

The volar plate forms the floor of the PIP and is composed of fibrocartilage. The volar plate is reinforced by cruciate (C1) and annular (A3) pulleys of the fibro-osseous flexor tendon sheath, and its distal lateral margins blend with the PCL at discrete junctures called the critical corners. Together, volar plate and PCL fibers insert into cortical bone of P2 via a fibrocartilage interface at these so-called critical corners. In contrast, the central 80% of the volar plate has a periosteal attachment to the palmar surface of P2. Moreover, the elongated proximal "check rein" ligaments also insert into periosteum on the palmar aspect of P1. The primary biomechanical role of the volar plate is to limit PIP hyperextension.

When the PIP is flexed, the volar plate and C1/A3 pulleys demonstrate redundancies, and the accessory collateral ligaments are lax. When the PIP is immobilized in flexion, these palmar capsular structures adapt by shortening with resultant limitations in active and passive PIP extension.

The present patient was treated with a combination of edema management, cohesive dressings, thermal modalities (to precondition soft tissues), joint mobilization of the PIP, and active and passive exercises. Intermittent dynamic splinting for PIP extension was also a useful adjunct.

The observed mismatch between active and passive IP flexion is attributable to frictional drag caused by joint edema, which is responsive to compression tape worn on the index finger at all times, except during performance of hygiene tasks. Blocked DIP flexion of the index finger, in which the patient supports the PIP in maximal available extension while actively flexing the DIP, serves to elongate volar structures: the volar plate, C1/A3 pulleys, ACL, and oblique retinacular ligament. This results in both increased PIP extension and DIP flexion.

Hand Therapy Pearls

1. The volar plate, C1/A3 pulleys of the fibro-osseous flexor tendon sheath, and ACL are redundant when the PIP is flexed. Splinting the PIP in flexion therefore results in adaptive shortening of these structures, with limited active and passive PIP extension. This is termed a capsular pattern of joint restriction.

2. The bony anatomy and soft tissues comprising the PIP contribute to rotatory and lateral stability as well as limit hyperextension. The PCL is the primary stabilizing restraint to lateral joint forces beyond 30° PIP flexion. The ACL is elongated at 10–15° PIP flexion through terminal extension, and together with the volar plate, contributes to lateral stability and minimizes hyperextension.

3. When immobilization of the PIP in flexion is indicated for interval protection, splint revisions of approximately 10°/week are desirable to maintain the resting lengths of the volar capsular structures.

REFERENCES

1. Bowers WH, Wolf JW, Nehil JL, et al: The proximal interphalangeal joint volar plate. I. An anatomical and biomechanical study. J Hand Surg 5A:79–88, 1980.
2. Dubousset JF: The digital joints. In Tubiana R (ed): The Hand, Vol. 1. Philadelphia, WB Saunders, 1981, pp 191–201.
3. Leibovic SJ, Bowers WH: Anatomy of the proximal interphalangeal joint. Hand Clin 10:169–178, 1994.
4. Williams EH, McCarthy E, Bickel KD: The histologic anatomy of the volar plate. J Hand Surg 23A:805–810, 1998.

PATIENT 65

A 32-year-old man with muscle weakness

A 32-year-old man described being thrown over the handlebars of his bicycle when the front tire struck a pothole in the road. He presented in the emergency department complaining of inability to straighten his fingers. With the exception of minor skin abrasions on his right forearm that were treated, his emergency department visit was unremarkable, and he is now referred to hand therapy for evaluation and treatment. The patient presents with his right upper extremity was immobilized in a sling.

Physical Examination: General: right wrist and fingers flexed. Palpation: soft tissues bounded by right proximal radius, lateral epicondyle, and cubital fossa tender. Skin: ecchymotic. Manual muscle testing: triceps 5/5; extensor carpi radialis longus (ECRL) 4/5; supinator (tested with right elbow in extension), extensor carpi radialis brevis (ECRB), extensor digitorum, extensor carpi ulnaris, extensor digiti minimi, abductor pollicis longus, extensor pollicis longus and brevis, and extensor indicis trace to 1/5; thumb opposition 5/5, thumb adduction 4/5. Musculoskeletal: when right wrist in 30° extension, active composite finger flexion complete to distal palmar crease; active finger extension resulted in intrinsic-plus pattern, characterized by composite IP extension of medial four fingers, with inability to extend the MCPs and thumb flexed (see figure). Neurologic: normal sensation of dorsum of right forearm and hand (Semmes-Weinstein 2.83 monofilament, equivalent to 68 mgf).

Questions: What is the affected anatomic structure? What is the best treatment option for this patient?

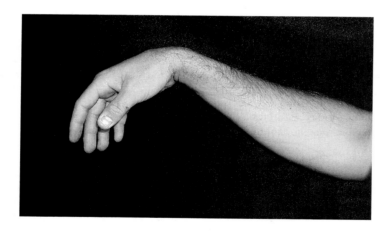

Answers: Posterior interosseous nerve. The best treatment option for this patient is dynamic splinting.

Discussion: Motor branches of the radial nerve proper supply the triceps and ECRL. After supplying the ECRL just proximal to the elbow, the radial nerve divides into two branches, superficial and deep. The superficial branch of the radial nerve is sensory and supplies the radial one-half of the dorsum of the hand. The deep branch of the radial nerve, the posterior interosseous nerve (PIN), is motor and supplies the ECRB. Passing dorsal in the forearm, the PIN then enters the supinator muscle, which it supplies. Upon emerging from the substance of the supinator, the PIN gives off multiple short motor branches supplying the extensor digitorum, extensor carpi ulnaris, and extensor digiti minimi. Long motor branches pass distally in the dorsal forearm, under cover of the aforementioned extensor muscles, and supply the abductor pollicis longus, extensor pollicis longus, extensor pollicis brevis, and extensor indicis.

Contusion of the dorsal proximal forearm can injure the PIN—*neuropraxia* is the term used to describe the resultant weakness of the extrinsic extensor/abductor muscles. Neuropraxia is defined as a localized conduction blockade, and while the axons and surrounding neural connective tissue envelopes retain their integrity, decreased or absent motor and/or sensory function can last momentarily or be of several months duration.

In the present patient, the triceps and ECRL, innervated by motor branches of the radial nerve proper, were spared, as was the superficial branch of the radial nerve. This was confirmed by normal results returned during motor and sensory testing. The supinator was tested with the elbow in extension to minimize participation of the biceps during forearm rotation. Decreased thumb adduction strength is accounted for by the fact that the EPL contributes to thumb adduction.

The acute injury described here resulted in frank mechanical deformation of the radial nerve characterized by ischemia and edema. The development of edema, coupled with oxygen deficiency, impairs the O_2-dependent ion pumps that are necessary for maintaining the electrochemical gradients across the neuron plasma membrane, and neurotransmission fails. A further consequence of nerve injury is activation of membrane phospholipases that initiate myelin breakdown, and fast-conducting, large-diameter motor axons are particularly susceptible to demyelination.

In this patient, active MCP extension, thumb CMC abduction/extension, and the normal tenodesis that permits balanced wrist extension and powerful finger flexion were lost with radial nerve injury. Treatment was therefore prioritized by fabrication of a custom, dorsal, forearm-based dynamic splint to substitute for weak extrinsic extensor/abductor musculature. The splint base ended proximal to the thumb CMC and the MCPs of the fingers. The wrist component was molded in approximately 30° of extension, which stabilized the wrist and permitted finger flexion. The wrist was also positioned in neutral with respect to radial and ulnar deviation, to balance the relatively strong ECRL.

Outriggers were attached to the splint base and finger loops with rubber-band traction were led to the proximal phalanges of all digits. Traction was adjusted to permit active composite flexion of the medial four fingers to the distal palmar crease, with dynamic-assist MCP return to approximately 15–30° flexion. Similarly, the thumb CMC was positioned near end-range abduction and in approximately 20° extension. Positioning the thumb in abduction and extension permitted clearance for the medial four fingers during fisting. Thumb traction was adjusted to permit opposition to the base of the small finger. The thumb intrinsics, innervated by the median and ulnar nerves, retain the ability to oppose and adduct the thumb, and to assist with thumb IP extension.

The duration of dynamic splint use is based on the return of motor function in the affected extrinsic extensor/abductor muscles. Weaning off the splint was indicated when muscle grades of ⅗ returned, demonstrating active motion through the available range against gravity.

Hand Therapy Pearls

1. Neuropraxia is characterized by localized conduction blockade in which the axons and surrounding neural connective tissue envelopes retain their integrity.

2. The deep branch of the radial nerve, the posterior interosseous nerve (PIN), innervates the extrinsic extensor/abductor muscles in the dorsal forearm.

3. The precise arborization of the radial nerve into superficial sensory and deep motor branches, as well as the innervation order of the muscles supplied by the PIN, are patient specific and therefore will vary.

4. The nature and extent of nerve injury can be determined through sensory and muscle testing. These empirical results guide the hand therapist's splint design.

REFERENCES

1. Abrams RA, Ziets RJ, Lieber RL, et al:. Anatomy of the radial nerve motor branches in the forearm. J Hand Surg 22A:232–237, 1997.
2. Colditz, JC: Splinting the hand with a peripheral nerve injury. In Hunter JM, Mackin EJ, Callahan AD (eds): Rehabilitation of the Hand: Surgery and Therapy, 4th ed. St. Louis, Mosby, 1995, pp 679–692.
3. Flynn CJ, Farooqui, AA, Horrocks LA: Ischemia and hypoxia. In Siegel GJ, Agranoff BW, Albers RW, et al (eds): Basic Neurochemistry, 4th ed. New York, Raven Press 1989, pp 783–795.
4. Smith KL: Nerve response to injury and repair. In Hunter JM, Mackin EJ, Callahan AD (eds): Rehabilitation of the Hand: Surgery and Therapy, 4th ed. St. Louis, Mosby, 1995, pp 609–626.

INDEX